Roeser's Audiology Desk Reference

Second Edition

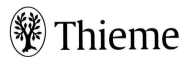

Roeser's Audiology Desk Reference

Second Edition

Ross J. Roeser, PhD, FAAA, CCC/A
Lois and Howard Wolf Professor in Pediatric Audiology
Executive Director Emeritus
Head, Doctor of Audiology (AuD) Program
Callier Center for Communication Disorders
University of Texas at Dallas
Dallas, Texas

Editorial Consultants:

Jackie L. Clark, PhD, FAAA, CCC/A
Deanna Meinke, PhD, FAAA, CCC/A
De Wet Swanepoel, PhD
Gary G. Wright, PhD

Thieme
New York · Stuttgart

Thieme Medical Publishers, Inc.
333 Seventh Ave.
New York, NY 10001

Executive Editor: Timothy Hiscock
Managing Editor: J. Owen Zurhellen IV
Editorial Assistant: Elizabeth Berg
Senior Vice President, Editorial and Electronic Product Development: Cornelia Schulze
Production Editor: Barbara A. Chernow
International Production Director: Andreas Schabert
Vice President, Finance and Accounts: Sarah Vanderbilt
President: Brian D. Scanlan
Compositor: Carol Pierson, Chernow Editorial Services, Inc.
Printer: Gopsons Papers Ltd.

Library of Congress Cataloging-in-Publication Data

Roeser, Ross J.
   Roeser's audiology desk reference / Ross J. Roeser. — 2nd ed.
     p. ; cm.
   Audiology desk reference
   Includes bibliographical references and index.
   ISBN 978-1-60406-398-1 — ISBN 978-1-60406-400-1 (eISBN)
   I. Title. II. Title: Audiology desk reference.
   [DNLM: 1. Audiology-Handbooks. WV 39]
   617.8—dc23   2012047826

Important note: Medical knowledge is ever-changing. As new research and clinical experience broaden our knowledge, changes in treatment and drug therapy may be required. The authors and editors of the material herein have consulted sources believed to be reliable in their efforts to provide information that is complete and in accord with the standards accepted at the time of publication. However, in view of the possibility of human error by the authors, editors, or publisher of the work herein or changes in medical knowledge, neither the authors, editors, nor publisher, nor any other party who has been involved in the preparation of this work, warrants that the information contained herein is in every respect accurate or complete, and they are not responsible for any errors or omissions or for the results obtained from use of such information. Readers are encouraged to confirm the information contained herein with other sources. For example, readers are advised to check the product information sheet included in the package of each drug they plan to administer to be certain that the information contained in this publication is accurate and that changes have not been made in the recommended dose or in the contraindications for administration. This recommendation is of particular importance in connection with new or infrequently used drugs.

Some of the product names, patents, and registered designs referred to in this book are in fact registered trademarks or proprietary names even though specific reference to this fact is not always made in the text. Therefore, the appearance of a name without designation as proprietary is not to be construed as a representation by the publisher that it is in the public domain.

Printed in India

5 4 3 2 1

ISBN 978-1-60406-398-1

Also available as an e-book:
eISBN 978-1-60406-400-1

Contents

Expanded Contents

2 Physical Acoustics • 117

4   Audiological Procedures / Materials • 145

6 Hearing Loss Prevention • 295

9   Psychosocial Aspects/Rehabilitation • 385

10   Deafness • 401

11   Organizations and Publications • 409

Preface to the Second Edition

The Internet has revolutionized the way we communicate, store, and retrieve knowledge and information, and the ease of information accessibility has affected virtually every aspect of our daily lives. Information is available at our fingertips. Those of us who have been through the transition from having to walk the stacks of the library to carry out our research, to now routinely conducting literature searches and the quest for information by clicking on a computer mouse realize the tremendous efficiency we have achieved in accessing information. We are now able to gain access to a world of facts on virtually any topic with a computer and Internet access to the World Wide Web. This efficiency has tremendous advantages, but the process lacks the important aspect of being able to hold a real book in one's hand and thumb through the pages to see what information is available. This is the reason why books are still valued as tools to provide information and knowledge.

The *Audiology Desk Reference* (ADR) is such a text. My publisher took a gamble when it was first published in 1996, because it was quite unique. Would audiologists value a compendium of information—an audiology desk reference—to the extent that they would want such a publication available on their bookshelves? Luckily, they did! In fact, the publishing life of the ADR seemed to be unusually long compared to that of other books. Typically, books are more in demand when they are first published and over time their popularity decreases. With the ADR the popularity of the text seems to have grown over the years, which is why we have waited more than 15 years to publish this second edition. Maybe the convenience of having computer access to information is being overshadowed by the need to have it in a hardcopy format. Only time will tell.

In the process of putting this edition together, I found one image that stood out and warrants specific comment. One of my University of Texas at Dallas/Callier Center faculty colleagues, Dr. Gary Wright, who has been studying cochlear anatomy and physiology for more than 40 years, showed me an impressive photo of the entire structure of an adult inner ear, including the cochlea, utricle/saccule, and semicircular canals, with a U.S. coin partially visible in the background (**Fig. 1**). My first guess was that the coin in the background was a 50-cent piece, but Dr. Wright said it was not. Was it a quarter? No. When Dr. Wright informed me that it was, in fact, a dime, I was stunned!

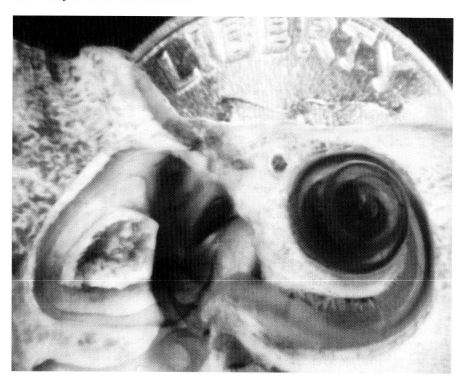

Figure 1 An adult inner ear showing the cochlea and semicircular canals. A U.S. coin in the background provides size perspective (see text for details).

The inner ear houses one of the most complicated sensory organs in the human body. It is a fluid-filled structure (about 100 microliters) housed 2 to 3 centimeters from the opening of the ear canal in one of the hardest bones in the human body—the petrous portion of the temporal bone (by the way, "petrous" comes from the name St. Peter: "And upon this rock I will build my church" [Matthew 16:18]). The cochlear partition alone has about 20,000 hair cells (12,000 to 16,000 outer hair cells and 2,000 to 3,000 inner hair cells) and over 24,000 neural fibers. Amazingly, this wondrous sensory system is housed within the circumference of a dime! Most of this text deals with this small structure that is responsible for transmitting acoustic energy into what we perceive as sound, as well as for helping us maintain our balance in and our orientation to our spatial world.

My hope is that readers will find the information in this second edition useful in their daily academic and clinical practice. I have tried to ensure that no errors have inadvertently crept in to the vast amount of material in this text. I urge readers to contact me at roeser@utdallas.edu should any be found so that they can be corrected in the next edition.

Acknowledgments

Any project of this magnitude requires the efforts of a village. My "village" started forming during the 2010 annual meeting of the American Academy of Audiology when Beth Campbell, an editor at Thieme, informed me that Thieme was interested in publishing a second edition of the *Audiology Desk Reference* (ADR). Following that meeting, Beth and I met regularly to review and develop ideas for the revision. After Beth took another position elsewhere, Emily Ekle, her successor, facilitated further work on the book. Elizabeth (Liz) D'Ambrosio, Emily's editorial assistant, transformed the raw material into publishable format and carried out the arduous task of obtaining all the permissions. Liz, I thank you wholeheartedly for your hard work.

One new aspect of this edition is that several of my close colleagues graciously agreed to function as editorial consultants. I thank Jackie L. Clark, Deanna Meinke, De Wet Swanepoel, and Gary G. Wright for their sage input and expert advice in selecting materials for this edition.

Finally, I want to thank two very special people, Lois and the late Howard Wolf, for championing my work and for their support of the field of pediatric hearing loss. Lois is passionate about helping people in general, as was Howard, and, partially because of Howard's hearing loss, they realized the severe impact that hearing loss has on human communication and achievement. They invested their philanthropic support in helping infants and children with hearing loss by creating the Lois and Howard Wolf Endowed Chair in Pediatric Hearing Loss that I am now so honored to hold. Their generosity will endure forever, and I am fortunate to honor their legacy of support for helping infants and children with hearing loss.

Editorial Consultants

Jackie L. Clark, PhD, FAAA, CCC/A
Callier Center for Communication Disorders
University of Texas at Dallas
Dallas, Texas
University of Witwatersrand
South Africa

Deanna Meinke, PhD, FAAA, CCC/A
Audiology and Speech-Language Sciences
University of Northern Colorado
Greeley, Colorado

De Wet Swanepoel, PhD
Department of Communication Pathology
University of Pretoria
South Africa
Callier Center for Communication Disorders
University of Texas at Dallas
Dallas, Texas

Gary G. Wright, PhD
Department of Otolaryngology–Head and Neck Surgery
University of Texas Southwestern Medical Center
Callier Center for Communication Disorders
University of Texas at Dallas
Dallas, Texas

1
Anatomy and Physiology

Basic Anatomy

The hearing and balance systems comprise the *peripheral receptor organs of the inner ear*, the *neural pathways*, and the *centers* within the central nervous system (CNS). Two main subdivisions can thus be distinguished:

- Peripheral part
  - External, middle, and inner ear
  - Vestibulocochlear nerve (cranial nerve VIII) with its two parts: the cochlear and the vestibular divisions
- Central part
  - Central hearing pathways
  - Subcortical and cortical auditory centers
  - Central balance mechanism

The anatomic boundary between the peripheral and central parts is the point of entry of cranial nerve VIII into the brainstem. The sensory organs of the membranous labyrinth develop from a structure known as the otic placode, which forms from the surface ectoderm of the early embryo. The bony capsule that surrounds the labyrinth is derived from embryonic connective tissue of mesodermal origin. The eustachian tube and the middle ear cavity arise from a diverticulum of the first pharyngeal pouch (endoderm). The malleus and incus develop from Meckel's cartilage, which arises from the first branchial arch and is supplied by the trigeminal nerve. The stapes arises from Reichert's cartilage, which arises from the second branchial arch and is supplied by the facial nerve.

The external meatus and the tympanic membrane develop from an ectodermal diverticulum between the first and second branchial arches (**Figs. 1.1** and **1.2**). Developmental disorders may cause deformities of the external and middle ears, which in some cases require corrective surgery. Bilateral lesions causing severe conductive deafness or a psychologically unacceptable deformity must be corrected for both aesthetic and functional reasons.

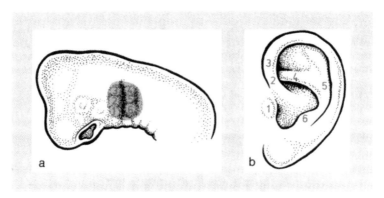

Fig. 1.1a,b Development of the external ear. (**a**) An 11-mm embryo, from the side. Outer ear development from six hillocks arising from the first and second branchial arches. (**b**) *1*, tragus; *2* crus helicis; *3*, helix; *4*, crus anthelicis; *5*, anthelix; *6*, antitragus.

External Ear

The *auricle* consists of a framework of elastic cartilage covered by skin, lying between the temporomandibular joint anteriorly and the mastoid process posteriorly. The skin adheres tightly to the perichondrium on the anterior surface but is more loosely attached posteriorly. For this reason contusions of the anterior surface often lead to detachment of the skin–perichondrial layer and to the formation of a *hematoma*.

The *external meatus* is approximately 3 cm long and consists of an outer cartilaginous part and an inner bony part. The cartilaginous meatus is curved and lies at an angle to the bony part. The tympanic membrane and the middle ear lying beyond it are thus protected from direct trauma.

> **Note:** In order for an otoscopic examination to be performed, the curved cartilaginous mobile part of the external auditory meatus must be drawn upward and posteriorly to bring it into the same axis as the bony part so that the otoscope can be introduced correctly.

The cartilaginous part is attached firmly to the rim of the *bony meatus* (os tympanicum) by connective tissue and is covered by a thin layer of skin that adheres to the periosteum. The skin of the bony meatus contains no accessory structures, in contrast to the cartilaginous part of the meatus that has numerous hair follicles and glands that form wax (epidermal squames, sebaceous matter, pigment).

The external meatus narrows medially so that foreign bodies often become impacted at the junction of the cartilaginous and bony meatus. The meatal cartilage does not form a closed tube but rather a channel closed superiorly by fibrous tissue. The cartilage contains several dehiscences (Santorini's clefts),

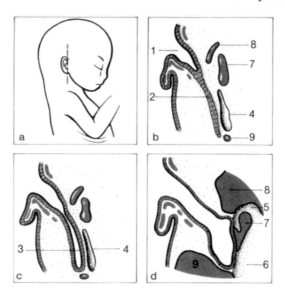

Fig. 1.2a–d Diagram of development of the external and middle ear. The first ectodermal branchial arch forms the primary anlage of the cartilaginous part of the external auditory meatus. The funnel-shaped tube is shown by **b**1. A string of epithelial cells grows mediocaudally toward the pharyngeal pouch (**b**2). The tympanic membrane (**c**3), the bony part of the external auditory meatus, the primitive middle ear cavity (**b**4 and **c**4), and the anlage of the tympanic plate (**b**9 and **d**9) develop later. The parts of the middle ear then begin to develop: the epitympanum (**d**5), the mesotympanum (**d**6), the malleus (**b** and **d**7), and the squamous part of the temporal bone (**b** and **d**8).

which provide a pathway for spread of severe bacterial infection to the parotid space, the infratemporal fossa, and the base of the skull. The so-called malignant otitis externa is often lethal.

The auricle and the cartilaginous meatus have a very rich *lymphatic drainage* to an extensive regional lymphatic network consisting of parotid, retroauricular, infraauricular, and superior deep cervical nodes. Infections of the external meatus with regional lymphadenitis can thus cause extensive swelling in these areas.

The *sensory innervation* is supplied by the trigeminal, great auricular, and vagus nerves and the sensory fibers of the facial nerve. The latter two branches respectively explain the cough reflex, which can be elicited from the posterior meatal wall, and the hypoesthesia of the posterosuperior meatal wall in patients with acoustic neuroma.

Relationships (Fig. 1.3)

The cartilaginous meatus abuts the parotid gland, thus allowing extension of infections or malignant tumors. The posterosuperior wall of the bony meatus forms a part of the *lateral attic wall* (the partition between external and auditory meatus and attic of the middle ear), the mastoid antrum, and the adjacent

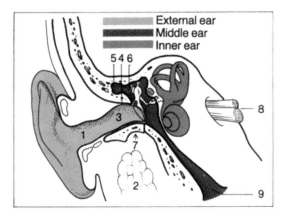

Fig. 1.3 Relationship of structures in the external auditory meatus and middle ear. *1*, cartilaginous part; *2*, parotid gland; *3*, bony meatus; *4*, lateral attic wall; *5*, mastoid antrum; *6*, attic; *7*, temporomandibular joint; *8*, facial, vestibular and auditory nerves; *9*, eustachian tube.

pneumatic system of the mastoid process. A middle ear infection can thus break through into the external auditory meatus causing sagging of the posterosuperior wall or fistula in acute mastoiditis. Equally, destruction of the lateral attic wall by cholesteatoma may form an open communication between the external auditory meatus and the attic or mastoid antrum. The anterior wall of the bony meatus forms part of the temporomandibular joint. There is thus a risk of fracture of the meatus as a result of a blow to the chin.

Middle Ear and Pneumatic System

The *middle ear cavity* consists of an extensive pneumatic system aerated by the eustachian tube. Its parts are as follows:

- Tympanic cavity
- Mastoid antrum
- Pneumatic system of the temporal bone

The *eustachian tube* consists of a mobile, cartilaginous portion (two thirds) suspended from the skull base, and a bony portion (one third). The bony portion, together with the tensor tympani muscle, forms the musculotubal canal in the temporal bone. This canal lies adjacent to the internal carotid artery. The funnel-shaped pharyngeal ostium of the cartilaginous part (torus tubarius) lies in the nasopharynx. The bony end opens into the middle ear.

The junction between the two parts of the eustachian tube is very narrow. This *isthmus* is the site of predilection for inflammatory stenosis of the tube. The tube serves to equalize air pressure between the middle ear and the nasopharynx, and thus to equalize the pressure on each side of the tympanic membrane. An increase in pressure in the tympanic cavity is usually compensated for passively via the eustachian tube to the nasopharynx, whereas a decrease in pressure usually requires active ventilation from the nasopharynx along the tube to the middle ear cavity. The tube opens and closes in response to movements of the neighboring muscles and differences of air pressure between the nasopharynx and the middle ear cavity, which tend to equalize spontaneously. The principal closing mechanism is the elastic recoil of the cartilage of the tube and the valvular action of the pharyngeal ostium of the tube. The tube is opened by contraction of the tensor palati and levator palati muscles. The mechanism is partially under the control of voluntary muscles, but the reflex movements on yawning and swallowing and the muscle tone are under autonomic control. Tension on the opening muscles is provided by the elastic recoil of the tubal cartilage and the pressure of the peritubal tissues, such as the pterygoid muscles, Ostmann's fatty bodies, the venous and lymphatic plexus of the tubal mucosa, and the pterygoid venous plexus.

The middle ear cavity is an air-containing space lying between the external ear and the inner ear. It is divided into three general parts (**Fig. 1.4**):

- Epitympanic recess or attic
- Mesotympanum
- Hypotympanic recess

Between the epi- and mesotympanum there is an anatomic constriction that can lead to retention of secretions during inflammation and to deficient aeration of the attic. This is due to the considerable narrowing of this area caused by the head of the malleus, the body of the incus, numerous ligaments, nerves (the chorda tympani), and mucosal folds and pockets. This is one of the causes of the chronic inflammation of the epitympanum (*chronic epitympanitis*), which is one of the causative factors of epitympanic cholesteatoma. A further narrow zone lies at the junction of the attic and the mastoid antrum (the *aditus ad antrum*), which may be closed by granulation tissue in chronic inflammation, leading to deficient aeration or drainage of the mastoid cell system. The lateral wall of the middle ear cavity is formed by the tympanic membrane. The hypotympanum is closely related to the bulb of the jugular vein.

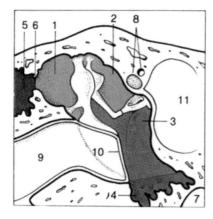

Fig. 1.4 Anatomy of the middle ear cavity. *1* and *2*, epitympanum; *3*, mesotympanum; *4*, hypotympanum; *5*, mastoid antrum; *6*, entrance to the antrum; *7*, internal jugular vein. The lower part of the attic (*2*) is markedly narrowed by the facial nerve and the horizontal semicircular canal (*8*). External meatus (*9*), tympanic membrane (*10*), and inner ear (*11*).

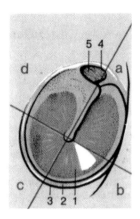

Fig. 1.5 Macroscopic appearance of the right tympanic membrane. *1*, pars tensa; *2*, anulus fibrosus; *3*, bony tympanic anulus; *4*, tympanic notch; *5*, pars flaccida. The visible part of the surface of the tympanic membrane is divided into four quadrants: anterosuperior (**a**), anteroinferior (**b**), posteroinferior (**c**), and posterosuperior (**d**).

The *tympanic membrane* consists of the pars tensa and the pars flaccida. The *pars tensa* forms the stiff vibrating surface of the membrane and is attached to a fibrous ring (the *anulus fibrosus*) lying in the tympanic sulcus of the tympanic part of the temporal bone. The *pars flaccida* is that part of the membrane in the area of the tympanic notch (of Rivinus) where the anulus fibrosus is discontinued (**Fig. 1.5**).

The microscopic appearance of the tympanic membrane is shown in **Fig. 1.6**. The epithelial or cuticular layer (stratum corneum) is similar in structure to the skin of the external auditory meatus, but the marginal zone bordering on the tympanic anulus shows extremely active proliferation due to papillary ingrowths of the stratum germinativum. This is a further important factor in the genesis of cholesteatoma, a disease in which skin invades the middle ear and causes bone erosion.

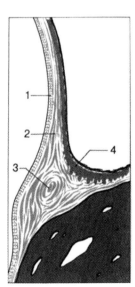

Fig. 1.6 Microscopic appearance of a sagittal section through the posteroinferior quadrant of the tympanic membrane. *1*, middle ear mucosa; *2*, middle fibrous layer; *3*, anulus fibrosus; *4*, epidermis layer with papillary downgrowths similar to the meatal skin bordering the tympanic membrane.

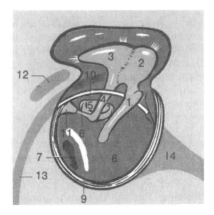

Fig. 1.7 Medial wall of the middle ear. Above the promontory (8) at the basal turn of the cochlea is the oval window niche with the stapes (5) whose footplate is held loosely in the oval window by the annular ligament. The long process of the incus (4) forms a joint by its lenticular process with the head of the stapes. The body of the incus (3) forms the joint surface for the head of the malleus (2). The malleus and incus vibrate as one body in the middle part of the frequency range. The round window (7) lies below the pyramidal eminence (11), which encloses the stapedius muscle whose tendon (6) runs to the head of the stapes. The bony facial canal (13) runs inferior to the horizontal semicircular canal (12). The handle and short process of the malleus (1) lie lateral to the chorda tympani (10). The pars tensa is anchored by the anulus fibrosus (9) in the bony niche of the anulus tympanicus. The middle ear cavity is aerated via the eustachian tube (14).

The keratinizing squamous epithelium regenerates not by superficial desquamation, as does the remaining part of the skin, but by migration of the epidermis from the center of the tympanic membrane to the periphery. This migration of the outer epidermal layer forms an important part of the self-cleaning mechanism of the external meatus.

The *lamina propria* has an external radial layer of fibers and an internal circular layer. The anulus fibrosus forms a thickening of the edge of the tympanic membrane and is formed by both layers of fibers. A lamina propria can also be seen in the *pars flaccid*, but it lacks the characteristic radial-circular structure described above, which provides the normal pars tensa with the necessary functional tension.

The *medial wall of the middle ear* also forms the lateral wall of the labyrinthine capsule (**Fig. 1.7**).

The *mucosa* that lines the middle ear space consists of pseudostratified ciliated epithelium around the mouth of the eustachian tube, becoming flattened peripherally to a stratified cuboidal epithelium. A few goblet cells and submucosal glands are normally present. The submucosa is very thin so that the mucosa lies directly on the periosteum to form a tightly bound unit, the *mucoperiosteum*. In pathological conditions such as tubal occlusion or chronic otitis media, the structure of the mucosa changes considerably to show hyperplasia of the glands, proliferation of the goblet cells, edema of the submucosa, vascular buds, and transformation of the flattened cuboidal epithelium to a columnar epithelium.

The middle ear mucosa forms several pouches and folds (*Prussak's space, von Troeltsch's pouch*) that are responsible for narrowing the junction between the attic and the rest of the middle ear and between the attic and the antrum. If embryonic connective tissue in this area does not involute properly after birth, the epitympanic recess remains as a narrow cleft. This "mesenchyme" can completely obliterate the epitympanum if a chronic hyperplastic inflammation follows an infection. The ventilation and drainage of the attic is then impeded by thickened masses of inflammatory tissue, despite normal tubal function. Deficient aeration and drainage of this small space favors the development of chronic *epitympanitis* and plays a considerable role in the pathogenesis of *chronic otitis media* and attic cholesteatoma.

The arterial blood supply is from branches of the internal and external carotid arteries and the subarcuate branch of the labyrinthine artery, which supplies the inner ear. The venous drainage of the middle ear is partly into the middle meningeal veins, partly into the venous plexus of the internal carotid artery and of the pharynx, and partly into the bulb of the internal jugular vein.

The nerve supply of the middle ear mucosa is provided in part by the tympanic branch of the glossopharyngeal nerve and partly by the auriculotemporal branch of the trigeminal nerve.

> **Note:** This joint sensory nerve supply of the oral and middle ear regions explains pain referred to the ear in diseases of the teeth and the jaws, and of the larynx and the pharynx.

Pneumatic System of the Temporal Bone

The air-containing cells of the mastoid process are in continuity with the air in the middle ear. These multiple interconnecting spaces arise from the mastoid antrum and show great variability in their degree of *pneumatization*. On the one hand, pneumatization may be well developed, extending to the temporal and occipital bones and the origin of the zygomatic arch. Acute infections of the mastoid may cause inflammatory swellings in these regions. On the other hand, the mastoid process may consist exclusively of compact bone if it is poorly pneumatized and the pneumatized cells are restricted to those in the immediate neighborhood of the antrum.

The mastoid process begins to develop after birth as a small tuberosity that is pneumatized synchronously with the growth of the mastoid antrum. In the first year of life it consists of spongy bone. Between the second and fifth years of life as pneumatization proceeds, it consists of mixed spongy and pneumatic bone. Pneumatization is complete between the sixth and the 12th years of life (**Figs. 1.8** and **1.9**).

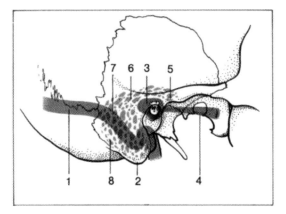

Fig. 1.8 Pneumatic system of the temporal bone. *1*, transverse sinus; *2*, mastoid process with tip cells; *3*, mastoid antrum; *4*, eustachian tube; *5*, zygomatic cells; *6*, cells of the squamous part of the temporal bone; *7*, sinodural angle, *8*, retrosinus cells.

Note: Characteristically, pneumatization of the temporal bone is reduced in chronic otitis media.

The better the temporal bone is pneumatized, the easier it is for infection to break through the thin cortical bone. In poor pneumatization (the so-called

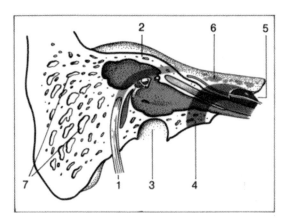

Fig. 1.9 Topographic relations of the middle ear cavity. *1*, facial nerve: inflammation and trauma often affect the mastoid segment; *2*, tegmen tympani, which is the site of predilection for a rupture of a mastoiditis into the middle cranial fossa; *3*, bulb of the internal jugular vein, which is the site of predilection for extension of a glomus tumor into the middle ear cavity; *4*, internal carotid artery (in petrositis, the inflammation can extend in the venous plexus around the carotid artery to set up a cavernous sinus thrombosis); *5*, cavernous sinus; *6*, apical cells (purulent infection in petrositis causes Gradenigo's syndrome); *7*, pneumatic system of the mastoid process.

dangerous mastoid process), the inflammatory process may be concealed in the depths and lead to unexpected complications.

Inner Ear, Peripheral Hearing, and Balance Organs

The inner ear, or labyrinth, which is embedded in the temporal bone, is divided into two functionally separate receptor mechanisms:

- The vestibular sensory organs (saccule, utricle, and semicircular ducts)
- The cochlea (the acoustic end organ)

The labyrinth can also be divided morphologically into a bony and a membranous part. The first is formed by the *labyrinthine capsule*, which arises by periosteal and enchondral ossification. It shows characteristic histopathological and chemical abnormalities in systemic bone diseases (e.g., Paget's disease and osteodystrophy) and in local diseases (e.g., otosclerosis). Both of these demonstrate continuous remodeling of bone.

The round and oval windows are openings to the labyrinth from the middle ear cavity. They are closed, respectively, by the round window membrane and the stapes footplate.

Bony and Membranous Labyrinths and Inner Ear Fluids (Fig. 1.10)

The bony labyrinth consists of a series of interconnected cavities in the temporal bone that are filled with fluid known as perilymph, which is similar in composition to cerebrospinal fluid. The perilymph is in fact in communication with the cerebrospinal fluid via the cochlear aqueduct, a bony channel that connects the basal end of the cochlea with the subarachnoid space surrounding the brain. Suspended within the bony labyrinth is the membranous labyrinth, a system of membranous sacs and ducts that enclose the inner ear sensory organs. The membranous labyrinth is filled with endolymph, a specialized fluid rich in potassium and low in sodium.

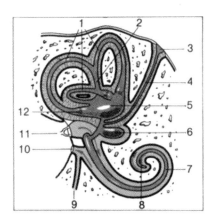

Fig. 1.10 Diagram of the inner ear. *1*, membranous semicircular ducts (horizontal, superior, and posterior); *2*, crus commune of the posterior and superior semicircular ducts; *3*, endolymphatic sac; *4*, endolymphatic duct; *5*, utricle; *6*, saccule; *7*, cochlear duct; *8*, helicotrema; *9*, cochlear aqueduct; *10*, round window; *11*, oval window; *12*, ampulla of the posterior semicircular duct.

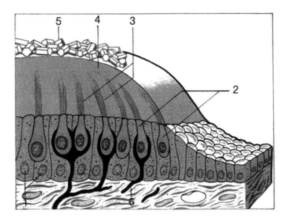

Fig. 1.11 Diagram of a vestibular macula. *1*, supporting cells; *2*, sensory cells; *3*, cilia; *4*, otoconial membrane; *5*, otoconia; *6*, afferent nerve fibers.

The perilymph is formed partly by filtration from the blood and partly by diffusion of cerebrospinal fluid via the cochlear aqueduct. The endolymph is a filtrate of perilymph, and its ionic composition (high potassium/low sodium) is kept constant by specialized epithelia located in the stria vascularis, the utricle, and the semicircular ducts.

Vestibular Sensory Organs

The peripheral vestibular system includes sensory receptors located in the saccule and utricle and in the three semicircular ducts (**Figs. 1.11, 1.12, 1.13, 1.14, 1.15**). All five of the vestibular sensory organs are stimulated by mechanical forces associated with acceleration, with the saccule and utricle being responsive to linear acceleration (straight line motion or the force of gravity) and the semicircular duct receptors responsive to angular acceleration (rotational motion). The neuroepithelia of all these organs contain sensory cells, known as hair cells, which are surrounded by supporting cells. The hair cells are equipped with cilia that project into an overlying accessory structure responsible for mechanical stimulation of the hair cells. In the saccule and utricle the accessory structure consists of a gelatinous sheet covered by calcium

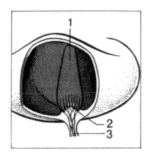

Fig. 1.12 Diagram of the ampulla of a semicircular duct. *1*, cupula; *2*, crista ampullaris; *3*, afferent nerve fibers.

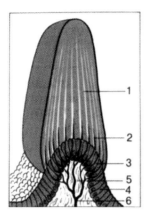

Fig. 1.13 Diagram of the crista ampullaris. *1*, cupula; *2*, cilia; *3*, sensory cells; *4*, supporting cells; *5*, crista ampullaris; *6*, afferent nerve fibers.

carbonate crystals called otoconia. Because of the inertial properties of the otoconia, the gelatinous sheet undergoes tiny displacements across the surface of the neuroepithelium (the macula) during linear acceleration, thereby deflecting the underlying cilia. These deflections produce electrical changes in the hair cells that alter the release of chemical neurotransmitters onto nerve

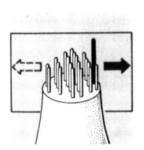

Fig. 1.14 Diagram of polarization of a vestibular sensory cell in the crista. Each sensory cell possesses one kinocilium *(black finger-like shape)* and approximately 60 stereocilia *(light finger-like shapes)*. Displacement of the cupula (and with it the cilia) toward the kinocilium causes a nerve stimulation by depolarization of the hair cell and increased neurotransmitter release. Displacement in the opposite direction hyperpolarizes the hair cell, resulting in decreased neural discharge. In the horizontal semicircular duct polarization is toward the utricle, but in the vertical ducts polarization is in the opposite direction, away from the utricle.

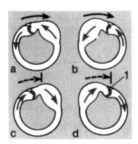

Fig. 1.15a–d The principle of function of the mechanoreceptors of the horizontal semicircular duct (see **Figs. 1.27** and **1.28**). Positive acceleration in a clockwise direction causes endolymph displacement in the opposite direction due to inertia, and utriculopetal deflection of the cupula in the right horizontal semicircular duct. (**b**) Utriculofugal deflection in the left horizontal semicircular duct (**a**). Neural discharge thus increases on the right side and decreases on the left side. Deceleration in a clockwise direction induces the opposite reaction: utriculopetal deflection on the left side (**c**) and utriculofugal deflection on the right side (**d**) with corresponding changes in neural activity. (*1*, cupula).

endings attached to the cells, thereby changing the flow of nerve impulses in the vestibular nerve.

The three semicircular ducts are attached to the utricle and each has an expansion at one end called the ampulla, which encloses a ridge of tissue (the crista) on which the hair cells and supporting cells are located. The cilia of the hair cells extend into a gelatinous mass called the cupula, which reaches to the roof of the ampulla. The cupula acts as a mobile partition that is deflected during angular acceleration, thereby stimulating the underlying hair cells (**Fig. 1.13**). Because the cupula has no otoconia, it has the same density as the surrounding endolymph and is unaffected by linear acceleration.

Cochlea (Acoustic End Organ)

The macro- and microscopic structure of the bony and membranous cochlea is shown in **Figs. 1.16** and **1.17**.

Functional Structure of Corti's Organ
The tallest cilia of the outer hair cells are in contact with the tectorial membrane. Radial forces are generated between the tectorial membrane and the basilar membrane when the latter vibrates. This exerts a shearing force on the cilia of the hair cells and defects them tangentially. The deflection of the inner hair cell stereocilia is believed to be due to fluid motion beneath the tectorial membrane as the basilar membrane vibrates. The mechanical stimulation is converted in the receptor organ to a neuronal stimulus via neurotransmitter release from the sensory cells. The inner hair cells form only one row, and each cell connects to multiple afferent nerve fibers. These constitute 95% of all afferent fibers in the acoustic nerve, whereas the outer hair cells, although they form three rows, converge in groups onto single afferent nerve fibers that form only 5% of the fibers of the auditory nerve. Each afferent fiber is associated with a specific frequency range.

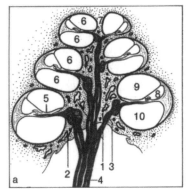 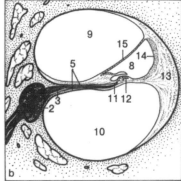

Fig. 1.16a,b Cochlear cross sections, showing the entire cochlea (**a**), and an enlarged section through a single cochlear turn (**b**).

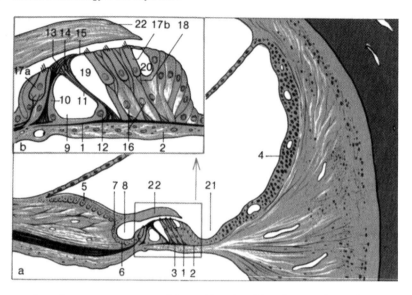

Fig. 1.17a,b   Schematic cross section of the cochlear duct (**a**) and organ of Corti (**b**).

The human cochlea is a spiral structure wound two and a half turns around a central bony axis called the modiolus (label **1** on **Fig. 1.16**), which lies in a nearly horizontal position when the head is upright. Its base is situated at the lateral end of the internal acoustic meatus and its apex (**7**) is directed antero-laterally toward the medial wall of the middle ear. The spiral ganglion, containing the cell bodies of the cochlear nerve (**2**), is located within the modiolus. The central processes of the ganglion cells (**3**) join together to form the trunk of the cochlear nerve (**4**). The osseous spiral lamina (**5**) is a bony plate or shelf that spirals around the modiolus from base to apex, much like the threads on a screw. The osseous lamina consists of two thin layers of bone between which nerve fibers pass from the spiral ganglion to reach the organ of Corti (**12**). The cochlear duct (**8**), filled with endolymph, lies between the scala vestibuli (**9**) and the scala tympani (**10**), both of which contain perilymph. The osseous lamina (**5**) and basilar membrane (**11**) separate the scala tympani from the scala vestibuli and cochlear duct. Reissner's membrane (**15**) separates the scala vestibuli from the cochlear duct. The stria vascularis (**14**) forms the lateral wall of the cochlear duct and contains numerous blood vessels. The stria maintains the high potassium concentration of the endolymph and the positive electrical potential (endolymphatic potential) of the cochlear duct. Adjacent to the stria vascularis and separating it from the bony cochlear wall is the spiral ligament, which plays an important role in movement of potassium ions between perilymph and endolymph (**13**).

The perilymphatic spaces of the cochlea (scala tympani and scala vestibuli) communicate with each other at the apex of the cochlea via an opening called the helicotrema (label **8** on **Fig. 1.10**). Scala vestibuli also communicates with the perilymphatic space of the vestibule, which contains the saccule and utricle of the vestibular system (labels **5, 6** on **Fig. 1.10**).

The basilar membrane (labels **1** and **3** on **Fig. 1.17**) is covered on its lower surface by cells (**2**) that line the scala tympani. The organ of Corti rests on the upper surface of the basilar membrane inside the cochlear duct. Medially, on the osseous spiral lamina, is the spiral limbus (**5**).

The tympanic lip (label **6** on **Fig. 1.17**) and the vestibular lip (**7**) of the limbus enclose the internal spiral sulcus (**8**). The stria vascularis (**4**) occupies the lateral wall of the cochlear duct. The inner tunnel (tunnel of Corti) (**9**) of the organ of Corti is bordered by the inner (**10**) and outer (**11, 12**) pillar cells, the upper parts of which (**13–15**) form portions of the reticular lamina at the upper surface of the organ of Corti. The inner (**17a**) and outer (**17b**) hair cells are situated on either side of the inner tunnel space. The inner hair cells are arranged in a single row, and there are three rows of outer hair cells supported by the Deiters' cells (**16, 18**). The outer hair cells are surrounded by Nuel's spaces (**19**) and the outer tunnel space (**20**). The fluid spaces inside the organ of Corti, including the inner tunnel, Nuel's spaces, and outer tunnel, are filled with a perilymph-like fluid known as Cortilymph. The fluid that fills the cochlear duct and surrounds the organ of Corti is endolymph. The external spiral sulcus (**21**) lies between the organ of Corti and the lateral wall of the cochlear duct. Extending from the surface of the spiral limbus is the tectorial membrane (**22**) that covers the organ of Corti and plays an important role in stimulation of the sensory cells during vibration of the basilar membrane.

Central Connections of the Auditory System (Fig. 1.18)

Cochlear nerve fibers from the spiral ganglion enter the brainstem at the lower border of the pons and terminate in the dorsal and ventral cochlear nuclei. Secondary neural projections from the ventral cochlear nuclei enter the ipsilateral and contralateral trapezoid nuclei. Fiber tracts from the trapezoid nuclei enter the lateral lemniscus to ascend to the auditory cortex via the inferior colliculus and medial geniculate body. Most fibers from the dorsal cochlear nuclei cross the midline to enter the lateral lemniscus where they ascend to the higher centers of the auditory pathway.

Central Connections of the Vestibular System (Fig. 1.19)

The bipolar neurons of the vestibular ganglion are divided into superior and inferior divisions that send their peripheral processes as two separate bundles of fibers to the sensory cells in the macula of the utricle, to the lateral and superior semicircular ducts (superior division), and to the posterior semicircular duct and the macula of the saccule (inferior division).

The central processes combine to form the vestibular division of cranial nerve VIII, which unites in the internal auditory meatus with the cochlear division to form the vestibulocochlear nerve. After entering the medulla oblongata, the vestibular division sends fibers to the brainstem vestibular nuclei and to the cerebellum. Major secondary pathways from the vestibular nuclei include the vestibulospinal tracts (which are important in regulating tone of

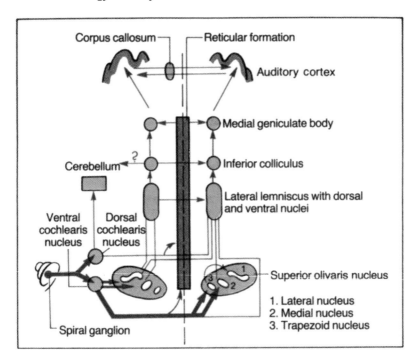

Fig. 1.18 Simplified diagram of the afferent auditory pathways. The pathways for one cochlea only are shown for the sake of simplicity.

postural muscles) as well as projections to the cerebellum, reticular formation and the nuclei of cranial nerves III, IV, and VI, which control the extraocular muscle. A vestibulocortical connection is provided via the thalamus. Vestibular information is projected to several areas of the cerebral cortex, where it is integrated with input from other systems, including visual and proprioceptive.

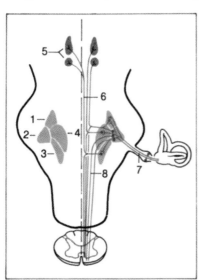

Fig. 1.19 Diagram of the central vestibular connections in the brainstem. *1*, superior vestibular nucleus of Bechterew; *2*, lateral vestibular nucleus of Deiters; *3*, inferior vestibular nucleus; *4*, medial vestibular nucleus of Schwalbe; *5*, centers for the eye muscles; *6*, medial longitudinal bundle; *7*, vestibular nerve; *8*, vestibulospinal tract.

Facial Nerve

Cranial nerve VII carries motor fibers for the muscles of facial expression and taste fibers and visceroefferent secretory neurons in a separate nerve bundle, the nervus intermedius. It also contains sensory fibers that supply the posterior wall of the external auditory meatus. This explains the reduced sensation of this area of skin in patients with acoustic neuroma (Hitselberger's sign) (**Figs. 1.20** and **1.21**).

The *motor fibers* originate from the facial motor nucleus in the floor of the fourth ventricle, run around the abducens nucleus (the internal "genu"), and leave at the lower border of the pons together with the *visceroefferent fibers* of the nervus intermedius arising from the superior salivatory nucleus. The *gustatory fibers* arise from the subcortical taste centers in the nucleus of the solitary tract. These branches form the *nervus intermediofacialis*, which first runs in the internal auditory meatus (the *meatal segment*). It enters the bony canal immediately adjacent to the labyrinth (the *labyrinthine segment*) and runs to the hiatus in the canal for the facial nerve. At this point the greater superficial petrosal nerve divides off from the main trunk. This branch goes to the lacrimal gland and also supplies fibers to the glands of the nasal mucosa. The first "genu" of the facial nerve lies at the level of the geniculate ganglion. The nerve then turns into the horizontal *tympanic segment* and then passes at the level of the entrance to the mastoid antrum, the second "genu," into the vertical *mastoid segment*. In this area it gives off fibers to the stapedius muscle and to the chorda tympani, which contains taste fibers for the anterior two

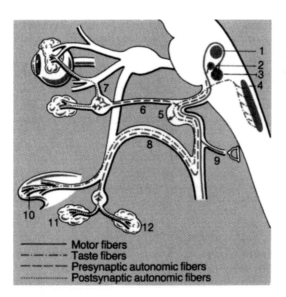

Fig. 1.20 Course of fibers in the facial nerve. *1*, abducens nucleus; *2*, secretory nucleus of the nervus intermedius; *3*, motor nuclei of the facial nerve; *4*, nucleus of the solitary tract; *5*, geniculate ganglion; *6*, greater superficial petrosal nerve; *7*, pterygopalatine ganglion with the lacrimal anastomosis; *8*, chorda tympani; *9*, stapedius nerve; *10*, taste fibers to the anterior two thirds of the tongue; *11*, sublingual gland; *12*, submandibular gland.

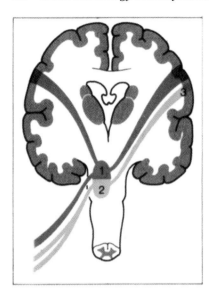

Fig. 1.21 Diagram of the bilateral corticobulbar innervations of the facial nucleus. This is important in the differential diagnosis of peripheral and central facial paralyses. The branch for the forehead (i.e., frontal) derives its fibers from the rostral facial nucleus (*1*), which is innervated by both cortices. The caudal nucleus (*2*), however, only receives fibers from the contralateral motor center (*3*). Therefore, the function of the fibers of the facial nerve for the forehead remains mainly intact in central paralysis because the facial nerve receives motor impulses from the intact homolateral cortical centers. In *peripheral and nuclear* facial paralyses all the fibers are paralyzed.

thirds of the tongue and visceroefferent fibers for the sublingual and submandibular glands. After leaving the mastoid process through the stylomastoid foramen, it divides into five extratemporal branches: temporal, zygomatic, buccal, marginal mandibular, and cervical to the platysma. There is great variability among these branches.

The facial nerve is surrounded in its course through the temporal bone by a tough fibrous sheath. Its individual fascicles are embedded in a well-developed *epineurium* of loose connective tissue that encloses the vessels and nerves. The fiber bundles are enclosed in perineurium. In repairing an injury of the nerve, the epineurium must be resected from the stump, and a perineural suture must be used so that the site of anastomosis can be adapted exactly, to prevent the formation of a scar tissue neuroma resulting from connective tissue infiltration of the anastomosis.

Physiology and Pathophysiology of Hearing and Balance

Physiology of Hearing

External and Middle Ear

The pinna and external auditory canal function to collect sound energy and transport the sound stimulus to the tympanic membrane. Due to their resonance properties, the concha and external canal increase the intensity of incoming sounds in the frequency range of 1500 to 7000 Hz by as much as 10 to 20 dB sound pressure level (SPL), thereby enhancing the transmission of the speech frequencies. In addition to its acoustic properties, the external ear canal helps to protect the tympanic membrane from mechanical trauma and from changes in temperature and humidity.

Sound waves transported by the external ear canal set the tympanic membrane into motion, and the vibrations of the membrane are transferred to the ossicular chain. The frequency of motion is the same as that of the vibrations in air, and its amplitude is proportional. The transmission of sound waves in air to the fluid of the inner ear is enhanced by the physical properties of the tympanic membrane and ossicular chain. Because fluid is denser than air, more pressure is required for the sound stimulus to be efficiently propagated in the cochlear fluids than in air. This mismatch in acoustic resistance (or impedance) is partially compensated for by the difference in surface area between the tympanic membrane and the stapes footplate and by the fact that the ossicular chain operates as a lever system. The functionally effective surface area of the tympanic membrane is approximately 55 mm^2. The area of the stapes footplate is approximately 3.2 mm^2. This difference in surface area (55/3.2) serves to increase the pressure on the footplate by a factor of 17. In addition, the pressure exerted by the stapes footplate is increased by a factor of 1.3 due to the lever action of the ossicular chain. The total pressure on the stapes footplate is therefore increased by approximately 22 times, or approximately 27 dB.

The prerequisite for normal transmission of sound to the inner ear is a tympanic membrane of normal position and mobility and a similar air pressure in the outer and middle ears. Impedance measurements at the tympanic membrane provide information about the function of the sound transmission apparatus, and this is used as a clinical method of testing called impedance audiometry. Sound energy reaches the cochlea first via the sound transmission system of the middle ear (air conduction) and secondarily through the bone of the skull, which is set in motion by the sound stimulus. The sound energy is thus transmitted directly to the cochlea via the labyrinthine capsule (bone conduction). Audiometry is used to measure the hearing threshold for both air and bone conduction.

The Cochlea

The cochlea functions to convert the mechanical energy of sound into electrical impulses that are conducted by the auditory nerve to the brain, a process called mechanoelectrical transduction. An important part of the transduction process is mechanical frequency analysis of the sound stimulus. Vibratory movements of the stapes footplate are transferred to the inner ear fluids, which in turn set the basilar membrane into motion. Because the basilar membrane is stiffer and less massive in the base of the cochlea than at the apex, the basal part of the basilar membrane begins to vibrate first in response to incoming sound, after which the progressively more massive parts of the membrane begin to move, giving rise to an apparent wave motion along the length of the membrane known as the "traveling wave." As the wave moves toward the cochlear apex its amplitude increases, and for any given frequency it reaches a maximum at a specific point along the basilar membrane. In the area of maximal amplitude the traveling wave causes a displacement of the surface of the organ of Corti relative to the overlying tectorial membrane so that the cilia of the hair cells are deflected at that location, thereby mechanically stimulating the sensory cells.

The region of maximal displacement of the traveling wave lies at a different location for each frequency; it is nearer the apex for lower frequencies and nearer the base for higher frequencies. Every frequency is thus represented at a particular point along the basilar membrane. This phenomenon provides a first analysis of the sound stimulus. However, it cannot fully account for the high level of sensitivity and frequency acuity observed in the cochlea. It is now believed that a metabolically active process is also at work that increases the cochlea's sensitivity to low-intensity sounds and sharpens its frequency response. That process is dependent on the outer hair cells of the organ of Corti, which have been shown to change their shape in response to sound stimulation in such a way as to alter the micromechanics of the organ of Corti and the basilar membrane. This active process, sometimes referred to as the cochlear amplifier, significantly contributes to the sensitivity and frequency selectivity of the inner ear.

As the basilar membrane vibrates, the stereocilia of the inner and outer hair cells are deflected in a back-and-forth manner. As the stereocilia are deflected outward, toward the lateral wall of scala media, ion channels near their tips are opened, allowing positively charged ions (mostly potassium) to flow inward, which depolarizes the sensory cells. This change in intracellular electrical potential triggers a series of events leading to release of neurotransmitter from the hair cells onto nerve endings of the auditory nerve, producing electrical impulses that are conducted from the cochlea to the CNS. The flow of potassium ions into the sensory cells is driven by the electrochemical gradient between the endolymph and the interior of the hair cells. That is, the endolymphatic compartment of scala media has a standing positive electrical potential (the endolymphatic potential [EP]) of approximately 80 millivolts, which is maintained by the stria vascularis. The combination of the EP and the high potassium concentration of the endolymph drives potassium ions into the hair cells when the stereocilia are appropriately deflected. The resulting reduction in the negative internal electrical potential of the cell (depolarization) then leads to generation of neural impulses as described above.

Nearly all the neural impulses that code information relating to auditory stimulation are generated by activity from the inner hair cells. Approximately 95% of spiral ganglion cell nerve fibers end on inner hair cells, with only 5% of the ganglion cell fibers reaching outer hair cells. Thus the inner hair cells are the principal sensory cells of the cochlea, whereas the outer hair cells have a primarily motor function, serving to alter cochlear micromechanics so as to more effectively stimulate specific groups of inner hair cells in response to sound stimulation. In addition to the afferent nerve fibers that carry information from the cochlea to the CNS, the inner ear also receives an efferent nerve supply that originates in the region of the superior olivary nuclei of the brainstem and projects peripherally to the organ of Corti, where it functions to modulate the responses of hair cells and afferent nerve fibers to auditory stimulation.

Physiology of Hearing: Retrocochlear Analysis of Acoustic Information

The pattern of sensory cell stimulation in the organ of Corti is converted in the peripheral cochlear neurons into the action potential pattern of the auditory nerve. The many parameters of the sound stimulus—such as frequency, intensity, temporal pattern, and periodicity of the action potentials—must be encoded to allow information analysis in the CNS:

- Sound frequency and sound intensity coding: These parameters play a very important role in the central analysis of the acoustic signal.
- Sound intensity coding by means of frequency modulation: With increasing sound intensity, the number of spikes in the sensory cell discharge increases.
- Sound frequency coding: Specific sensory cell groups in Corti's organ are stimulated depending on the sound frequency. Tonotopy (see below) allows these locally circumscribed stimulus patterns produced on the basilar membrane to be conducted without distortion by the auditory nerve to the higher centers.
- Tonotopy: This is a point-to-point connection between the sound receptors and the neurons analyzing the signal. Each cochlear neuron has a so-called best frequency that responds preferentially to an acoustic stimulus whose frequency is identical with the frequency assigned to it (tonotopy).

The acoustic system can process the duration, intensity, and frequency parameters of the acoustic signal in the following ways:

- With increasing intensity and constant frequency the action potential rate in the nerve fibers increases and the number of stimulated afferent neurons also increases, corresponding to the extent of the deflected area of the basilar membrane.
- At constant intensity and variable frequency, the deflected area of the basilar membrane is displaced into the appropriate segment of Corti's organ within the cochlea so that frequency is determined by point analysis. Furthermore, changes occur in the periodicity of the action potential series within the individual nerve fibers, which are analyzed by means of periodicity analysis. This provides another means of frequency determination.
- A further means of differentiation is provided by the temporal stimulus pattern. The sound frequency-adjustment is based on the relation of several frequency-sensitive neurons. These are characterized by a tuning

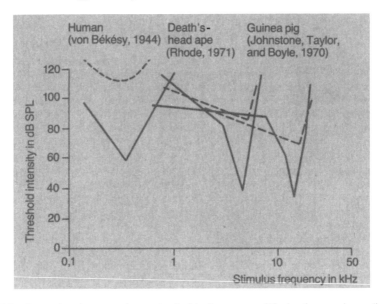

Fig. 1.22 Comparison between the mechanical tuning curves of the basilar membrane *(broken lines)* and the corresponding tuning curves of individual nerve fibers *(solid lines)*. The curves are recorded for the actual measured intensity area.

curve that encompasses the entire stimulus range of the neurons. The lowest point of the curve is the actual threshold, and it indicates the best sound frequency of the appropriate neuron (**Fig. 1.22**). This neuronal tuning curve is not to be confused with the mechanical tuning curve, which shows how the stimulus intensity must be changed relative to frequency so that a particular point on the basilar membrane always has the same deflection amplitude (**Fig. 1.22**).

- Frequency analysis by means of local pattern scanning, appreciation of intensity by frequency modulation, and time-periodicity analysis by combined time and place pattern evaluation also proceed in the higher hearing centers thanks to tonotopy.

Pathophysiologic Basis of Hearing Disorders

Conductive or middle ear deafness is caused by lesions of the stimulus transport system. A characteristic symptom of this type of hearing loss is that bone conduction functions better than the air conduction. The depression of the hearing threshold for air conduction is associated with an increase of acoustic impedance, for example, as a result of stapes fixation due to otosclerosis.

Sensory deafness is caused by lesions in the cochlea or in the auditory nerves.

Disorders of sound perception are caused by lesions in the subcortical or cortical auditory centers and by pathological processes involving the central auditory pathway. As a result, the acoustic signals are falsely coded, stimulus patterns are wrongly analyzed, and acoustic information can no longer be integrated. The patient may hear but not understand.

Central hearing disorders are characterized by a loss of integrative functions of the hearing centers. Differences in level of tone, differences in loudness, and temporal differences of acoustic stimulus pattern can no longer be analyzed. The *redundancy* is also reduced in that the information content is reduced due to loss of secondary and tertiary cochlear neurons. These disorders affect the understanding of speech (whereas hearing for pure tones may be preserved), directional hearing, and speech intelligibility.

Recruitment

In certain forms of unilateral sensorineural deafness, the loudness perception rises quickly with increasing loudness intensity so that, despite different hearing thresholds, both ears hear the tone with the same loudness once a certain threshold is reached. This phenomenon is called *recruitment.*

The pathophysiological basis of recruitment is not entirely clear. Because it is an abnormal phenomenon of loudness sensitivity, it is probably associated with the coding of loudness. At present, *positive recruitment* is generally regarded as a sign of a cochlear lesion, whereas *absent recruitment* indicates a retrocochlear lesion localized to the first or second neuron.

There is a hypothesis about the cause of recruitment. Damaged sensory cells and afferent neurons of lower frequency selectivity require very high sound pressure for excitation compared with healthy hair cells and neurons of higher frequency selectivity. As soon as the stimulus intensity rises above the pathologically raised threshold, the number of sensory cells and their associated afferent neurons that are stimulated increases due to spread of the stimulus to neighboring neurons with a similar best frequency (the summation principle.) Subjectively, this declares itself by a disproportionately rapid increase of sound sensitivity once that pathologically raised hearing threshold has been exceeded. Very loud sounds are uncomfortable for the deaf patient because he experiences distortion and even pain, as the *dynamic hearing range* (i.e., the difference between the threshold of hearing and that for pain) is reduced.

Physiology of the Balance System

Balance is maintained by coordination of visual, proprioceptive, and vestibular regulatory mechanisms. The vestibular sensory organs of the inner ear respond to physical stimuli related to movement and orientation of the head in three-dimensional space (**Figs. 1.12, 1.13, 1.14, 1.15, 1.16**). In response to mechanical forces acting on the inner ear, neural messages regarding head motion and head position are generated by the vestibular apparatus and relayed to the brain. That information, along with visual and proprioceptive

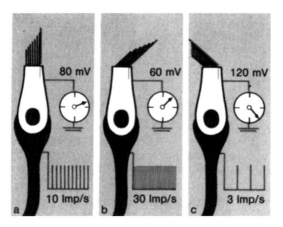

Fig. 1.23a–c Diagram of the bioelectrical activity of the vestibular sensory cells at rest, and in response to stimulation. (**a**) At rest. (**b**) Deflection of the stereocilia toward the kinocilium causes depolarization and increase of the neural discharge frequency. (**c**) Bending in the opposite direction causes hyperpolarization and inhibition of the resting activity (see **Fig. 1.14**). Imp/s, impulses per second.

input, is used by the CNS to help maintain clear vision during head movement, to control muscles responsible for maintaining body posture, and to provide a sense of orientation with respect to the surrounding environment.

The afferent nerve fibers connected to the vestibular sensory cells transmit a steady stream of impulses to the CNS even when the sensory epithelia are not under active stimulation. As shown in **Fig. 1.23,** this "spontaneous" or resting discharge may be increased or decreased by changes in intracellular electrical potential that occur when a stimulus is applied to the receptor cells. Because the spontaneous discharge may be modulated either up or down, the system shows directional sensitivity. Movement of the cupula or otoconial membrane in one direction increases the neural discharge, whereas movement in the opposite direction decreases the discharge.

Function of the Saccule and Utricle

Neural impulses resulting from linear acceleratory stimulation of the saccule and utricle are relayed to the brainstem, activating the maculo-ocular reflex, which produces compensatory eye movements that ensure appropriate positioning of the eyes in response to linear movement and changes of head position relative to the gravitational field. Maculospinal reflexes are also evoked, which influence the musculature of the trunk and limbs to stabilize body position during linear movement. Because the saccule and utricle are constantly acted on by the force of gravity, even when the head is not moving, they continuously generate neural input to the CNS that is important in regulation of postural muscle tone and awareness of body position in space.

Function of the Semicircular Ducts

A positive or negative angular acceleration causes displacement of endolymph within the semicircular ducts lying in the plane of the applied force. The stimulus always affects the semicircular ducts of both sides; the cupula on one side is deflected toward the utricle (utriculopetal stimulation) and on the other side in the opposite direction (utriculofugal stimulation). If the stimulus is affecting the cristae of the horizontal semicircular ducts, then the resting neural discharge of the crista whose cupula is deflected toward the utricle will increase (depolarization effect), whereas the discharge rate will decrease on the opposite side (hyperpolarization effect). For a stimulus applied to either of the vertical semicircular ducts, the opposite effects occur because cupular deflection toward the utricle produces hyperpolarization of the sensory cells in the cristae of the vertical ducts.

The change in neural discharge induced by angular acceleration is relayed to the brainstem nuclei responsible for control of eye movement, and the extraocular muscles will draw the eyes in a direction opposite to the direction of rotation (**Fig. 1.24**). This response is the vestibulo-ocular reflex, which serves to stabilize the visual field on the retina as the head moves, thereby reducing visual blurring during head motion, which helps to maintain clear vision as the body moves. When the eyes reach their limit of motion within the orbits, they quickly reset to the midline before moving again in the direction opposite

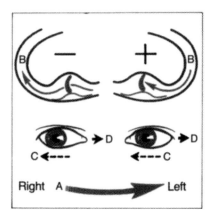

Fig. 1.24 Diagram of the vestibuloocular reflex. Angular acceleration from right to left *(A)* causes displacement of the endolymph to the right because of the inertia of the inner ear fluid. Deflection of the cupula causes depolarization on the left side and hyperpolarization on the right. This results in increased bioelectric activity in the left vestibular sensory organ *(B)* and the ipsilateral vestibular centers. Innervation of the left oculomotor nerve and the right abducens nerve via the medial longitudinal bundle (see **Fig. 1.19**). This induces a slow conjugated eye movement to the right in the direction opposite to the direction of rotation. This is the slow component of nystagmus *(C)*. Once maximal ocular deviation has been achieved there is a fast eye movement in the same direction as that of the rotation *(D)*, i.e., the fast component of nystagmus. The eyes are thus returned to the neutral position. *The direction of nystagmus is always defined as that of the fast component.*

to that of the head rotation. This repeated pattern of eye movement, in which the eyes move relatively slowly in one direction and then quickly return to the midline, is called nystagmus. The initial, slower phase of the nystagmic beat is controlled by the vestibular system, whereas the quick return to midline is under control of the brainstem reticular formation. Because the quick return is the most obvious part of the nystagmic beat, it is the direction of eye movement during that phase that said to be the direction of nystagmus. The assessment of nystagmus is an important part of the clinical evaluation of vestibular function.

In addition to its connections with the brainstem nuclei that control the extraocular muscles, important CNS neural projections of the vestibular system include the vestibulospinal tracts, reciprocal connections with the cerebellum, the brainstem reticular formation, and vestibular projections via the thalamus to the cerebral cortex.

Pathophysiological Basis of Functional Vestibular Disorders

A vestibular disorder manifests itself in the following ways:

1. *Vertigo*, partial or complete loss of spatial orientation, for example, an apparent movement of the environment as a result of spontaneous vestibular nystagmus (**Fig. 1.25**)
2. A *disturbance of balance*, with inability to maintain balance, to stand upright, or to walk properly (ataxia)

Vestibular disorders may be *peripheral*, caused by sudden unilateral failure of one labyrinth or by a unilateral lesion of the vestibular nerve, or may be *central*, caused by a lesion of the vestibular centers or their central connections to the cerebellum and reticular formation.

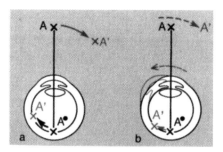

Fig. 1.25a,b Diagram of production of apparent movement of the visual field during nystagmus and induction of rotatory dizziness. (**a**) If the visual field moves on the retina with fixed gaze (Ax-xA′), the environment appears to move in the direction of displacement of the visual field, as a result of displacement of the image on the retina in the opposite direction (A•x–xA′) (**b**) If the visual field is stationary and the eyes move in conjugation (nystagmus), a subjective impression of movement of the environment also occurs caused by displacement of the visual image on the retina (A•x-A′). This is accompanied by a subjective sensation of rotator vertigo in the same direction as the fast phase of the nystagmus (A-A′).

Functional disturbance in a vestibular end organ causes unequal activity in the higher vestibular centers. This central imbalance produces initially a disturbance of vestibular physiology. The multisensory spatial orientation can thus no longer function because vestibular information, on the one hand, and visual somatosensory information, on the other hand, contradict each other. This causes disturbance of orientation, which in turn causes dizziness. If the central imbalance in the vestibular centers influences the main neighboring coordination centers for eye movements in the reticular formation of the brainstem, spontaneous abnormal eye movements occur that have the characteristics of nystagmus.

The direction of the sense of rotation is almost always the same as that of the fast phase of the nystagmus (**Fig. 1.25**).

Peripheral functional failure is compensated centrally by adjustment to altered peripheral input in the central vestibular centers and by substitution of visual and somatosensory regulatory mechanisms for the loss of peripheral vestibular function. This process is called *central vestibular compensation*. Central vestibular disorders are only incompletely compensated by the above mechanisms (or not at all) because the multisensory connections to the vestibular centers are damaged.

Survey of the Brainstem and Cranial Nerves

(In this survey section, the citations in parentheses refer to the labels on the figures cited in the headings. For example, **c1** in the Brainstem subsection refers to label **1** on part c of **Fig. 1.26**, and **ad5** refers to label **5** on parts **a** and **d**.)

Brainstem (Fig. 1.26)

The **brainstem (truncus cerebri)** may be divided into three sections: the *medulla oblongata* (**c1**), the *pons* (**c2**), and the *mesencephalon (midbrain)* (**c3**). This is the part of the brain that lies above the chorda dorsalis (notochord) during embryonic development and from which several true peripheral (cranial) nerves emerge. The cerebellum, which belongs to it ontogenetically, is discussed separately because of its special structure.

The **medulla oblongata**, between the pyramidal decussation and the lower margin of the pons, forms the transition from the spinal cord to the brain. The *anterior median fissure* extends as far as the pons, interrupted by the pyramidal decussation (**a4**), and is paralleled on both sides by the *anterior lateral sulcus* (**ad5**). The anterior funiculi become thicker below the pons and form the *pyramids* (**a6**). On both sides the *olives* bulge lateral to them (**ad7**).

The **pons**, or bridge (**a**), forms a wide, arching bulge with marked transverse fibers. It switches descending pathways from the cerebrum onto fibers leading to the cerebellum.

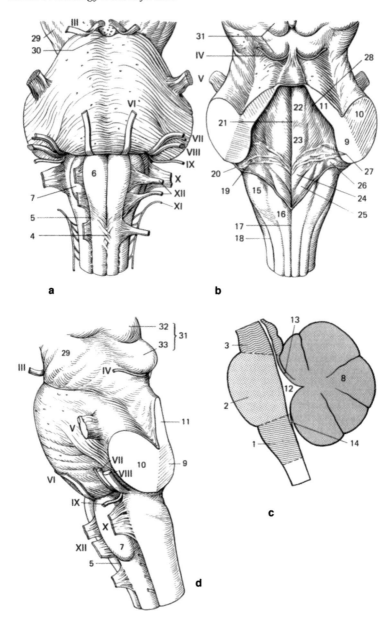

Fig. 1.26a–d   (**a**) Basal view of the brainstem. (**b**) Dorsal view of the brainstem, rhomboid fossa. (**c**) Subdivisions of the brainstem. (**d**) Lateral view of the brainstem.

The dorsal surface of the brainstem is covered by the *cerebellum* (**c8**). Upon removal of it, the three *cerebellar peduncles* on each side are cut through: the *inferior cerebellar peduncle (restiform body)* (**bd9**), *medial cerebellar peduncle (brachium pontis)* (**bd10**), and the *superior cerebellar peduncle (brachium conjunctivum)* (**bd11**). This exposes the *fourth ventricle* (**c12**), whose tent-shaped roof is formed by the *superior medullary velum* (**c13**) and in the *inferior medullary velum* (**c14**). The floor of the fourth ventricle, the *rhomboid fossa* (**b**), is now exposed. The medulla and the pons, which together are known as the **rhombencephalon**, are named after it. On each side the posterior funiculi thicken to form the *tuberculum nuclei cuneati* (**b15**) and the *gracilis* (**b16**), which are bordered in the midline by the *posterior median sulcus* (**b17**), and on both sides by the *posterior lateral sulcus* (**b18**).

The **fourth ventricle** forms bilaterally the *lateral recess* (**b19**), which communicates with the external cerebrospinal fluid space by *the lateral aperture (Luschka's foramen)* (**b20**). An unpaired opening lies under the inferior medullar velum *(median aperture, foramen of Magendie)*. The floor of the rhomboid fossa shows bulges near the *median sulcus* (**b21**) over the nuclei of the cranial nerves: *medial eminence* (**b22**), *facial colliculus* (**b23**), *trigone of the hypoglossal nerve* (**b24**), *trigone of the vagus nerve* (**b25**), and the *vestibular area* (**b26**). The rhomboid fossa is crossed by myelinated nerve fibers, the *striae medullares* (**b27**). The pigmented nerve cells of the locus coeruleus (**b28**) glimmer with a blue color through the floor of the rhomboid fossa. They are mostly noradrenergic and project to the hypothalamus, the limbic system and the neocortex. The locus coeruleus also contains peptidergic neurons (encephalin, neurotensin).

The ventral surface of the **mesencephalon** is formed by the *cerebral peduncles* (**ad29**) (descending cerebral tracts). The *interpeduncular fossa* (**a30**) lies between the two peduncles. Its floor is perforated by large numbers of blood vessels, *the posterior perforated substance*. On the dorsal surface of the mesencephalon lies the *quadrigeminal plate, lamina tecti,* (**bd31**), with two upper and two lower hillocks, the *superior* (**d32**) and *inferior* (**d33**) *colliculi*.

Organization (Fig. 1.27)

The longitudinal organization of the *neural tube* (**a1**) is still recognizable in the brainstem, although it is altered by the enlargement of the central canal into the fourth ventricle (**a2** and **a3**).

The ventrodorsal arrangement of the motor basal plate (**a4**), the visceromotor region (**a5**), the viscerosensory region (**a6**), and the *sensory alar plate* (**a7**) is changed to a mediolateral arrangement by flattening and opening out of the neural tube on the floor of the rhomboid fossa (**a2**): the *somatomotor zone* lies medially, next to it is the visceromotor zone, and the *viscerosensory* and *somatosensory zones* are displaced laterally. The cranial nerve nuclei in the medulla oblongata are arranged according to this basic pattern (**a3**).

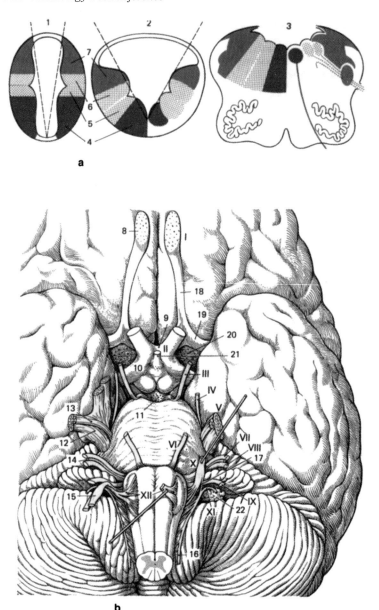

Fig. 1.27a,b (**a**) Longitudinal organization of the medulla oblongata. (**b**) Cranial nerves, base of the brain.

Cranial Nerves

According to the classical anatomists, there are 12 pairs of cranial nerves, although the first two are not true nerves. The **olfactory nerve** (**I**) consists of bundles of processes of sensory cells of the olfactory epithelium, which together form the olfactory nerves and enter the olfactory bulb (**b8**). The **optic nerve** (**II**) is a cerebral nerve pathway. The retina, the origin of the optic nerve fibers, like the pigmentary epithelium of the eyeball is developmentally a derivative of the diencephalon. *Optic chiasm* (**b9**), *optic tract* (**b10**).

The nerves that supply the muscles of the eye are somatomotor nerves: the **oculomotor nerve** (**III**) leaves the brain in the floor of the *interpeduncular fossa* (**b11**); the **trochlear nerve** (**IV**) emerges from the dorsal surface of the midbrain and runs to the basal surface around the cerebral peduncles (IV) (**Fig. 1.26b,d**); the **abducens nerve** (**VI**) emerges from the lower margin of the pons.

Five nerves have developed from the branchial arch nerves of lower vertebrates: **trigeminal nerve** (**V**), **facial nerve** (**VII**), **glossopharyngeal nerve** (**IX**), **vagus nerve** (**X**), and **accessory nerve** (**XI**). The muscles supplied by these nerves are derived from the branchial arch muscles of the foregut. Originally they were visceromotor nerves. In mammals the branchial arch muscles became the striated muscles of the pharynx, mouth, and face. They differ from other striated muscles by not being entirely under voluntary control (emotionally dependent, mimic reactions of the facial muscles). The vestibular part of the *vestibulocochlear nerve* (**VIII**) has a phylogenetically old association with the balance apparatus, which is already present in lower vertebrates.

The trigeminal nerve (**V**) emerges from the lateral part of the pons. Its *sensory branch* runs to the *trigeminal ganglion (semilunar ganglion, gasserian ganglion)* (**b12**); its *motor branch* (**b13**) bypasses the ganglion. The facial nerve (**VII**) and the vestibulocochlear nerve (**VIII**) leave the medulla at the cerebellopontine angle. Taste fibers in the facial nerve emerge as an independent nerve, the **intermedius nerve** (**b14**). The glossopharyngeal (**IX**) and vagus (**X**) nerves arise dorsal to the olive. *Superior ganglion of the vagus nerve* (**b15**). The cervical fibers of the accessory nerve (**XI**) join to form the radix spinalis (**b16**). The superior fibers, radix cranialis, which emerge from the medulla oblongata, run a short course in the nerve as the *internal branch* (**bl7**) and then join the vagus nerve.

The **hypoglossal nerve** (**XII**), a somatomotor nerve, is developmentally a remnant of several cervical nerves that have secondarily become included in the cerebral area and have lost their sensory roots.

Olfactory tract (**b18**), lateral olfactory stria (**b19**), anterior perforated substance (**b20**), hypophysial stalk (**b21**), choroid plexus (**b22, d12**).

Base of the Skull (Figs. 1.28 and 1.29)

The base of the skull carries the brain. The basal surface of the brain on each side corresponds to three bony fossae: the basal surface of the frontal lobe lies

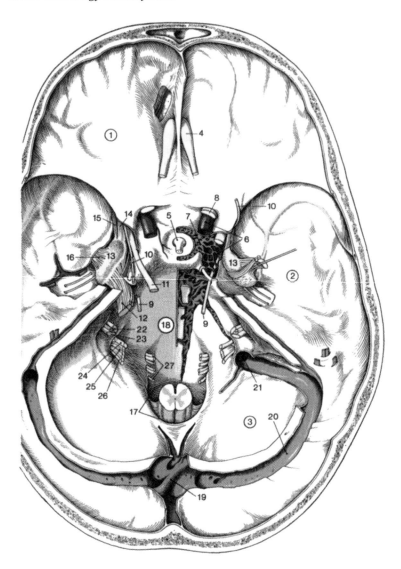

Fig. 1.28 View of the base of the skull from above.

in the *anterior cranial fossa* (**1**), the base of the temporal lobe in the *middle cranial fossa* (**2**), and the lower surface of the cerebellum in the *posterior cranial fossa* (**3**). The inner surface of the skull is covered by the *dura mater*. It consists of two layers that form the covering of the brain and the periosteum. The large venous trunks run between the two layers. Nerves and blood vessels run through the numerous foramina at the base of the skull.

Near the midline, in the floor of the anterior cranial fossa, the *olfactory nerves* pass to the olfactory bulbus (**4**) through the openings of the thin *lamina*

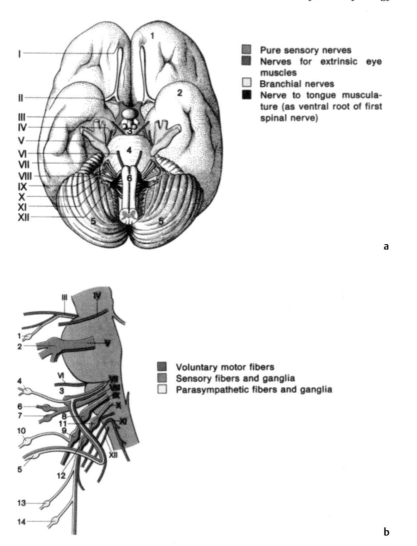

I

II

III
IV
V
VI
VII
VIII
IX
X
XI
XII

■ Pure sensory nerves
■ Nerves for extrinsic eye
  muscles
☐ Branchial nerves
■ Nerve to tongue musculature (as ventral root of first
  spinal nerve)

a

■ Voluntary motor fibers
■ Sensory fibers and ganglia
☐ Parasympathetic fibers and ganglia

b

Fig. 1.29a,b   (**a**) Cranial nerves, basal view. *1, 2, cerebrum; 1*, frontal lobe; *2*, temporal lobe; *3-6, brainstem; 3*, infundibulum with hypophysis; *4*, pons; *5*, cerebellar hemispheres; *6*, medulla oblongata. (**b**) Nerve fiber components and ganglia of cranial nerves III to XII and their branching, view from left side. *1*, ciliary ganglion (*III*); *2*, trigeminal ganglion (*V*); *3*, geniculate ganglion (*VII*); *4*, pterygopalatine ganglion (*VII*); *5*, submandibular ganglion (*VII*); *6*, vestibular ganglion (*VIII*); *7*, cochlear ganglion (*VIII*); *8*, superior ganglion (*IX*); *9*, inferior ganglion (*IX*); *10*, otic ganglion (*IX*); *11*, superior ganglion (*X*); *12*, inferior ganglion (*X*); *13, 14*, autonomic ganglia in thorax and abdomen.

cribrosa. The sella turcica rises between the two middle cranial fossae and contains the *hypophysis* (**5**), which is attached to the floor of the diencephalon. The *internal carotid artery* (**6**) runs into the skull through the *carotid canal,* lateral to the sella. Its S-shaped course runs through the *cavernous sinus* (**7**). In the medial part of the fossa, the **optic nerve** (**8**) enters the skull through the optic canal, and the nerves to the muscles of the eye leave through the orbital fissure. The paths taken by the **abducens** (**9**) and **trochlear** (**10**) **nerves** are characterized by an intradural course. The abducens nerve penetrates the dura at the middle part of the clivus and the trochlear nerve runs along the edge of the clivus at the attachment of the tentorium. The **oculomotor nerve** (**11**) and the trochlear nerve run through the lateral wall of the cavernous sinus, and the abducens nerve runs through the sinus laterobasal to the internal carotid artery. The **trigeminal nerve** (**12**) runs beneath a bridge of dura in the middle cranial fossa, where the **trigeminal ganglion** (**13**) lies in the trigeminal cave, a pocket formed by two layers of the dura. The three branches of the trigeminal nerve leave the interior of the skull through different foramina: the **ophthalmic nerve** (**14**), after passing through the wall of the cavernous sinus, leaves with its branches through the orbital fissure. The **maxillary nerve** (**15**) leaves through the foramen rotundum, and the **mandibular nerve** (**16**) through the foramen ovale.

The two posterior cranial fossae surround the *foramen magnum* (**17**), to which the *clivus* (**18**) descends steeply from the sella. The brain stem lies on the clivus. The cerebellar hemispheres lie in the basal fossae. The *transverse sinus* (**20**) arises from the *confluent sinus* (**19**), runs round the posterior fossa and opens into the *internal jugular vein* (**21**). The **facial** (**22**) and **vestibulocochlear** (**23**) **nerves** run together to the posterior aspect of the petrous bone, to the *terminal acoustic meatus.* Basal to the meatus, the **glossopharyngeal** (**24**), **vagus** (**25**), and **accessory** (**26**) **nerves** run through the anterior part of the *jugular foramen.* The fiber bundles of the **hypoglossal nerve** (**27**) pass through the hypoglossal canal to the nerve.

Cranial Nerve Nuclei (Fig. 1.30)

As in the spinal cord, where the origin of the motor fibers is in the anterior horn and the termination of the sensory fibers is in the posterior horn, in the medulla are found cell aggregations with efferent fibers (**nuclei originis**) and cell aggregations (**nuclei terminales**) upon which terminate the afferent fibers whose pseudounipolar cells lie in sensory ganglia outside the brainstem.

The somatomotor nuclei lie near the midline: nucleus of the *hypoglossal nerve* (**ab1**) (tongue muscles), *nucleus of the abducens* (**ab2**), *nucleus of the trochlear nerve* (**ab3**), and *nucleus of the oculomotor nerve* (**ab4**) (eye muscles).

Laterally follow the visceromotor nuclei: the true visceromotor nuclei of the parasympathetic system, and the former visceromotor nuclei of the now transformed branchial arch musculature. The parasympathetic nuclei include

Table 1.1   Fiber components and peripheral organization of cranial nerves

Sequence and Designation	SS	VS	VM	Sepc. VM	SM	Peripheral Organization
I. Olfactory	(+)					Olfactory epithelium (nerve of smell)
II. Optic	(+)					Retina (nerve of sight)
III. Oculomotor					(+)	Extrinsic eye muscles
I.			+			Intrinsic eye muscles
IV. Trochlear					(+)	Extrinsic eye muscles
V. Trigeminal	+	+				Face and head up to crown, nasal, eye, oral cavities
I.				+		Mandibular arch muscles
VI. Abducens					(+)	Extrinsic eye muscles
VII. Facial		+				Taste fibers (anterior half of tongue)
I.				+		Hyoid arch muscles
I.			+			Salivary, lacrimal glands
VIII. Vestibulocochlear	(+)					Labyrinth organ (nerve of hearing and balance)
IX. Glossopharyngeal		+				Taste fibers (posterior half of tongue, pharynx)
I.				+		Pharynx
I.			+			Parotid gland
X. Vagus	+					Part of external acoustic meatus
I.		+				Laryngeal taste buds
I.				+		Larynx
I.			+			Intestinal canal up to transverse colon, lungs, bronchial tubes, heart
XI. Accessory				+		Trapezius, sternocleidomastoid
XII. Hypoglossal					+	Tongue musculature

Abbreviations: SS, somatosensory; VS, viscerosensory; VM, visceromotor; Spec. VM, special visceromotor; SM, somatomotor.

the *dorsal nucleus of the vagus nerve* (**ab5**) (viscera), the *inferior salivatory nucleus* (**ab6**) (preganglionic fibers to the parotid), the *superior salivatory nucleus* (**ab7**) (preganglionic fibers to the *submandibular* and *sublingual glands*), and the *Edinger-Westphal nucleus* (**ab8**) (preganglionic fibers to the *pupillary sphincter* and *ciliary muscle of the eye*).

   The row of motor nuclei of the branchial arch nerves begins caudally with the *spinal nucleus of the accessory nerve* (**ab9**) (shoulder muscles), which extends into the cervical cord as the *nucleus of the spinal root of the accessory nerve*. It extends cranially with the *nucleus ambiguus* (**ab10**), the motor nucleus of the *vagus nerve* and of the *glossopharyngeal nerve* (pharyngeal and laryngeal muscles), and the *nucleus of the facial nerve* (**ab11**) (facial muscles). The nucleus of the facial nerve lies deeply, as do all the motor nuclei of the

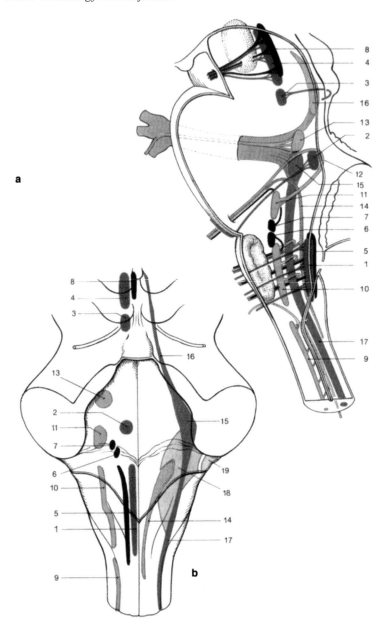

Fig. 1.30a,b (**a**) Cranial nerve nuclei; medial view of a midline section through the medulla oblongata. (**b**) Dorsal view of the rhomboid fossa showing the cranial nerve nuclei.

branchial arch nerves. Its fibers run a dorsally arched course, in the floor of the rhomboid fossa *(colliculus facialis)*, around the abducens nucleus *(facial knee, genu internum of the facial nerve* [**a12**]), and then they turn downward to the inferior margin of the pons, where they leave the medulla. The most cephalic motor nucleus of the branchial arch nerves is the *motor nucleus of the trigeminal nerve* (**ab13**) (masticatory muscles).

The sensory nuclei lie laterally: the most medial is the viscerosensory *nucleus of the tractus solitarius* (**ab14**), in which end sensory fibers from the *vagus* and *glossopharyngeal nerves,* and all taste fibers. Further laterally extends the region of the nuclei of the trigeminal nerve, which, with the *pontine nucleus of the trigeminal nerve (principal nucleus)* (**ab15**), the *mesencephalic nucleus of the trigeminal nerve* (**ab16**), and the *spinal nucleus of the trigeminal nerve* (**ab17**), forms the largest expanse of all the cranial nerve nuclei. All fibers of exteroceptive sensation from the face, mouth, and sinuses end in this area. Finally, lying most laterally is the area of the *vestibular* (**b18**) and *cochlear* (**b19**) *nuclei,* in which end the fibers of the vestibular *root* (organ of equilibrium) and the *cochlear root* (auditory organ) of the vestibule cochlear nerve.

Medulla Oblongata (Fig. 1.31)

Level of the Hypoglossal Nerve (a)

These semischematic illustrations of brainstem cross sections show cell staining on the left and nerve fiber staining on the right.

In the dorsal part, the *tegmentum,* the cranial nerve nuclei can be seen, and the ventral portion shows the *olive* (**ab1**) and the *pyramidal tract* (**ab2**).

Medially in the tegmentum lies the large-celled *nucleus of the hypoglossal nerve* (**ab3**) and dorsal to it the *dorsal nucleus of the vagus nerve* (**ab4**) and the *nucleus solitarius* (**ab5**), which contains a large number of peptidergic neurons. Dorsolaterally the posterior funiculi of the spinal cord end in the *nucleus gracilis* (**a6**) and the *cuneate nucleus* (**ab7**), from which arises the secondary sensory pathway, the *lemniscus medialis.* The nucleus of the spinal trigeminal root, the *nucleus spinalis n. trigemini* (**ab8**), lies ventral to the cuneate nucleus. The large cells of the *nucleus ambiguus* (**ab9**) stand out in the center of this area; they lie in the region of the reticular formation, of which only the somewhat denser *lateral reticular nucleus* (**ab10**) is designated. The *olive* (**a1**), whose fibers pass toward the cerebellum, is accompanied by two accessory nuclei, the *dorsal olivary nucleus* (**ab11**) and the *medial olivary nucleus* (**ab12**). At the ventral surface of the pyramids appears the *arcuate nucleus* (**ab13**) in which collaterals of the pyramidal tract synapse.

The fibers of the *hypoglossal nerve* (**a14**) cross the medulla to their exit between the pyramid and the olive. Dorsal to the hypoglossal nucleus lies the *dorsal longitudinal fasciculus* (**ab15**), laterally the *tractus solitarius* (**ab16**), and ventrally the *medial longitudinal fasciculus* (**ab17**). The *internal arcuate fibers* (**a18**) radiate broadly from the nuclei of the posterior funiculus into the *medial*

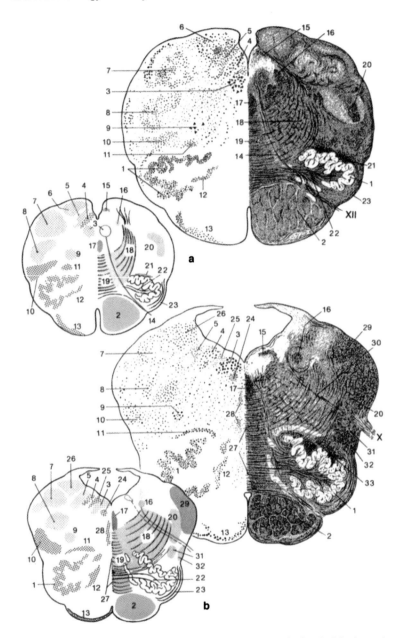

Fig. 1.31a,b (**a**) Cross section through the medulla oblongata at the level of the hypoglossal nerve. (**b**) Cross section through the medulla oblongata at the level of the vagus nerve.

lemniscus (**a19**). The spinal tract of the *trigeminal nerve* (**a20**) runs laterally, and dorsal to the main olivary nucleus the *central tegmental tract* (**a21**) (extrapyramidal motor tract) passes downward. Fibers of the *olivocerebellar tract* (**a22**) run through the hilum of the olive, and around the lateral margin pass the *superficial arcuate fibers* (**a23**) (nucleus arcuatus, cerebellum). The ventral region is occupied by the *pyramidal tract* (**a2**).

Level of the Vagus Nerve (b)

The fourth ventricle has become enlarged. The same nuclear columns are found in its floor as in **a**. Ventral to the *hypoglossal nucleus* (**b3**) is *Roller's nucleus* (**b24**), and dorsally the *intercalate nucleus of Staderini* (**b25**); the fiber connections of these two nuclei are not known. In the lateral field the posterior funicular nuclei are mostly disappearing and are being replaced by the *vestibular nuclei (medial vestibular nucleus* [**b26**]). Decussating fibers in the midline of the medulla form a *raphe* (**b27**). On both sides of this raphe lie the small cell groups of the *raphe nucleus* (**b28**) whose serotoninergic neurons project to the hypothalamus, the olfactory cortex, and the limbic system. The raphe nuclei are also rich in peptidergic neurons (vasoactive intestinal peptide [VIP], encephalin, neurotensin, and thyroliberin). The spinal fibers that run to the cerebellum aggregate laterally in the *inferior cerebellar peduncle* (**b29**). Fibers that enter and leave the *vagus nerve* (**b30**) traverse the medulla. Ventral to them, on the lateral border of the medulla, are the ascending *spinothalamic* (**b31**) and *spinocerebellar* (**b32**) *tracts*. Dorsal to the olive, the *olivocerebellar fibers* (**b33**) collect to extend toward the inferior cerebellar peduncle.

Pons (Fig. 1.32)

Level of the Genu of the Facial Nerve (a)

Semischematic; cell staining on the left, fiber staining on the right.

Beneath the floor of the rhomboid fossa lie the large cells of the nucleus of the *abducens nerve* (**a1**) and ventrolateral to it the *facial nerve nucleus* (**a2**). Between the abducens and the facial nerve nuclei lies the visceral efferent *superior salivatory nucleus* (**a3**). The lateral field contains the *vestibular* and *trigeminal nuclei*: the *medial vestibular nucleus* (**a4**), *lateral vestibular nucleus* (**a5**), and the spinal nucleus of the trigeminal root (**a6**).

Fibers of the facial nerve bend around the abducens nucleus (**a1**) to form the *facial colliculus* (**a7**). We distinguish in this bundle of fibers an ascending (**a8**) limb and a descending limb, which lies cranial to the level of the section illustrated. Its vertex is the *genu of the facial nerve* (**a9**). Fibers of the *abducens nerve* (**a10**) run downward through the medial part of the tegmentum. Medial to the abducens nucleus lies the *medial longitudinal fasciculus* (**ab11**) and dorsal to it the *dorsal longitudinal fasciculus* (**ab12**). The *central tegmental* (**ab13**) and *spinothalamic* (**a14**) *tracts* lie deep in the tegmentum of the pons. Second-

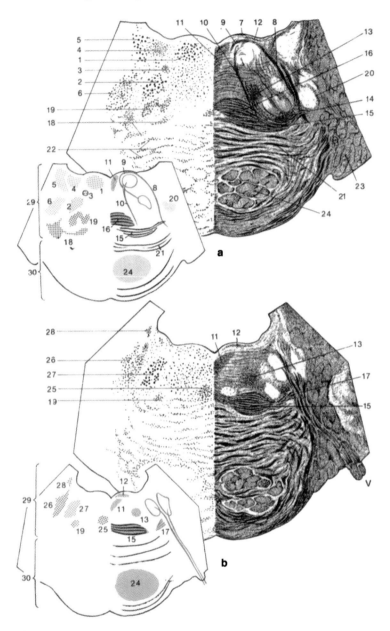

Fig. 1.32a,b (**a**) Transverse section through the pons at the level of the genu of the facial nerve. (**b**) Transverse section through the pons at the level of the trigeminal nerve.

ary fibers of the auditory tract collect in a broad band, the *corpus trapezoideum* (**ab15**), and cross to the opposite side ventral to the *medial lemniscus* (**a16**), where they ascend in the *lateral lemniscus* (**b17**). They synapse partly in the adjacent *nuclei of the trapezoid body–ventral* (**a18**) and *dorsal* (superior olive) (**ab19**). The spinal *tract of the trigeminal nerve* (**a20**) lies in the lateral field.

The base of the pons is formed by the *transverse pontine fibers* (**a21**). These are corticopontine fibers, which synapse in the *pontine nuclei* (**a22**), and pontocerebellar fibers, which are postsynaptic and extend to the cerebellum in the *medial cerebellar peduncle (brachium pontis)* (**a23**). In the middle of the longitudinally cut fiber bundle lie the transversely cut fibers of the *pyramidal tract* (**a24**).

Level of the Trigeminal Nerve (b)

The medial zone of the tegmentum of the pons contains the tegmental nuclei. The nuclei, of which only the inferior central tegmental nucleus (nucleus papiliformis) (**b25**) can readily be distinguished, belong to the reticular formation. In the lateral region the trigeminal complex is most extensive: laterally the *pontine nucleus of the trigeminal nerve* (**b26**), medial to it the *motor nucleus of the trigeminal nerve* (**b27**), and dorsally the nucleus of the mesencephalic trigeminal root (**a28**). The afferent and efferent fibers together form a thick trunk that leaves at the ventral surface of the pons.

The *lateral lemniscus* (**b17**) and the *trapezoid body* (**b15**), with the adjacent *dorsal nucleus of the trapezoid body* (**b19**), are situated ventral to the trigeminal nuclei. The *dorsal longitudinal* (**b12**) and the *medial longitudinal* (**b11**) *fasciculi* and the *central tegmental tract* (**b13**) may be distinguished among the descending and ascending tracts. *Tegmentum of the pons* (**ab29**), *base of the pons* (**ab30**).

Hypoglossal Nerve (Fig. 1.33)

Cranial nerve XII is a purely somatomotor nerve for the muscles of the tongue. Its nucleus (**b1**) forms a column of large, multipolar nerve cells in the floor of the rhomboid fossa *(trigone of the hypoglossal nerve)*. It consists of several cell groups, each of which supplies a particular tongue muscle. The nerve fibers leave between the pyramid and the olive and form two bundles that combine into a nerve trunk.

The nerve then leaves the skull through the *hypoglossal canal* (**b2**) and passes downward, lateral to the vagus nerve and the internal carotid artery. It describes a loop, the **arcus n. hypoglossi** (**a3**), and reaches the root of the tongue a little above the hyoid bone, between the *hyoglossal* and *mylohyoid muscles,* where it divides into its terminal branches.

The fibers of cranial nerves I and II adhere to the hypoglossal nerve. They form the **ansa cervicalis profunda** (branches to the infrahyoid muscles), where they branch off again as the **superior root** (**a4**) and join the **inferior**

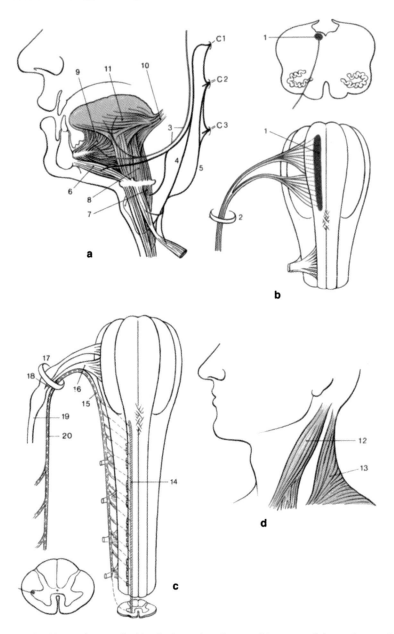

Fig. 1.33a–d (**a**) Muscles supplied by the hypoglossal nerve. (**b**) Region of the nucleus and exit of the hypoglossal nerve. (**c**) Region of the nucleus and exit of the accessory nerve. (**d**) Muscles supplied by the accessory nerve.

root (**a5**) (cranial nerves II and III). The cervical fibers for the *geniohyoid muscle* (**a6**) and the **thyroid muscle** (**a7**) extend further in the hypoglossal nerve. The hypoglossal nerve gives off branches, the **rami linguales**, to the *hyoglossal muscle* (**a8**), *genioglossal muscle* (**a9**), *styloglossal muscle* (**a10**), and the intrinsic muscles of the tongue (**a11**). The nerve supply to the tongue musculature is strictly unilateral.

> **Clinical tips:** Damage to the hypoglossal nerve produces hemiatrophy of the tongue. When the tongue is thrust out, it deviates to the damaged side because the action of the genioglossus muscle that moves the tongue forward predominates on the intact side.

Accessory Nerve

Cranial nerve XI is purely motor. Its external branch supplies the **sternocleidomastoid muscles** (**d12**) and the **trapezius muscle** (**d13**). Its nucleus, the *spinal nucleus of the accessory nerve* (**c14**), forms a narrow column of cells from C1 to C5 or C6. The large, multipolar nerve cells lie on the lateral margin of the anterior horn. Cells in the caudal part supply the trapezius muscle and those in the cranial part supply the sternocleidomastoid muscle. The nerve fibers leave at the lateral surface of the cervical cord between the anterior and posterior roots and combine to form a single trunk that enters the skull as the **external** (spinal) **branch** (**c15**) through the foramen magnum, alongside the spinal cord. Here, fiber bundles from the caudal part of the *nucleus ambiguus* join the nerve as the **internal** (cranial) **branch** (**c16**). Both components pass through the *jugular foramen* (**c17**). Immediately after their exit, the fibers from the nucleus ambiguus form the **internal branch** (**c18**) and join the vagus nerve (**c19**). The fibers from the cervical cord form the **external branch** (**c20**), which supplies the sternocleidomastoid and trapezius muscles as the *accessory nerve*. It passes through the sternocleidomastoid muscle and its terminal branches reach the trapezius muscle.

> **Clinical tips:** Damage to the nerve results in a tilted position of the head and the arm cannot be lifted above the horizontal.

Vagus Nerve (Fig. 1.34)

Cranial nerve X not only supplies regions of the head, as do the other cranial nerves, but also descends into the thorax and abdomen where it divides into

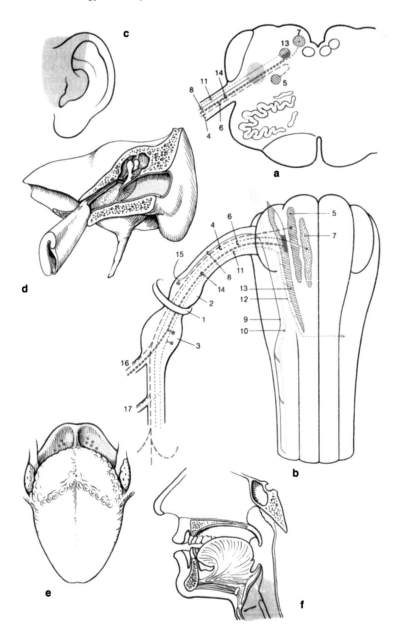

Fig. 1.34a–f (**a**) Nuclear region of the vagus nerve. (**b**) Exit of the vagus nerve. (**c**) Sensory supply of the external ear. (**d**) Sensory supply of the external auditory meatus. (**e**) Tongue, sensory supply, and taste. (**f**) Sensory supply of the throat.

a plexus for the viscera. It is the largest **parasympathetic nerve** of the vegetative nervous system and thus the most important **antagonist of the sympathetic nervous system.** It has the following components: motor fibers (branchial arch muscles), *exteroceptive sensory* fibers, *visceromotor* and *viscerosensory* fibers, and *taste fibers.* The fibers leave just behind the olive, combine into the nerve trunk, and leave the skull through the *jugular foramen* (**b1**). In the foramen the nerve forms the **superior ganglion** *(jugular ganglion)* (**b2**) and after its exit the considerably larger **inferior ganglion** *(ganglion nodosum)* (**b3**).

Fibers to the branchial arch muscles (**ab4**) come from the large multipolar nerve cells of the **nucleus ambiguus** (**ab5**). The visceromotor fibers (**ab6**) arise in the small-celled **dorsal nucleus of the vagus nerve** (**ab7**), which lies lateral to the hypoglossal nerve nucleus in the floor of the rhomboid fossa. The exteroceptive sensory fibers (**ab8**) stem from nerve cells in the *superior ganglion.* They descend with the *spinal trigeminal root* (**b9**) and terminate in the **nucleus of the spinal tract of the trigeminal nerve** (**b10**). Cells of the viscerosensory fibers (**ab11**) lie in the *inferior ganglion.* The fibers run caudally as part of the **tractus solitarius** (**B12**) and terminate at various levels in the **nucleus solitarius** (**ab13**). The nucleus contains many peptidergic neurons (VIP, corticoliberin, dynorphin). Taste fibers (**ab14**) also arise from cells of the *inferior ganglion* and end in the cranial part of the *nucleus solitarius.*

Head Region

In addition to the *meningeal branch* (sensory supply to the dura in the posterior cranial fossa), the vagus nerve gives off an **auricular branch** (**b15**). It branches off at the superior ganglion and runs through the *mastoid canaliculus* and reaches the external auditory meatus through the *tympanomastoid fissure.* It supplies the skin of the dorsal and caudal region of the meatus and a small area on the lobe of the ear *(exteroceptive sensory* component of the nerve) (**c,d**).

Cervical Part

The nerve descends in the neck in a common connective tissue sheath with the common carotid artery and internal jugular vein and passes with them through the superior aperture of the thorax. It gives off the following branches:

1. **Pharyngeal branches** (**b16**) at the level of the inferior ganglion. They join in the pharynx with fibers from the *glossopharyngeal nerve* and the *sympathetic* chain to form the **pharyngeal plexus.** On the external surface of the muscles and in the submucosa of the pharynx this forms a network of small fibers and groups of nerve cells. The vagal fibers provide the sensory supply to the mucous membrane of the trachea and the esophagus, including the epiglottis (**e,f**). The taste buds that lie on the epiglottis are also supplied by the vagus nerve. Superior laryngeal nerve (**b17**).

Vagus Nerve, Cervical Region (Fig. 1.35)

Pharyngeal branches. Motor fibers of the vagus nerve innervate the muscles of the soft palate and the pharynx: the muscles of the tonsillar niche, the *levator veli palatini muscle,* and the *constrictor muscles of the pharynx* (**b1**).

    2. **Superior laryngeal nerve** (**a2**). It arises below the inferior ganglion and divides at the level of the hyoid bone into an *external branch* (motor supply to

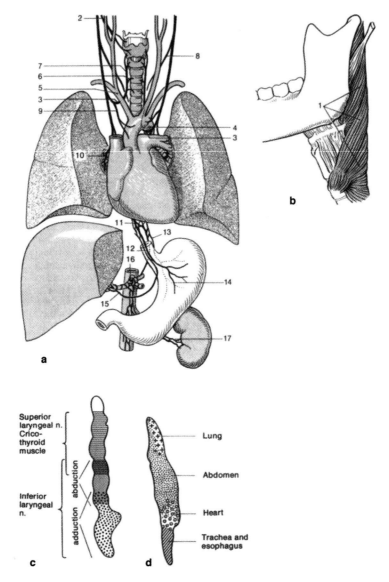

Fig. 1.35a–d (a) Thoracic and abdominal parts of the vagus nerve. (b) Muscles supplied by the vagus nerve. (c) Somatotopic organization of the nucleus ambiguus. (d) Somatotopic organization of the dorsal nucleus of the vagus nerve.

the cricothyroid muscle) and an *internal branch* (sensory supply to the mucous membrane of the larynx down to the vocal cords).

3. **Recurrent laryngeal nerve** (**a3**). It branches off in the thorax, after the vagus has deviated to the left across the *arch of the aorta* (**a4**), or to the right across the *subclavian artery* (**a5**). It passes on the left around the aorta and the ligamentum arteriosum and on the right around the subclavian artery and then ascends again on their posterior side. Between the trachea and the esophagus, to which it gives off **tracheal** (**a6**) and **esophageal branches**, it passes to the larynx. Its terminal branch, the **inferior laryngeal nerve** (**a7**), supplies the motor innervation to all laryngeal muscles, apart from the cricothyroid muscle, and the sensory innervation to the laryngeal mucous membrane below the vocal cords.

The motor fibers stem from the **nucleus ambiguus** (**c**), whose cell groups show a topographic arrangement: from the cranial part arise the fibers of the *glossopharyngeal nerve,* including those for the *superior laryngeal nerve,* and caudally fibers for the *inferior laryngeal nerve.* The nerves responsible for abduction and adduction of the vocal cords are arranged one below the other.

4. **Cervical cardiac branches** (*preganglionic parasympathetic fibers*). The *superior branches* (**a8**) are given off at various levels and pass with the large vessels to the heart, where they terminate in the parasympathetic ganglia of the *cardiac plexus.* In one branch run viscerosensory fibers, which carry information about aortic wall tension. Stimulation results in a fall of blood pressure (*"depressor nerve"*). The *inferior cervical cardiac rami* (**a9**) are given off from the recurrent laryngeal nerve, or from the main trunk, and terminate in the ganglia of the *cardiac plexus.*

Thoracic and Abdominal Parts

Here the vagus loses its identity as a single nerve and expands as a visceral nerve network. It forms the *pulmonary plexus* (**a10**) at the hilum of the lung, the *esophageal plexus* (**a11**) from which the anterior vagal trunk (**a12**) and the *posterior vagal trunk* (**a13**) extend toward the anterior and posterior surfaces of the stomach, the *anterior* (**a14**) and *posterior gastric branches. Hepatic branches* (**a15**) pass to the *hepatic plexus, celiac branches* (**a16**) to the *celiac plexus,* and the *renal branches* (**a17**) to the *renal plexus.*

The *visceromotor (preganglionic parasympathetic)* fibers arise from the **dorsal nucleus of the vagus nerve** in which a topographic arrangement of the supply to the viscera (**d**) can be demonstrated.

> **Clinical tips:** If the vagus nerve is damaged, there is impairment of function in the throat and the larynx; unilateral paralysis of the *levator veli palatini muscle* (**f18**) causes the soft palate and the uvula to be displaced to the intact side. The vocal cord on the affected side (**f19**) will remain immobile in the *cadaver position (recurrent laryngeal nerve palsy)* as a result of paralysis of the internal laryngeal muscles.

Glossopharyngeal Nerve (Fig. 1.36)

Cranial nerve IX supplies the sensory innervation of the *middle ear* and parts of the *tongue* and *pharynx,* and motor fibers to the muscles of the pharynx. It contains *motor, visceromotor, viscerosensory,* and *taste fibers.* Behind the olive it emerges from the medulla immediately above the vagus nerve and then leaves the skull together with the vagus nerve through the **jugular foramen** (**b1**). In the foramen it forms the **superior ganglion** (**b2**) and, after passage through the foramen, the larger **inferior ganglion** *(ganglion petrosum)* (**b3**). Lateral to the internal carotid artery and the pharynx it arches toward the root of the tongue, where it divides into several terminal branches.

The motor fibers (**ab4**) stem from the cranial part of the **nucleus ambiguus** (**ab5**), and the visceroefferent (secretory) fibers (**ab6**) from the **inferior salivary nucleus** (**ab7**). The cells of the viscerosensory fibers (**ab8**) and the taste fibers (**ab9**) lie in the *inferior ganglion* and the fibers descend in the **tractus solitarius** (**b10**) to terminate at specific levels of the **nucleus solitarius** (**ab11**).

The first branch, the **tympanic nerve** (**b12**), arises from the inferior ganglion with viscerosensory and preganglionic secretory fibers in the petrosal fossa. It passes through the *inferior tympanic canaliculus* into the *middle ear,* where it receives sympathetic fibers from the plexus of the internal carotid artery via the *caroticotympanic nerve,* and forms the **tympanic plexus.** It supplies sensory fibers to the mucous membrane of the middle ear and the *auditory (eustachian) tube.* Secretory fibers extend to the otic ganglion as the lesser petrosal nerve.

In addition to connections with the vagus nerve, the facial nerve and the sympathetic system, the inferior ganglion gives off the **branch to the carotid sinus** (**b13**) *(viscerosensory),* which descends to the bifurcation of the common carotid artery and terminates in the wall of the *carotid sinus* (**b14**) and in the *carotid body* (**b15**).

The nerve conducts impulses from the *mechanoreceptors* of the sinus and the *chemoreceptors* of the carotid body to the medulla, and via the collaterals to the dorsal nucleus of the vagus (afferent limb of the sinus reflexes). From the nucleus of the vagus, preganglionic fibers pass to groups of nerve cells in the cardiac atria, whose axons (postganglionic parasympathetic fibers) end on the sinoatrial and atrioventricular nodes (efferent pathway of the sinus reflexes). This system registers and regulates blood pressure and pulse rate.

Pharyngeal branches (**b16**) are also given off and together with part of the vagus nerve they form the pharyngeal plexus, which takes part in the sensory (**e**) and motor supply to the pharynx. A motor branch, the *branch to the stylopharyngeal muscle* (**b17**), innervates the *stylopharyngeal muscle,* and a few sensory **tonsillar branches** (**d18**) run to the tonsils and the soft palate. Below the tonsils, the nerve divides into the **lingual branches** (**d19**), which supply the posterior third of the tongue, including the vallate papillae, with sensory and taste fibers (**d20**).

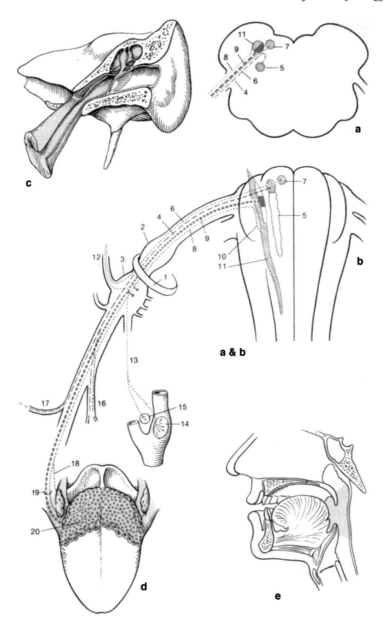

Fig. 1.36a–e (**a,b**) Region of the nucleus and root of the glossopharyngeal nerve. (**c**) Sensory supply of the middle ear. (**d**) Tongue, sensory supply, and taste nerves. (**e**) Sensory supply of the pharynx.

Vestibulocochlear Nerve (Fig. 1.37)

Cranial nerve VIII is an afferent nerve made up of two parts: the cochlear branch from the organ of hearing and the vestibular branch from the organ of equilibrium.

Cochlear Division (a)

The nerve fibers arise from the bipolar neurons of the **spiral ganglion** (**a1**), a band of cells that follows the spiral course of the cochlea. The peripheral processes of the cells end on the hair cells of *Corti's organ;* the central processes form small bundles that combine as the *tractus spiralis foraminosus* (**a2**) and join on the floor of the *internal acoustic meatus* to form the **cochlear nerve** (**a3**). This runs through the *internal acoustic meatus* into the cranial cavity together with the **vestibular nerve**, surrounded by a common connective tissue sheath. At the entrance of cranial nerve VIII into the medulla at the cerebello-pontine angle, the cochlear component lies dorsally and the vestibular component ventrally.

The cochlear fibers terminate in the **ventral** (**a4**) and **dorsal** (**a5**) **cochlear nuclei.** Secondary fibers from the ventral nucleus cross to the opposite side (**corpus trapezoideum** (**a6, Fig. 1.32**) (ab15) and ascend, partly synapsing in the *trapezoid nuclei*, as the **lateral lemniscus** (**a7**) (central auditory tract). Fibers that arise from the dorsal cochlear nucleus cross, partly as **dorsal acoustic striae**, close below the floor of the rhomboid fossa and likewise ascend in the lateral lemniscus.

Vestibular Division (b)

The nerve fibers arise from bipolar cells of the **vestibular ganglion** (**b8**), which lies in the internal acoustic meatus. The peripheral cell processes terminate in the sensory epithelia of the *semicircular ducts* (**b9**), the *sacculus* (**b10**), and the *utriculus* (**b11**). Their central processes join to form the vestibular nerve (**b12**) and, after dividing into ascending and descending branches, terminate in the vestibular nuclei of the medulla oblongata. Only a few extend directly over the inferior cerebellar peduncle into the cerebellum.

The vestibular nuclei lie in the floor of the rhomboid fossa beneath the lateral recess: **superior nucleus** *(Bekhterev)* (**b13**), **medial nucleus** *(Schwalbe)* (**b14**), **lateral nucleus** *(Deiters)* (**b15**), and the **inferior nucleus** (**b16**). The majority of primary vestibular fibers end in the medial nucleus. Secondary fibers from the vestibular nuclei pass to the cerebellum, to the nuclei of the nerves of the eye muscles, to the reticular formation, and into the spinal cord (**vestibulospinal tract [b17]**).

The function of the vestibular apparatus is of decisive importance for balance and maintenance of upright posture. These functions are subserved particularly by the tracts to the cerebellum and the spinal cord. The vestibulo-spinal tracts influence muscle tone in various parts of the body. The vestibular

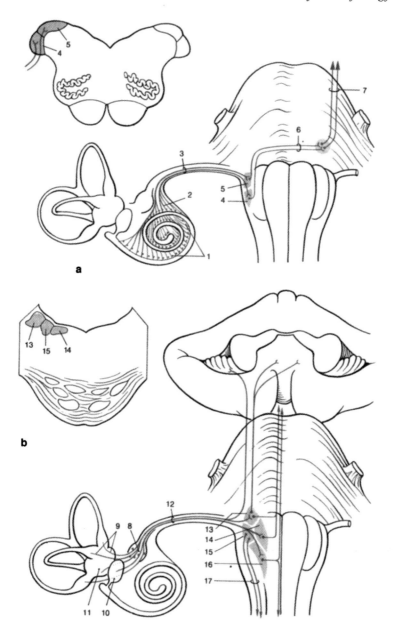

Fig. 1.37a,b (**a**) Vestibulocochlear nerve; region of the nuclei and projections of the cochlear part. (**b**) Vestibulocochlear nerve; region of the nuclei and entrance of the vestibular branch.

apparatus is particularly concerned with the control of movements of the head and the fixation of vision during movement (tracts to the eye muscle nuclei).

Facial Nerve (Figs. 1.38 and 1.39)

Cranial nerve VII contains motor fibers to the mimetic muscles of the face and in the *intermediate nerve,* which arises from the brainstem as a *separate bundle, taste,* and *visceroefferent (secretory)* fibers. The motor fibers (**ab1**) stem from the large, multipolar nerve cells of the **facial nerve nucleus** (**ab2**). They bend around the *abducens nucleus* (**ab3**) *(genu of the internal facial nerve)* and exit from the lateral surface of the medulla at the lower border of the pons. The cells of the preganglionic secretory fibers (**ab4**) form the **superior salivatory nucleus** (**ab5**). The taste fibers (**ab6**), whose pseudounipolar cells of origin lie in the **geniculate ganglion** (**bC7**), terminate in the cranial part of the **nucleus solitarius** (**ab8**). Visceroefferent and gustatory fibers do not bend around the abducens nucleus but join the descending limb of the nerve and emerge as the **intermediate nerve** (**b9**), between the facial and the vestibulo-cochlear nerves.

Both parts of the nerve pass through the *internal acoustic meatus* (petrosal part of the temporal bone, porus acusticus internus), and enter the *facial canal* as a single trunk. At the bend of the nerve in the petrous bone *(external facial genu)* lies the *geniculate ganglion* (**bc7**). The canal then runs in the medial wall of the tympanic cavity and turns caudally to the **stylomastoid foramen** (**bc10**), through which the nerve leaves the skull. It divides into its terminal branches in the *parotid gland* (**parotid plexus [e11]**).

Within the facial canal, the nerve gives off the **greater petrosal nerve** (**bc12**), the **stapedius nerve** (**bc13**), and the **chorda tympani** (**bc14**). The *greater petrosal nerve* (preganglionic secretory fibers to the lacrimal glands, nasal glands, and palatal glands) separates off from the geniculate ganglion, extends through the *hiatus of the canal for the greater petrosal nerve* and into the cranial cavity across the anterior surface of the petrous bone, across the foramen lacerum, and finally through the *pterygoid canal* to the *pterygopalatine ganglion* (**c15**). The *stapedius nerve* supplies the stapedius muscle in the middle ear. The *chorda tympani* (taste fibers to the anterior two thirds of the tongue [**d**] and preganglionic fibers to the submandibular and sublingual glands) branches off above the stylomastoid foramen, runs beneath the mucous membrane through the middle ear cavity and through the petrotympanic fissure, finally to join the *lingual nerve* (**c16**).

Before it enters the parotid gland, the facial nerve gives off the **posterior auricular nerve** (**e17**) and branches to the posterior belly of the *digastric muscle* (**ce18**) and to the *stylohyoid muscle* (**c19**). The parotid plexus gives off the *temporal branches* (**e20**), *zygomatic branches* (**e21**), *buccal branches* (**e22**), the *marginal mandibular branch* (**e23**), and the *cervical branch* (**e24**) for the *platysma.* These branches supply all the mimetic muscles.

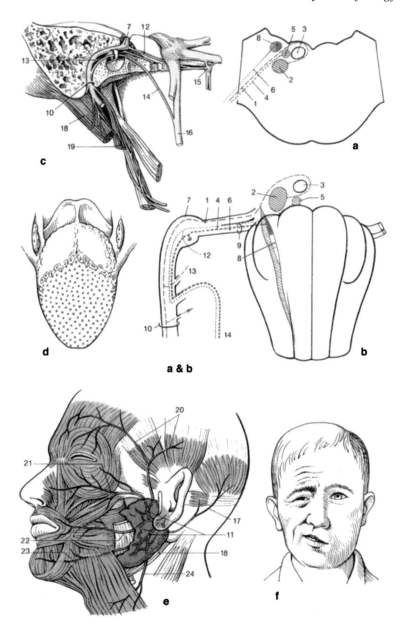

Fig. 1.38a–f (**a,b**) Region of the nucleus and course of the facial nerve. (**c**) Course taken in the petrous bone. (**d**) Tongue, taste. (**e**) Muscles supplied by the facial nerve. (**f**) Left-sided facial nerve paralysis.

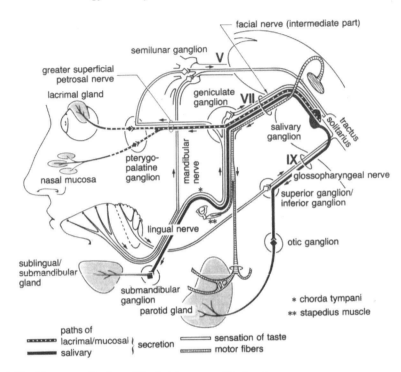

Fig. 1.39 Diagrammatic view of the facial nerve and its functions.

The ramifications of the cervical branch beneath the platysma form a *plexus* by anastomosing with branches of the sensory transverse cervical nerve, the *ansa cervicalis superficialis.* The small branches given off by this plexus are mixed sensorimotor nerves. Terminal twigs from the temporal and buccal branches and the marginal branch of the mandible form similar plexuses with branches of the trigeminal nerve.

> **Clinical tips:** Damage to the nerve results in flaccid paralysis of all the muscles on the affected side of the face. The corner of the mouth hangs down, the eye cannot be closed (**f**), and hyperacusis, increased sensitivity to sound, is suffered.

Trigeminal Nerve (Fig. 1.40)

Cranial nerve V contains *sensory* fibers for the skin and mucous membrane of the face, and *motor* fibers for the muscles of mastication, the mylohyoid, and the anterior belly of the digastric muscles, and probably also for the tensor veli

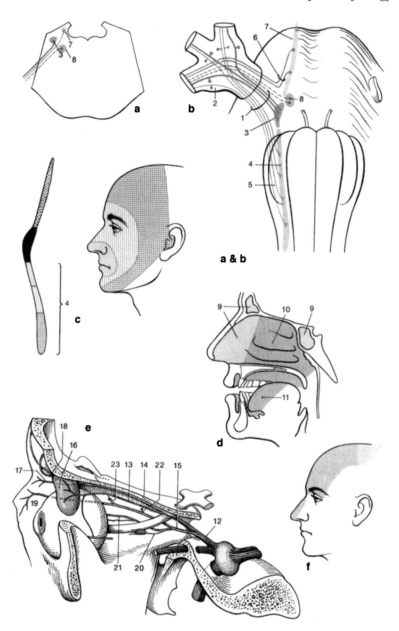

Fig. 1.40a–f   (**a,b**) Region of the nuclei and the exit of the trigeminal nerve. (**c**) Somatotopic distribution in the spinal trigeminal nucleus. (**d**) Sensory supply of the mucous membrane. (**e**) Ophthalmic nerve. (**f**) Area of skin supplied by the ophthalmic nerve.

palatini and the tensor tympani muscles. It leaves the pons as a thick trunk with a larger **sensory root** *(major part)* and a thinner **motor root** *(minor part)* and passes anteriorly over the petrous bone, on the anterior surface of which it lies in a flat sulcus, the *trigeminal impression.* The *trigeminal ganglion (semilunar ganglion of Gasser)* lies in a dural pouch, the *cavum trigeminale,* and gives off three main branches: the *ophthalmic, maxillary,* and *mandibular* nerves.

The sensory fibers (**b1**) stem from the pseudounipolar cells of the trigeminal ganglion (**b2**), whose central processes end in the sensory trigeminal nucleus. Fibers of *epicritic* sensation terminate primarily in the pontine nucleus of the trigeminal nerve **(principal nucleus)** (**ab3**), whereas fibers of *protopathic* sensation end mainly in the **spinal nucleus of the trigeminal nerve** (**bc4**). As the **spinal tract** (**b5**) the fibers descend as far as the upper cervical cord, where they end in a somatotopic arrangement (**c**): fibers for the perioral region terminate cranially and fibers for the adjacent cutaneous areas terminate further caudally ("onion-skin" arrangement of central sensory supply). The mesencephalic tract (**b6**) carries *proprioceptive sensory* impulses from the muscles of mastication.

The mesencephalic nucleus of the trigeminal nerve (**ab7**) consists of pseudounipolar nerve cells, whose processes run through the trigeminal ganglion without interruption. These are the only sensory fibers whose cells of origin do not lie in a ganglion outside the CNS, but in a nucleus of the brainstem which, so to speak, represents a sensory ganglion within the brain.

The motor fibers arise from large multipolar nerve cells of the **motor nucleus of the trigeminal nerve** (**ab8**).

Nerve Supply of the Mucous Membrane

The *ophthalmic nerve* supplies the frontal and sphenoidal sinuses and the wall of the nasal septum (**d9**); the *maxillary nerve* supplies the maxillary sinuses, nasal conchae, palate, and gingiva (**d10**); and the *mandibular nerve* supplies the lower part of the oral cavity and the cheeks (**d11**).

Ophthalmic Nerve (e12)

This nerve gives off a recurrent, *tentorial branch* and divides into *lacrimal* (**e13**), *frontal* (**e14**), and *nasociliary* (**e15**) *nerves.* These branches pass through the superior orbital fissure into the orbital fossa; the nasociliary nerve passes through the medial part of the fissure and the other branches through its lateral part.

The **lacrimal nerve** runs to the lacrimal gland (**e16**) to supply the skin at the lateral corner of the eye. Postganglionic parasympathetic secretory fibers from the *zygomatic nerve* pass through a communicating branch to innervate the lacrimal gland.

The **frontal nerve** divides into the **supratrochlear nerve** (**e17**) (medial corner of the eye) and the **supraorbital nerve** (**e18**), which runs through the *supraorbital notch* (the conjunctiva, upper eyelid, and skin of the forehead as far as the vertex).

The **nasociliary nerve** passes to the medial corner of the eye, which it supplies with its terminal branch, the **infratrochlear nerve** (**e19**). It gives off the following branches: a communicating branch to the *ciliary ganglion* (**e20**), the **long ciliary nerves** (**e21**) to the eyeball, the **posterior ethmoidal nerve** (**e22**) (sphenoidal sinus and ethmoidal cells), and the **anterior ethmoidal nerve** (**e23**), which runs through the *ethmoid foramen* to the ethmoid plate, which it penetrates to enter the nasal cavity. Its terminal branch, the *external nasal branch,* supplies the skin of the alae and tip of the nose.

Trigeminal Nerve (Continued) (Fig. 1.41)

Maxillary Nerve (a1)

This nerve, after it has given off a *meningeal branch,* passes through the *foramen rotundum* (**a2**) into the pterygopalatine fossa, where it divides into the *zygomatic nerve,* the *ganglionic branches (pterygopalatine nerves),* and the *infraorbital nerve.*

The **zygomatic nerve** (**a3**) passes through the inferior orbital fissure onto the lateral wall of the orbit. It gives off a communicating branch (postganglionic, parasympathetic secretory fibers to the lacrimal gland from the pterygopalatine ganglion) to the lacrimal nerve and divides into a **zygomaticotemporal branch** (**a4**) (temple) and a **zygomaticofacial branch** (**a5**) (skin over the zygomatic arch).

The **ganglionic branches** (**a6**) are two to three fine twigs that extend down to the pterygopalatine ganglion. The fibers carry a sensory supply to the upper pharynx, the nasal cavity, and the hard and soft palates.

The **infraorbital nerve** (**a7**) passes through the inferior orbital fissure into the orbit, and through the infraorbital canal (**a8**) to the cheek, where it supplies the skin between the lower eyelid and the upper lip (**b**). It gives off the **posterior superior alveolar nerves** (**a9**) (to the molars), the **medial superior alveolar nerve** (**a10**) (to the premolars), and the **anterior superior alveolar nerve** (**a11**) (to the canine and incisors). Above the alveoli, these nerves form the **superior alveolar plexus**.

Mandibular Nerve (c)

After its passage through the *foramen ovale,* and after giving off a *meningeal branch* (**c12**), in the infratemporal fossa the nerve divides into the *auriculotemporal, lingual,* and *inferior alveolar nerves,* the *buccal nerve,* and the purely *motor branches.*

The pure **motor branches** leave the mandibular nerve shortly after it has passed through the foramen: the **masseteric nerve** (**c13**) to the masseter muscle (**f14**), the **deep temporal nerves** (**c15**) to the temporalis muscle (**f16**),

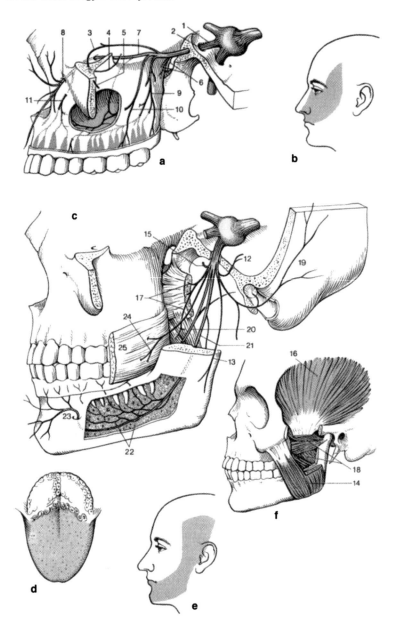

Fig. 1.41a–f (**a**) Maxillary nerve. (**b**) Region of the skin supplied by the nerve. (**c**) Mandibular nerve. (**d**) Sensory supply to the tongue. (**e**) Cutaneous innervations. (**f**) Muscles of mastication innervated by the mandibular nerve.

and the **pterygoid nerves** (**c17**) to the pterygoid muscles (**f18**). Motor fibers to the tensor tympani and tensor veli palatini muscles run to the otic ganglion (**ab1**) and leave as the **nerve to the tensor tympani muscle** and the **nerve to the tensor veli palatini muscle.**

The **auriculotemporal nerve** (**c19**) (to the skin of the temporal region, external auditory meatus, and tympanic membrane) usually arises from two roots, which surround the middle meningeal artery and then join to form the nerve. The **lingual nerve** (**c20**) descends in an arch to the base of the tongue and supplies the sensory innervation to the anterior two thirds of the tongue (**d**). It receives taste fibers from the chorda tympani (facial nerve). The **inferior alveolar nerve** (**c21**) carries motor fibers for the mylohyoid muscle and the anterior belly of the digastric muscle, in addition to sensory fibers that enter the mandibular canal and give off numerous **inferior dental branches** (**c22**) to the teeth of the lower jaw. The cutaneous branch of the nerve, the **mental nerve** (**c23**), exits through the mental foramen and provides the sensory supply for the chin, the lower lip, and the skin over the body of the mandible (**e**). The **buccal nerve** (**c24**) runs through the buccinator muscle (**c25**) to supply the mucous membrane of the cheek.

Parasympathetic Ganglia (Fig. 1.42)

Fibers from the visceroefferent nuclei, both motor and secretory, synapse in parasympathetic ganglia to form postganglionic fibers. In addition to the parasympathetic root (preganglionic fibers), each ganglion has a sympathetic root, fibers of which have their synapses in the ganglia of the sympathetic chain, and a sensory root, whose fibers run straight through the ganglion without interruption. Thus, all branches leaving the ganglion contain sympathetic, parasympathetic, and sensory fibers.

Ciliary Ganglion (ab1)

This is a small, flat body that lies lateral to the optic nerve in the orbit. Its parasympathetic fibers, which arise from the Edinger-Westphal nucleus in the midbrain, run in the oculomotor nerve (**ab2**) and cross to the ganglion as the *oculomotor root* (**ab3**) (parasympathetic root). The preganglionic sympathetic fibers arise in the lateral horn of the spinal cord, C8-T2 (**ciliospinal center [b4]**) and synapse in the *superior cervical ganglion* (**b5**). The postganglionic fibers ascend in the carotid plexus (**b6**) and pass to the ganglion as the *sympathetic root* (**b7**). Sensory fibers arise from the *nasociliary nerve* (nasociliary root) (**ab8**).

The **short ciliary nerves** (**ab9**) run to the eyeball from the ganglion and penetrate the sclera to reach the interior of the bulb of the eye. Their parasympathetic fibers innervate the *ciliary muscle* (accommodation) and the *sphincter muscle of the pupil*, and their sympathetic fibers innervate the *dilatator muscle of the pupil*.

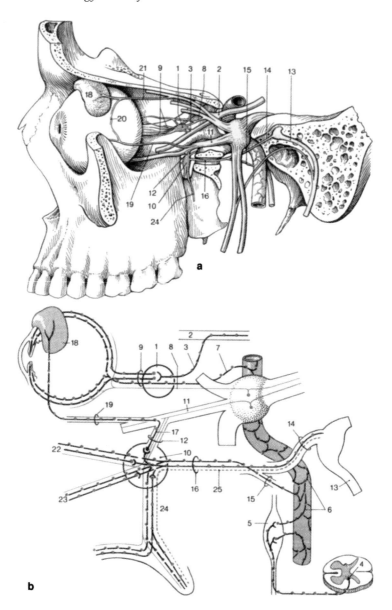

Fig. 1.42a,b (a) Topography of the ciliary ganglion and pterygopalatine ganglion. (b) Conduction pathways of the ciliary ganglion and the pterygopalatine ganglion. *Blue line*, sensory fibers; *blue dots*, parasympathetic fibers; *red dots*, sympathetic fibers; *blue dashed line,* taste fibers.

> **Clinical tips:** The pupil is antagonistically innervated by parasympathetic (papillary constriction) and sympathetic (papillary dilatation) nerve fibers. Damage to the ciliospinal center or to the spinal roots C8, T1 (paralysis of the lower plexus) produces ipsilateral papillary constriction.

Pterygopalatine Ganglion (ab10)

The ganglion lies on the anterior wall of the pterygopalatine fossa below the maxillary nerve (**ab11**), which gives off the **ganglionic branches** *(pterygopalatine nerves)* (**ab12**) to the ganglion (sensory root). The parasympathetic secretory fibers from the superior salivatory nucleus travel in the facial nerve (intermedius nerve) (**ab13**) to the genu of the facial nerve, where they separate as the **greater petrosal nerve** (**ab14**). This nerve passes through the *foramen lacerum* in the base of the skull and through the *pterygoid canal* to the ganglion (parasympathetic root). Sympathetic fibers from the carotid plexus form the **deep petrosal nerve** (**ab15**) (sympathetic root) and join with the greater petrosal **nerve to form the nerve of the pterygoid canal** (**ab16**).

The branches that are given off supply secretory fibers to the lacrimal gland and the glands of the nose. The parasympathetic fibers (**b17**) to the lacrimal gland (**ab18**) synapse in this ganglion. The postganglionic fibers run in the ganglionic rami (**b12**) to the maxillary nerve (**b11**) and reach over the zygomatic nerve (**ab19**) and its anastomosis (**a20**) to the lacrimal nerve (**A21** to the lacrimal gland.

The remaining parasympathetic secretory fibers run in the **orbital branches** (**b22**) to the posterior ethmoid bone cells, in the **lateral posterior nasal branches** (**b23**) to the nasal conchae, in the **nasopalatine** (incisivus) **nerve** over the wall of the nasal septum and through the incisor canal to the anterior part of the palate, and in the **palatine nerves** (**ab24**) to the hard and soft palates.

Taste fibers (**b25**) for the soft palate run in the palatine and greater petrosal nerves.

Parasympathetic Ganglia (Continued) (Fig. 1.43)

Otic Ganglion (ab1)

The ganglion is a flat body lying below the foramen ovale on the medial side of the *mandibular nerve* (**a2**), from which sensory and motor fibers (*sensorimotor root* [**ab3**]) enter the ganglion and pass through without synapsing. The preganglionic parasympathetic fibers stem from the *inferior salivatory nucleus.* They run in the glossopharyngeal nerve and pass with the tympanic nerve from the inferior ganglion of the glossopharyngeal nerve in the petrosal fossa to the tympanic cavity. The fibers leave the tympanic cavity as a slender branch, the **lesser petrosal nerve** (**ab4**) *(parasympathetic root)* through the *hiatus canal* for the lesser petrosal nerve. The nerve extends beneath the dura

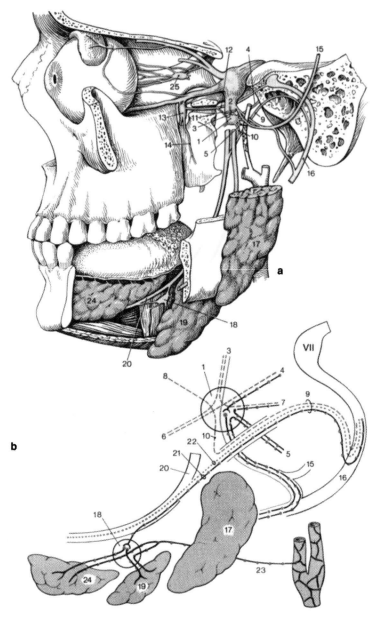

Fig. 1.43a,b (**a**) Topography of the otic and submandibular ganglia. (**b**) Conduction pathways of the otic and submandibular ganglia. *Red dashed line,* motor fibers; *blue dashed line,* taste fibers; *blue dots,* parasympathetic fibers; *red dots,* sympathetic fibers.

on the surface of the petrous bone, and after its passage through the foramen ovale it reaches the otic ganglion. The fibers of the *sympathetic root* (**ab5**) arise from the plexus of the middle meningeal artery.

Motor fibers in the motor root of the trigeminal nerve, which pass through the ganglion, leave it in the **tensor veli palatine nerve** (**b6**) (soft palate) and in the **tensor tympani nerve** (**b7**) (for the tensor tympani muscle, which tenses the tympanic membrane). *Motor fibers* (**b8**) from the facial nerve VII for the *levator veli palatini muscle* run in the chorda tympani (**ab9**) and join the ganglion through the *communicating branch of the chorda tympani* (**ab10**). They pass through it without synapsing and run through a communicating branch (**a11**) to the greater petrosal nerve (**a12**), with which it reaches the pterygopalatine ganglion (**al3**). They reach the palate in the palatine nerves (**a14**).

The postganglionic parasympathetic secretory fibers together with sympathetic fibers cross into the *auriculotemporal nerve* (**ab15**), and from this nerve via an additional anastomosis into the *facial nerve* (**ab16**). With branches of the latter they ramify in the *parotid gland* (**ab17**). In addition to the parotid gland they supply the buccal and labial glands via the *buccal* and *inferior alveolar nerves.*

Submandibular Ganglion (ab18)

The ganglion and a few small subsidiary ganglia lie in the floor of the mouth above the *submandibular gland* (**ab19**) on the inferior side of the *lingual nerve* (**ab20**), with which it is connected by several ganglionic branches. Its preganglionic parasympathetic fibers (**b21**), which stem from the *superior salivatory nucleus,* run in the facial nerve (intermedius nerve) and leave it with the taste fibers (**b22**) in the *chorda tympani* (**b9**). They pass in the latter to the lingual nerve (**b20**) and with that nerve to the floor of the mouth, where they are transferred to the ganglion. Postganglionic sympathetic fibers from the plexus of the external carotid artery reach the ganglion through the *sympathetic branch* (**b23**), which arises from the plexus of the facial artery and runs through it without synapsing.

The postganglionic parasympathetic and sympathetic fibers pass partly in *glandular branches* to the submandibular gland and partly further in the lingual nerve to the *sublingual gland* (**ab24**) and to the glands in the anterior two thirds of the tongue. Ciliary ganglion (**a25**).

Midbrain (Fig. 1.44)
Structure

The brainstem has a uniform structure with certain modifications in the *medulla oblongata* (**a1**), *pons* (**a2**), and *mesencephalon* (**a3**). The phylogenetically old part of the brainstem, which is common to all three regions and which contains the cranial nerve nuclei, is the *tegmentum* (**a4**). At the level of the medulla and the pons it is overlaid by the cerebellum and in the midbrain by the

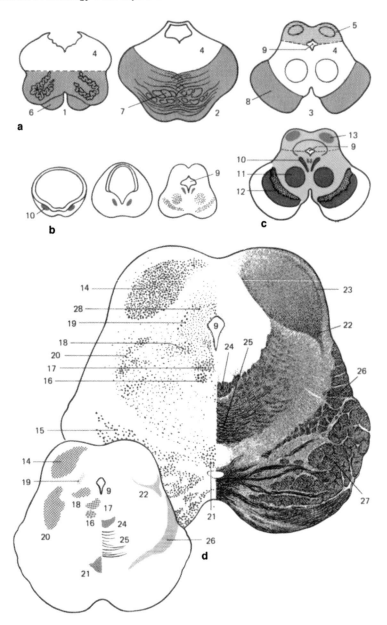

Fig. 1.44a–d **(a)** Structure of the medulla oblongata, pons, and midbrain. **(b)** Development of the midbrain. **(c)** Organization in the basal and alar plates. **(d)** Transverse section through the midbrain at the level of the posterior colliculi; myelin stain and cell stain.

tectum, the *quadrigeminal plate* (**a5**). The basal part contains principally the large descending tracts from the telencephalon; in the medulla they form the *pyramids* (**a6**), in the pons the *pontine bulb* (**a7**), and in the mesencephalon, the **cerebral peduncles** (**a8**).

In the midbrain the ventricular system is greatly narrowed and forms the **cerebral aqueduct** (of *Sylvius*) (**abcd9**). The lumen of the neural tube becomes increasingly narrowed during development through the increase in volume of the midbrain tegmentum (**b**). The primitive structure of the neural tube remains intact: ventrally lie the motor parts of the basal plate, the *oculomotor nerve nucleus* (**bC10**), the *trochlear nerve nucleus* (extraocular muscles), the *red nucleus* (**c11**), and the *substantia nigra* (**c12**) (extrapyramidal motor system); and dorsally lie the sensory derivatives of the alar plate, *lamina tecta* (**c13**) (synaptic relay station for acoustic and optic tracts).

Section Through the Midbrain (d)

This is the level of the two inferior colliculi. Dorsally lies the *inferior colliculus* with its nucleus (**d14**) (a relay station for the central auditory tract). Basally lies the zone of transition between the pons and the cerebral peduncles and the most caudal cell groups of the *substantia nigra* (**d15**). In the midzone of the tegmentum below the aqueduct is the conspicuous large-celled *nucleus of the trochlear nerve* (**d16**), above which lies the *dorsal tegmental nucleus* (**d17**). Further laterally lie the cells of the *locus coeruleus* (**d18**) (a pontine respiratory center with adrenergic neurons extending into the midbrain. Above this nucleus are scattered the relatively large cells of the *mesencephalic nucleus of the trigeminal nerve* (**d19**). The lateral field is occupied by the *pedunculopontine tegmental nucleus* (**d20**). At the lower margin of the tegmentum lies the *interpeduncular nucleus* (**d21**), which contains many peptidergic neurons (especially *encephalin*). In it terminates the habenulopeduncular tract (retroflex tract of Meynert), descending from the *habenular nucleus neurons.*

The *lateral lemniscus* (**Fig. 1.37**) spreads out into the ventral part of the inferior collicular nucleus (**d14**). At the lateral margin the fibers of the *peduncle of the inferior colliculus* (**d23**) aggregate before they pass to the *medial geniculate body* (central auditory tract). In the medial field the *medial longitudinal fasciculus* (**d24**) and the *decussation of the superior cerebellar peduncle* (**d25**) are visible. Laterally lies the fiber tract of the *medial lemniscus* (**d26**). The fibers of the *cerebral peduncle* (**d27**) are cut transversely and are interrupted by a few longitudinal fibers of the pons. Periaqueductal gray, *griseum centrale* (**d28**).

Midbrain (Continued) (Fig. 1.45)

Section Through the Superior Colliculi (a)

Dorsally both *superior colliculi* (**a1**) have been sectioned. In the lower vertebrates they are the most important optic center, with several cell and fiber

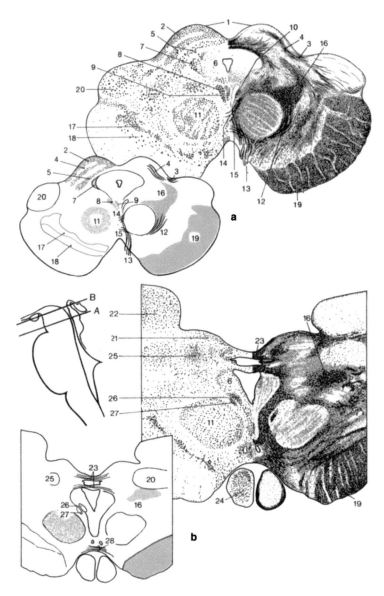

Fig. 1.45a,b (**a**) Transverse section through the midbrain at the level of the superior colliculi. (**b**) Transverse section through the midbrain at the level of the pretectal region.

layers, but in humans they are only a synaptic relay station for reflex movements of the eye and for pupillary reflexes. They possess a rudimentary layered structure. In the superficial gray layer *(stratum griseum superficiale)* (**a2**) fibers from the occipital fields of the cerebral cortex, *corticotectal tract* (**a3**), terminate. The *stratum opticum* (**a4**), which consists of fibers of the optic tract in lower vertebrates, consists in humans of fibers from the lateral geniculate body. The deeper cell and fiber layers may be grouped together as the *stratum lemnisci* (**a5**), in which end the spinotectal tract, fibers from the medial and lateral lemnisci, and fiber bundles from the inferior colliculi.

The aqueduct is surrounded by the periaqueductal gray, *griseum centrale* (**ab6**). It contains a large number of peptidergic neurons (VIP, encephalin, cholecystokinin, etc.). Lateral to it lies the *mesencephalic nucleus* of the trigeminal nerve (**a7**), and ventral is the **oculomotor nerve nucleus** (**a8**) and the Edinger-Westphal nucleus (**a9**). Dorsal to both nuclei passes the *dorsal longitudinal fasciculus* and ventral the *medial longitudinal fasciculus* (**a10**). The chief nucleus in the tegmentum is the **red nucleus** (**ab11**), which is delimited by a capsule of afferent and efferent fibers, among others the *dentatorubral fasciculus* (**a12**). The fiber bundles of the *oculomotor nerve* (**a13**) run ventrally at its medial border. Tectospinal (pupillary reflex) and tectorubral fibers cross the midline in the *superior tegmental decussation (Meynert)* (**a14**), and tegmentospinal fibers cross in the *inferior decussation (Forel's decussation)* (**a15**). The lateral field is occupied by the medial lemniscus (**ab16**).

Ventrally, the tegmentum borders on the **substantia nigra** *(pars compacta* [**a17**] and *pars reticulata* [**a18**]). On both sides the base is formed by the corticofugal fiber mass of the **cerebral peduncles** (**ab19**). *Medial geniculate body* (**ab20**).

Section Through the Pretectal Region

The **pretectal region** (**b21**), which lies in front of the superior colliculi, represents the transition between the midbrain and the diencephalon. The section, therefore, shows already some features of the diencephalon: on both sides lies dorsally the *pulvinar* (**b22**), in the center the *posterior commissure* (**b23**), and at the base the *corpora mamillaria* (**b24**). Dorsolaterally lies the pretectal region with the **principal pretectal nucleus** (**b25**). It is an important synaptic region for the pupillary light reflex and in it the fibers of the optic tract and the occipital cortical fields terminate. An efferent pathway from the nucleus extends across the posterior commissure to the Edinger-Westphal nucleus. Ventral to the aqueduct lie **Darkshevich's nucleus** (**b26**) and the **interstitial nucleus** *(Cajal's nucleus)* (**b27**), relay stations for the medial longitudinal fasciculus.

Animal experiments have shown that the *interstitial nucleus of Cajal* and the more orocaudally situated *prestitial nucleus* are important relay stations for the control of automatic movements within the extrapyramidal motor system. The interstitial nucleus and the prestitial nucleus contain the essential synapses for rotation of the body about its long axis, and the prestitial nucleus contains the essential synapses for raising the head and the upper part of the body. Supramamillary commissure (**b28**).

Red Nucleus and Substantia Nigra (Fig. 1.46)

Lateral View of the Brainstem

The two large nuclei project far toward the diencephalon. The **substantia nigra** (**ab1**) extends from the oral part of the *pons* (**a2**) to the *pallidum* (**ab3**) in the diencephalon. Both nuclei are important relay stations of the extrapyramidal system.

Red Nucleus (ab4)

In a fresh brain section the nucleus appears reddish (high iron content). It consists of small-celled *(neorubrum)* and large-celled *(paleorubrum)* parts. The paleorubrum is a small, ventrocaudally situated region.

Afferent connections: (1) The *dentatorubral fasciculus* (**b5**) from the *dentate nucleus* (**b6**) of the cerebellum runs in the *superior cerebellar peduncle* and ends in the contralateral red nucleus. (2) The *tectorubral tract* (**b7**) from the superior colliculi ends on the homolateral and contralateral paleorubrum. (3) The *pallidorubral tract* (**b8**), pallidotegmental bundle, from the inner segment of the pallidum. (4) The *corticorubral tract* (**b9**) from the frontal and precentral cortex terminates in the homolateral red nucleus.

Efferent connections: (1) The *rubroreticular* and *rubro-olivary fibers* (**b10**) run in the *central tegmental tract* and end for the most part in the olive (neuronal circuit: dentate nucleus–red nucleus–olive–cerebellum). (2) The *rubrospinal tract* (**b11**) (poorly developed in humans) crosses in Forel's tegmental decussation and terminates in the cervical cord.

The red nucleus is a relay and control station for cerebellar, pallidal, and corticomotor impulses, which are important for muscle tone, body posture, and walking. Damage to the nucleus causes a tremor at rest, alteration in muscle tone and choreiform-athetoid movements.

Substantia Nigra

This consists of the dark compact part (**pars compacta**—nerve cells with black melanin pigment [**c**]) and the reticular part (**pars reticularis**—with a reddish color, rich in iron). The tracts of the substantia nigra consist of fine fibers in loose bundles that cannot readily be identified.

Afferent connections: The anterior part receives (1) fibers from the caudate nucleus *(fasciculus strionigralis)* (**b12**), (2) fibers from the frontal cortex (areas 9 to 12)—*fibrae corticonigrales* (**b13**). (3) The fibers from the putamen (**b14**) and (4) fibers from the precentral cortex (areas 4 and 6) (**b15**) terminate in the caudal part of the nucleus.

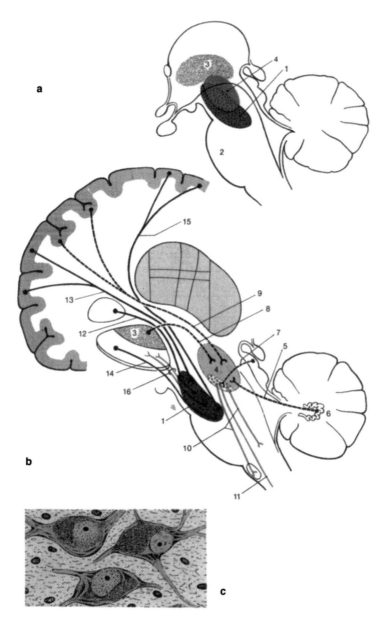

Fig. 1.46a–c (**a**) Position of the red nucleus and the substantia nigra in the brainstem: lateral view. (**b**) Connections of the tracts of the red nucleus and the substantia nigra. (**c**) Melanin-containing nerve cells of the substantia nigra.

Efferent connections: (1) **Nigrostriatal fibers (b16)** pass from the pars compacta to the striatum, and (2) fibers from the pars reticularis to the thalamus.

The majority of efferent fibers ascend to the striatum, with which the substantia nigra is closely associated functionally through the nigrostriatal system. Along the axons of the *dopaminergic* nigral neurons (pars compacta), dopamine passes into the putamen and is stored there in boutons terminaux. Cutting through the nigrostriatal tract causes a fall in the dopamine content of the putamen. There is a topistic relationship between the substantia nigra and the putamen: the cranial and caudal parts of the nucleus nigra are associated with the corresponding parts of the caudate nucleus and the putamen.

The substantia nigra is of particular importance for the control of involuntary coordinated movements and the rapid onset of movement *(starter function)*. Damage to it causes tremor at rest, loss of coordinated movements, and a *masklike* face.

Nerves to the Muscles of the Eye (Fig. 1.47)

Abducens Nerve (c1)

Cranial nerve VI is a *somatomotor nerve* that innervates the **lateral rectus muscle** (**e2**). Its fibers arise from the large, multipolar nerve cells of the **nucleus of the abducens nerve** (**c3**), which lies in the pons in the floor of the rhomboid fossa (**Fig. 1.32** [**a1**]). The fibers emerge at the lower margin of the pons, above the pyramid. After running a long intradural course, the nerve passes through the cavernous sinus and leaves the cranial cavity through the *superior orbital fissure.*

Trochlear Nerve (bc4)

Cranial nerve IV (a pure *somatomotor nerve)* supplies the *superior oblique muscle* (**e5**). Its fibers arise from the large multipolar neurons of the **trochlear nerve nucleus** (**bc6**), which lies in the midbrain below the aqueduct at the level of the inferior colliculi. The fibers ascend dorsally in an arch, cross above the aqueduct, and leave the midbrain at the lower margin of the inferior colliculi. The nerve is the only cranial nerve to leave the brainstem on its dorsal surface. It descends to the base of the skull in the subarachnoid space, where it enters the dura at the margin of the tentorium and extends further through the lateral wall of the cavernous sinus. It enters the orbit through the superior orbital fissure.

Oculomotor Nerve (ac7)

Cranial nerve III contains *somatomotor* and *visceromotor* (**a8**) fibers. It innervates the remaining external ocular muscles, and its visceromotor part supplies the internal ocular muscles. Its fibers leave from the floor of the interpeduncular fossa at the medial margin of the cerebral peduncles in the oculomotor

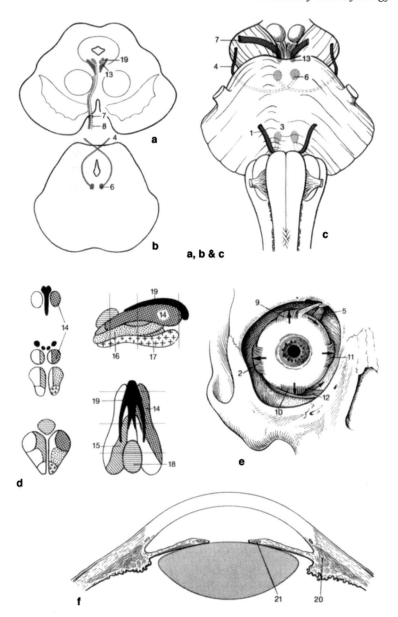

Fig. 1.47a–f (**a–c**) Abducens nerve, trochlear nerve, and oculomotor nerve; regions of the nuclei and emergence of the nerves. (**d**) Somatotopic arrangement of the neurons in the oculomotor nucleus. (**e**) External ocular muscles. (**f**) Internal ocular muscles.

sulcus. Lateral to the sella, the nerve penetrates the dura, runs through the roof and the lateral wall of the cavernous sinus, and enters the orbit through the *superior orbital fissure.* There it divides into a *superior branch,* which supplies the *levator palpebrae superior muscle* and the *superior rectus muscle* (**e9**), and an *inferior branch* to the *inferior rectus muscle* (**e10**), the *medial rectus muscle* (**e11**), and the *inferior oblique muscle* (**e12**).

The somatomotor fibers arise from large, multipolar nerve cells in the **oculomotor nerve nucleus** (**ac13**), which lies in the midbrain beneath the aqueduct, at the level of the superior colliculi.

The cell groups of this nucleus are arranged longitudinally and supply particular muscles: cells for the inferior rectus muscle (**d14**) lie dorsolaterally, those for the superior rectus muscle (**d15**) lie dorsomedially, and below them are cells for the inferior oblique muscle (**d16**)—ventrally are those for the medial rectus muscle (**d17**), and dorsocaudally are neurons for the levator palpebrae superioris muscle (**d18**) (central caudal oculomotor nucleus). In the middle third between the two paired main nuclei, there is usually an unpaired group of cells, the *nucleus of Perlia,* which is important in convergence.

Preganglionic parasympathetic visceromotor fibers stem from the small-celled **Edinger-Westphal** accessory oculomotor nucleus (**ad19**). They pass from the oculomotor nerve to the ciliary ganglion, where they synapse. The postganglionic fibers enter through the sclera into the eyeball and supply the *ciliary muscle* (**f20**) and the *pupillary sphincter muscle* (**f21**).

Long Tracts (Fig. 1.48)

Corticospinal Tract, Corticonuclear Fibers

The pyramidal tract, also called the corticospinal tract, extends through the basal part of the brainstem, where it occupies the middle of the cerebral peduncle; in the pons it forms several fiber bundles that have been cut transversely, and in the medulla oblongata it forms the pyramids proper.

Some pyramidal tract fibers terminate in cranial motor nerve nuclei (**corticonuclear fibers**): (1) *bilaterally* in the oculomotor nucleus III, the motor trigeminal nucleus V, the caudal part of the facial nucleus VII (forehead muscles), and the nucleus ambiguus X; (2) *crossing* to the contralateral nucleus: abducens nucleus VI, the rostral part of the facial nucleus VII (facial muscles with the exception of the forehead muscles), and the hypoglossal nucleus XII; and (3) *uncrossed* on the homolateral nucleus: trochlear nucleus IV.

> **Clinical tips:** In *central facial paralysis,* in which the paralysis of the facial musculature results from damage to the corticobulbar fibers, there is retention of movement of the forehead muscles because of their bilateral innervations.

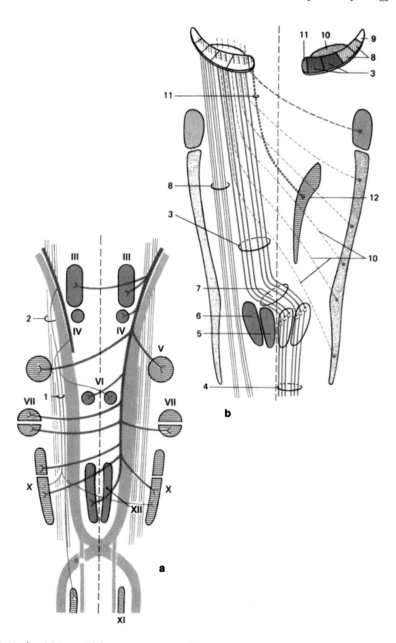

Fig. 1.48a,b (**a**) Pyramidal system; corticonuclear tract and corticobulbar fibers. (**b**) Ascending tracts of the medial lemniscus.

Aberrant fibers *(Déjérine)* (**a1**): at various levels in the midbrain and pons, fine fiber bundles branch from the corticonuclear tract and combine to form the *aberrant mesencephalic tract* and the *aberrant pontine tract*. Both descend in the medial lemniscus (**a2**) and end in the contralateral abducens VI and hypoglossal nuclei XII, in both ambigui nuclei X, and in the spinal accessory nucleus XI.

Medial Lemniscus

This fiber system includes the most important ascending tracts in the spinal cord and brainstem for exteroceptive sensation. It is divided into the *spinal* and *trigeminal lemnisci*. The spinal lemniscus contains the sensory tracts for the trunk and the extremities (*bulbothalamic, spinothalamic,* and *spinotectal tracts*), and the trigeminal lemniscus carries the sensory fibers that supply the face *(ventral tegmental fasciculus)*.

1. **Bulbothalamic tract** (**b3**). The fibers are an extension of the posterior funiculi of the spinal cord (**b4**) (epicritic sensibility). They originate in the nucleus gracilis (**b5**) and the nucleus cuneatus (**b6**), cross as arcuate fibers (decussation of the lemnisci [**b7**]), and form the medial lemniscus in the true sense (p. 40 [a19]). At first the cuneate fibers lie dorsal to the gracilis fibers, whereas in the pons and the midbrain they lie medial to them. They terminate in the thalamus.

2. **Spinothalamic tract** *(lateral and ventral)* (**b8**). The fibers (protopathic sensibility: pain, temperature, and coarse touch sensation) have already crossed to the opposite side at various levels of the spinal cord and form somewhat scattered, loose bundles in the medulla *(spinal lemniscus)*. They only become attached to the medial lemniscus in the midbrain (**Fig. 1.44**).

3. **Spinotectal tract** (**b9**). Its fibers run together with those of the lateral spinothalamic tract. In the midbrain, they form the lateral point of the lemniscus and they terminate in the superior colliculi (pupillary response to pain).

4. **Ventral tegmental fasciculus** *(Spitzer)* (**b10**). The fibers (protopathic and epicritic sensibility in the face) cross to the opposite side *(trigeminal lemniscus)* in small bundles from the *spinal nucleus of the trigeminal nerve* and from the *pontine nucleus of the trigeminal nerve*, and attach themselves to the medial lemniscus at the level of the pons. They end in the thalamus.

5. **Secondary taste fibers** (**b11**). They arise from the rostral part of the nucleus solitarius (**b12**), probably cross to the opposite side, and occupy the medial edge of the lemniscus. They end in the thalamus.

Long Tracts (Continued) (Fig. 1.49)

Medial Longitudinal Fasciculus

The *medial longitudinal bundle* is not a uniform fiber tract but contains several different fiber systems that enter and leave at various levels. It extends from the rostral part of the midbrain down into the spinal cord and connects several

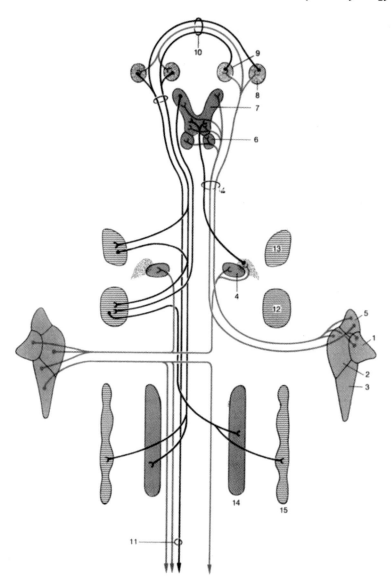

Fig. 1.49 Medial longitudinal fasciculus.

brainstem nuclei with each other. A transverse section through the brainstem shows it in the center of the tegmentum ventral to the periventricular gray (**Figs. 1.31**, **1.32**, **1.33**).

Vestibular part: Crossed and uncrossed fibers from the lateral (**1**), medial (**2**), and inferior (**3**) vestibular nuclei travel in the longitudinal fasciculus to the abducens nucleus (**4**) and the motor anterior horn cells of the cervical cord. Fibers to the homolateral trochlear (**6**) and oculomotor nuclei (**7**) ascend from the superior vestibular nucleus (**5**). Vestibular fibers finally terminate homolaterally and contralaterally in the interstitial nuclei of Cajal (**8**) and in Darkshevich's nucleus (**9**) (crossing in the posterior commissure [**10**]). The longitudinal bundle connects the vestibular apparatus to the oculomotor and cervical muscles and to the extrapyramidal system.

Extrapyramidal part: The interstitial nucleus of Cajal and Darkshevich's nucleus are intercalated in the course of the longitudinal fasciculus. They receive fibers from the striatum and pallidum and crossed fibers from the cerebellum. They send a fiber bundle, the *interstitiospinal fasciculus* (**11**), into the longitudinal fasciculus to the caudal brainstem and the spinal cord.

Internuclear part: This consists of communicating fibers between the cranial motor nerve nuclei: between the abducens (**4**) and the oculomotor nuclei (**7**), the facial nucleus (**12**) and the oculomotor nucleus, the facial nucleus and the motor trigeminal nucleus (**13**), and the hypoglossal nucleus (**14**) and the nucleus ambiguus (**15**).

The connection between the motor cranial nerve nuclei enables certain muscle groups to function together, for example, the coordination of the ocular muscles in movements of the eyeball, of the eyelid muscles during opening and closing of the eyes, and of the muscles of mastication and of the tongue and pharynx during swallowing and speech.

Internuclear Association of the Trigeminal Nuclei

Only a few secondary trigeminal fibers enter the medial longitudinal fasciculus. The majority, generally uncrossed, travel in the dorsolateral region of the tegmentum to the motor cranial nerve nuclei and form the basis for numerous important reflexes. Crossed and uncrossed fibers pass to the facial nucleus as the basis for the corneal reflex. There is a connection with the superior salivary nucleus for the lacrimal reflex. Fibers to the hypoglossal nucleus, the nucleus ambiguus, and the anterior horn cells of the cervical cord (cells of origin of the phrenic nerve) form the basis of the sneezing reflex. The reflexes of swallowing and regurgitation depend on fiber connections to the nucleus ambiguus, the dorsal nucleus of the vagus, and the motor nucleus of the trigeminus. The tract for the oculocardiac reflex (slowing down of the heart beat following pressure on the eyeballs) is associated with the dorsal nucleus of the vagus.

Long Tracts (Continued) (Fig. 1.50)

Central Tegmental Tract (a)

The *central tegmental tract* is the most important efferent pathway of the extrapyramidal motor system. It runs from the midbrain down to the inferior **olive** (**a1**), where the main portion ends. The remainder is thought to extend via short neurons, which synapse one after another *(reticuloreticular fibers [**a2**])* as far as the spinal cord. In the caudal midbrain the tract lies dorsolateral to the decussation of the superior cerebellar peduncle; in the pons it forms in

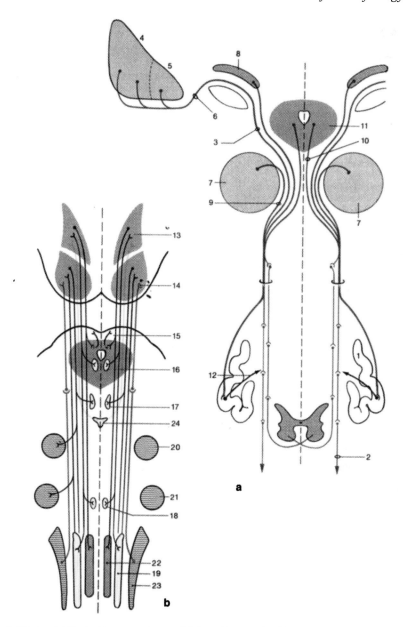

Fig. 1.50a,b (**a**) Central tegmental tract. (**b**) Dorsal longitudinal fasciculus.

the midpart of the tegmentum a large, indistinctly demarcated fiber plate (**Fig. 1.32 [ab12]**).

It consists of three components:

1. **Pallido-olivary fibers** (**a3**) from the *striatum* (**a4**) and the *pallidum* (**a5**), which pass in the pallidotegmental bundle (**a6**) to the capsule of the red nucleus (**a7**), and then to the olive. It is joined by fibers from the *zona incerta* (**a8**).
2. **Rubro-olivary fibers** (**a9**) from the small-celled part of the red nucleus, which forms in humans a large fiber tract, the *rubro-olivary fasciculus (Probst-Gamper),* the most important descending tract from the red nucleus.
3. **Reticulo-olivary fibers** (**a10**) enter the tegmental tract at various levels: from the region of the red nucleus, the periaqueductal gray (**a11**), and from the reticular formation of the pons and medulla.

Impulses that reach the olive from the extrapyramidal motor centers, and probably also from the motor cortex, are conveyed to the cerebellar cortex through *olivocerebellar fibers* (**a12**).

Dorsal Longitudinal Fasciculus (b)

The *dorsal longitudinal fasciculus (Schütz's bundle)* contains ascending and descending fiber systems that connect the hypothalamus with various brainstem nuclei and provide connections between the visceroefferent, parasympathetic nuclei. The majority of the fibers are peptidergic (somatostatin).

The fibers arise, or end, in the *septum,* the *oral hypothalamus,* the *tuber cinereum* (**b13**), and the *corpora mamillaria* (**b14**). They collect in the midbrain beneath the ependymal lining of the aqueduct and form the dorsal longitudinal fasciculus, which extends beneath the ependymal lining of the floor of the fourth ventricle as far as the lower medulla (**Fig. 1.31 [ab15]**, **Fig. 1.32 [ab12]**).

Fibers are given off to the two *superior colliculi* (**b15**) and the parasympathetic nuclei: *Edinger-Westphal nucleus* (**b16**), *superior salivatory nucleus* (**b17**), *inferior salivatory nucleus* (**b18**), and the *dorsal nucleus of the vagus* (**b19**). Other fibers end in cranial nerve nuclei: in the motor *nucleus of the trigeminal nerve* (**b20**) and the *facial* (**b21**) and *hypoglossal nerve nuclei* (**b22**). Fibers are also exchanged with the nuclei of the reticular formation.

Olfactory impulses reach the *dorsal longitudinal fasciculus* through the dorsal tegmental nucleus (via the habenular ganglion, interpeduncular nucleus, and dorsal tegmental nucleus).

Long ascending tracts: fibers from the nucleus solitarius (**b23**), probably taste fibers, ascend to the hypothalamus after synapsing in the ventral tegmental nucleus. Fibers of serotoninergic neurons may be followed by fluorescence microscopy from the *nucleus of the dorsal raphe* (**b24**) as far as the septal region.

In addition to other impulses, the dorsal longitudinal fasciculus receives hypothalamic, olfactory, and gustatory impulses that are passed on to the motor and secretory nuclei of the brainstem (reflex movements of the tongue, salivary secretion).

Reticular Formation (Fig. 1.51)

The scattered neurons of the tegmentum and their network of communicating processes are known as the reticular formation. It lies in the midpart of the tegmentum and extends from the medulla to the rostral midbrain. Several regions of different structure may be distinguished (**a**). In the medial region there are large-celled nuclei from which arise long ascending and descending tracts. The small-celled lateral strips are supposed to be association areas.

Many nerve cells have long ascending or descending axons or axons that divide into an ascending and a descending branch. Golgi impregnation methods show that from one such cell (**b1**) fibers reach both caudal cranial nerve nuclei (**b2**) and diencephalic nuclei (**b3**). The reticular formation contains a large number of peptidergic nerve cells (e.g., encephalin, neurotensin).

Afferent connections: Input from all types of sensations reaches the reticular formation. Sensory spinoreticular fibers terminate in the medial part of the medulla and pons, as do secondary fibers from the trigeminal and vestibular nuclei. Collaterals from the lateral lemniscus carry acoustic impulses and fibers of the tectoreticular fasciculus carry optic impulses. Stimulation experiments show that reticular neurons are activated more by sensory (pain), acoustic, and vestibular stimuli than by optic stimuli. Other afferent fibers arise from the cerebral cortex, the cerebellum, the red nucleus, and the pallidum.

Efferent connections: The **reticulospinal tract** runs from the medial region of the medulla and pons into the spinal cord. Bundles from the **reticulothalamic fasciculus** ascend to the nonspecific nuclei of the thalamus (truncothalamus). Fiber bundles from the midbrain terminate in the oral hypothalamus and septum.

Respiratory and circulatory center: Groups of nerve cells regulate respiration, heartbeat, and blood pressure (changes due to physical work or emotion). The inspiratory neurons lie in the midpart of the lower medulla (**c4**), whereas expiratory neurons lie more dorsally and laterally (**c5**). The pons contains superimposed synaptic centers for inhibition and facilitation *(locus coeruleus)* of respiration. The vegetative nuclei of the glossopharyngeal and vagus nerves are involved in the regulation of heart rate and blood pressure. Electrical stimulation of the caudal midpart of the medulla leads to lowering of blood pressure *(depressor center* [**d6**]), whereas stimulation of other parts of the reticular formation of the medulla causes an increase (**d7**).

Influence on the motor system: The spinal motor system is affected in various ways by the reticular formation. In the medial area of the medulla lies an inhibitory center, stimulation of which lowers muscle tone, extinguishes

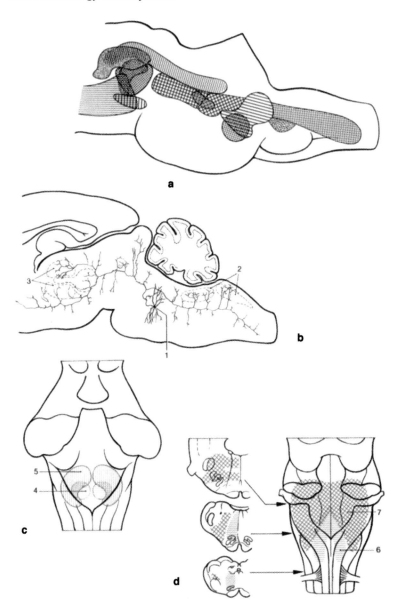

Fig. 1.51a–d (**a**) Extent and organization of the reticular formation in humans. (**b**) Nerve cell with dendritic branches; reticular formation of the rat. (**c**) Respiratory center, brainstem of the monkey. (**d**) Circulatory center, brainstem of the cat.

reflexes, and prevents any response from the motor cortex on electrical stimulation. The reticular formation of the pons and midbrain, on the other hand, enhances the activity of the motor system.

Ascending activation system: Through its connections with the nonspecific nuclei of the thalamus, the reticular formation influences the state of consciousness. If strongly aroused by sensory or cortical afferent stimuli, the organism suddenly becomes fully alert, a necessary state for attention and perception. Electrical stimulation of the reticular formation enables an objective assessment of this arousal activity by changes in the electrical activity of the brain (electroencephalogram [EEG]).

Pictorial Anatomy of the Auditory and Vestibular Systems

The letters following the text point to the figure parts where the concepts can be found using the numbers. (Abbreviations: a., artery; aa., arteries; m., muscle; mm., muscles; n., nerve; nn., nerves; v., vein; vv., veins.)

(Fig. 1.52)

1 **VESTIBULOCOCHLEAR ORGAN,** "organum vestibulocochleare." Sensory apparatus, in temporal bone, concerned with perception of sounds, balance, and position.

2 **INTERNAL EAR,** "auris interna." Portion of statoacoustic organ in petrosal bone.

3 **Membranous labyrinth,** "labyrinthus membranaceus." Complex system of canaliculi and dilatations with sensory epithelia; suspended by connective tissue in osseous labyrinth.   **a**

4 **Endolymph,** "endolympha." Fluid within membranous labyrinth.

5 **Perilymph,** "perilympha." Fluid in space between membranous and osseous labyrinths.

6 **Vestibular labyrinth,** "labyrinthus vestibularis." Content of labyrinth, including semicircular ducts.

7 **Endolymphatic duct,** "aqueductus vestibuli, ductus endolymphaticus." Small canal passing from saccule through osseous vestibular aqueduct to endolymphatic sac.   **a**

8 **Endolymphatic sac,** "saccus endolymphaticus." Blind sac on posterior wall of petrosal bone between the two dural sheets.   **a**

9 **Utriculosaccular duct,** "ductus utriculosaccularis." Small duct from lower end of endolymphatic duct to utricle.   **a**

10 **Utricle,** "utriculus." Small sac, 2.5 to 3.5 mm in diameter, serving as base for three semicircular ducts.   **a**

11 **Semicircular ducts,** "ductus semicirculares." Membranous semicircular canals, which, in osseous semicircular canals, describe three arcs perpendicular to each other; each corresponds to about two thirds of the arc of a circle.

12 *Anterior semicircular duct,* "ductus semicircularis anterior." Rises vertically and is approximately perpendicular to axis of petrosal bone.   **a**

13 *Posterior semicircular duct,* "ductus semicircularis posterior." Rises approximately vertically in a plane parallel to longitudinal axis of petrosal bone.   **a**

14 *Lateral semicircular duct,* "ductus semicircularis lateralis." Located most laterally; courses horizontally and may bulge tympanic cavity wall.   **a**

15 **Membrane propria of semicircular duct,** "membrana propria ductus semicircularis." Layer beneath basement membrane composed at first of rather densely packed fibers; continues into loose meshwork of perilymphatic space.   **c**

16 **Basal membrane of semicircular duct,** "membrana basalis ductus semicircularis." Basement membrane directly beneath epithelium; appears homogeneous under light microscope.   **c**

17 **Epithelium of semicircular duct,** "epithelium ductus semicircularis." Simple epithelial lining of membranous semicircular ducts with flat cells that become cuboidal on concave surface.   **c**

18 **Membranaceous ampullae,** "ampullae membranaceae." Dilatation of semicircular ducts near utricle.

19 *Anterior membranaceous ampulla,* "ampulla membranacea anterior." Dilatation of anterior semicircular duct, located anteriorly near lateral ampulla.   **a**

20 *Posterior membranaceous ampulla,* "ampulla membranacea posterior." Dilatation of posterior semicircular duct, located far from other two ampullae.   **a**

21 *Lateral membranaceous ampulla,* "ampulla membranacea lateralis." Dilatation of lateral semicircular duct, located near anterior ampulla.   **a**

22 **Ampullary sulcus,** "sulcus ampullaris." Notch beneath ampullary crest for entry of branch from ampullary n. to ampullary crest.   **b**

23 **Ampullary crest,** "crista ampullaris." Crescent-shaped ridge protruding into lumen of ampulla, covered with sensory epithelium and a base of n. fibers and connective tissue.   **b**

24 *"Neuroepithelium."* Sensory epithelium of ampulla composed of supporting and sensory cells that do not completely reach base; cilia on their upper surface protrude into cupula.   **b**

25 *"Cupula."* Gelatinous body suspended above epithelial crest, extending to roof of ampulla; penetrated by cilia of sensory cells.   **b**

26 **Membranous crura,** "crura membranacea." Ends of crura of semicircular ducts opening into utricle.

27 *Simple membranous crus,* "crus membranaceum simplex." Posterior end or crus of lateral semicircular duct, which empties solely into utricle.   **a**

28 *Ampullary membranous crura,* "crura membranacea ampullaria." Part of semicircular duct between ampullae and utricle.   **a**

29 *Common membranous crus,* "crus membranaceum commune." Common opening of anterior and posterior semicircular ducts into utricle.   **a**

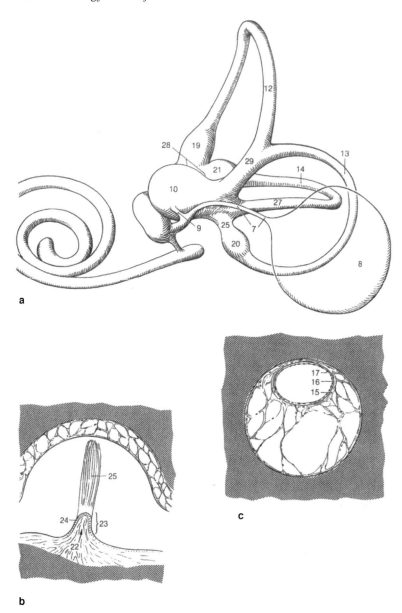

Fig. 1.52a–c (**a**) Membranous labyrinth. (**b**) Ampulla of semicircular duct. (**c**) Semicircular duct, cross section.

(Fig. 1.53)

1 **Hensen's duct,** "ductus reuniens." Tubular connection between saccule and cochlear duct. **b**

2 **Saccule,** "sacculus." Rounded sac, 2 to 3 mm long, supplied with sensory field. **b**

3 **Maculae staticae.** Sensory fields for perception of head position in space. **ab**

4 *Macula of utricle,* "macula utriculi." Sensory field, approximately 2.3 to 3 mm in size, located horizontally on floor of utricle. **b**

5 *Macula of saccule,* "macula sacculi." Vertically placed, curved sensory field at medial wall of sacculus, approximately 1.5 mm wide. **b**

6 *Otoconia,* calcium particles up to 25 μm in size, lying on a gelatinous substance together with sensory hairs. **a**

7 *Otoconial membrane,* "membrana statoconiorum." Accessory structure covering the maculae, composed of gelatinous ground substance covered by otoconia. **a**

8 *"Neuroepithelium."* Sensory epithelium of maculae composed of supporting and sensory cells. Hair-like extensions of sensory cells, approximately 20 to 25 μm long, extend into statoconial membrane. **a**

9 **Endolymph,** "endolympha." Fluid within membranous labyrinth.

10 **Perilymph,** "perilympha." Fluid in space surrounding the membranous labyrinth.

11 **Labyrinth of cochlea,** "labyrinthus cochlearis." Content of bony cochlea. **c**

12 **Perilymphatic space,** "spatium perilymphaticum." Spaces, including scala tympani and scala vestibuli, subdivided by connective tissue trabeculae, containing perilymph. **ab**

13 *Vestibular scala,* "scala vestibuli." Space above osseous spiral lamina and cochlear duct. **c**

14 *Tympanic scala,* "scala tympani." Perilymphatic duct beneath osseous spiral lamina and basilar lamina. **c**

15 *Perilymphatic duct,* "ductus perilymphaticus, aquaeductus cochleae." Communication between the perilymphatic and subarachnoid spaces. Opens near tympanic canaliculus. **b**

16 **Cochlear duct,** "ductus cochlearis." Duct, triangular in cross section, spiraling to apex of cochlea in 2½ to 2¾ turns; contains sensory epithelium for perception of sound. **bce**

17 **Cupular cecum,** "cecum (cecum) cupulare." Blind end of cochlear duct in apex of cochlea. **b**

18 Vestibular cecum, "cecum (cecum) vestibulare." Blind end of cochlear duct facing vestibule. **b**

19 **Tympanic wall of cochlear duct,** "paries tympanicus (membrana spiralis), ductus cochlearis." Inferior wall located above scala tympani. **e**

20 **Spiral or Corti's organ,** "organum spirale." Sensory epithelium on basilar membrane for transformation of sound waves into nerve impulses. **d**

21 **Basilar membrane,** "lamina basilaris." Connective tissue partition between cochlear duct and scala tympani: extends between tympanic lamella of bony spiral lamina and spiral ligament. **e**

22 **Spiral ligament of cochlea,** "crista spiralis (lig. spirale)." Connective tissue lateral to cochlear duct adjacent to bony cochlear wall.   **e**

23 **"Foramina nervosa."** Apertures in basilar lamina for passage of acoustic n. fibers in their course from hair cells to spiral ganglion.   **d**

24 **"Limbus laminae spiralis osseae."** Mound of tissue on upper surface of spiral lamina to which tectorial membrane is attached.   **e**

25 **Vestibular lip,** "labium limbi vestibulare." Upper, shorter extension of limbus; point of attachment for tectorial membrane.   **e**

26 **Tympanic lip,** "labium limbi tympanicum." Lower, longer extension of limbus, on basilar lamina.   **de**

27 **Tectorial membrane,** "membrana tectoria." Gelatinous membrane above Corti's organ, attached by narrow strip to vestibular lip; ends freely beyond external row of hair cells.   **de**

28 **"Dentes acustici."** Cell rows forming small ridges along upper surface of vestibular lip; tectorial membrane anchored in this region.   **d**

29 **Internal spiral sulcus,** "sulcus spiralis internus." Groove between vestibular and tympanic lips.   **de**

30 **External spiral sulcus,** "sulcus spiralis externus." Groove on external wall of cochlear duct between spiral prominence and Corti's organ.   **e**

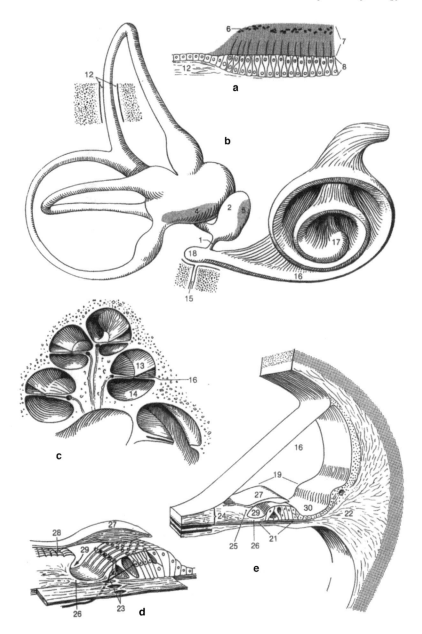

Fig. 1.53a–e (**a**) Macula of saccule or utricle. (**b**) Membranous labyrinth. (**c**) Cochlea, opened. (**d**) Corti's organ. (**e**) Cochlear duct.

(Fig. 1.54)

1. **Reticular membrane,** "membrana reticularis." Upper surface of Corti's organ composed of upper terminal plates of pillar cells and Deiters' cells.   **b**

2. **"Vas spirale."** Small blood vessel running in tympanic layer of basilar membrane, under tunnel.   **a**

3. **Vestibular wall of cochlear duct,** "paries vestibularis ductus cochlearis (membrane vestibularis Reissneri)." Superior wall of cochlear duct, about 3 μm thick.   **a**

4. **External wall of cochlear duct,** "paries externus ductus cochlearis." Lateral wall.   **a**

5. **Basal crest,** "crista basalis." Pointed extension of spiral lig. continuing into basilar membrane.   **a**

6. **Spiral prominence,** "prominentia spiralis." Ridge above external spiral sulcus composed of connective tissue and a single blood vessel.   **a**

7. **"Vas promineus."** Blood vessel of spiral prominence.   **a**

8. **"Stria vascularis."** Broad, highly vascularized band above spiral prominence with specialized epithelial cells important in regulating composition of endolymph.   **a**

9. **Spiral ganglion,** "ganglion spirale cochleae." Cluster of bipolar ganglion cells in spiral canal of modiolus; peripheral branches that come from organ of Corti. Central axons form cochlear branch of vestibulocochlear n.   **c**

10. **Vessels of internal ear**, "vasa auris internae."   **c**

11. **Labyrinthine artery,** "a. labyrinthi." Emerges from basilar a. in front of anterior inferior cerebellar a.; accompanies vestibulocochlear n. through internal acoustic meatus into petrosal bone, where it divides to supply inner ear.   **c**

12. *Vestibular branches,* "rami vestibulares." Supply ampullae, maculae, semicircular ducts and lower third of basal turn of cochlea.   **c**

13. *Cochlear branch,* "ramus cochlearis." Runs in cochlear axis and sends branches out to spiral ganglion and cochlear ducts and their content, except for lower third of basal turn.   **c**

14. *Glomeruli of cochlear arteries,* "glomeruli arteriosi cochleae." Spiral arterial network accompanying spiral vein.   **c**

15. **Labyrinthine veins,** "vv. labyrinthi." Accompany labyrinthine a.; pass through internal acoustic meatus and open either into inferior petrosal sinus or directly into internal jugular vein.   **c**

16. *Spiral vein of modiolus,* "v. spiralis modioli." Spiral v. of cochlear axis; opens into labyrinthine vein.   **c**

17. *Vestibular veins,* "vv. vestibulares." Emerge from semicircular ducts in region of utricle and saccule; empty into labyrinthine vein and vein of vestibular aqueduct.   **c**

18. *Vein of vestibular aqueduct,* "v. aquaeductus vestibuli." Accompanies endolymphatic duct; empties into inferior petrosal sinus.   **c**

19. *Vein of cochlear aqueduct,* "v. aquaeductus cochleae." Accompanies perilymphatic duct; provides major venous drainage for cochlea.   **c**

20. **Osseous labyrinth,** "labyrinthus osseous." Bony capsule containing membranous labyrinth.   **d**

21 **Vestibule,** "vestibulum." Perilymphatic space containing utricle and saccule.   **d**

22 **Spherical recess,** "recessus sphericus." Rounded depression in medial vestibular wall containing saccule.   **d**

23 **Elliptical recess,** "recessus ellipticus." Depression in medial vestibular wall containing superior portion of the utricle.   **d**

24 **Crest of vestibule,** "crista vestibuli." Ridge between spherical and elliptical recesses.   **d**

25 **Pyramid of vestibule,** "pyramis vestibuli." Upper, broader part of crest of vestibule.   **d**

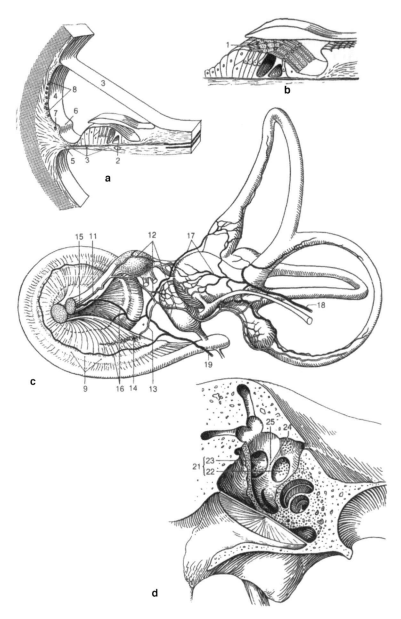

Fig. 1.54a–d (**a**) Cochlear duct. (**b**) Corti's organ. (**c**) Vessels of labyrinth. (**d**) Bony labyrinth, posterior wall.

(Fig. 1.55)

1 **Cochlear recess,** "recessus cochlearis." Depression below and in front of spherical recess; contains lower end of cochlear duct.   **c**

2 **"Maculae cribrosae."** Perforated bony areas for passage of fibers from vestibulocochlear n.

3 *"Macula crib rosa superior."* Perforated bony area for passage of utriculoampullary n. fibers.   **c**

4 *"Macula cribrosa media."* Perforated bony area near base of cochlea for passage of saccular n. fibers.   **c**

5 *"Macula cribrosa inferior."* Perforated bony area in wall of posterior osseous ampulla for passage of posterior ampullary n. fibers.   **c**

6 **Osseous semicircular canals,** "canales semiculares ossei." Bony canals housing semicircular ducts.   **c**

7 *Anterior semicircular canal,* "canalis semicircularis anterior." Shares a common limb with posterior semicircular canal; stands vertically, approximately perpendicular to axis of petrosal bone.   **b**

8 *Posterior semicircular canal,* "canalis semicircularis posterior." Located posteriorly and inferiorly; almost parallel to axis of petrosal bone.   **b**

9 *Lateral semicircular canal,* "canalis semicircularis lateralis." Lies horizontally and may bulge medial wall of tympanic cavity.   **b**

10 **Osseous ampullae,** "ampullae osseae." Enlargements of semicircular canals near their bases, containing membranaceous ampullae.   **c**

11 *Anterior osseous ampulla,* "ampulla ossea anterior." Ampulla of anterior semicircular canal located anteriorly, close to lateral ampulla.   **b**

12 *Posterior osseous ampulla,* "ampulla ossea posterior." Ampulla of posterior semicircular canal located below level of lateral semicircular canal.   **b**

13 *Lateral osseous ampulla,* "ampulla ossea lateralis." Ampulla of lateral semicircular canal located close to anterior ampulla.   **b**

14 **Osseous crura,** "crura ossea." Bony limbs of semicircular canals.

15 *Common osseous crus,* "crus osseum commune." Located posteriorly and formed by union of crura of anterior and posterior osseous semicircular canals.   **b**

16 *Simple osseous crus,* "crus osseum simplex." Crus of lateral semicircular canal located posteriorly; opens separately on vestibular canal.   **b**

17 *Ampullary osseous crura,* "crura ossea ampullaria." Enlargements of semicircular canals containing ampullae of membranous labyrinth.   **b**

18 **"Cochlea."** Consists in humans of 2½ to 2¾ turns. Base is 8 to 9 mm wide, height 4 to 5 mm.   **b**

19 **Apex,** "cupula cochleae." Top of cochlea directed anteriorly, slightly inferiorly and laterally.   **b**

20 **Base,** "basis cochleae." Surface faces approximately in direction of internal acoustic meatus.   **a**

21 **Spiral canal,** "canalis spiralis cochleae." Separated into three canals by bony spiral lamina and basilar membrane and by vestibular membrane.   **a**

22 **"Modiolus."** Conical axis of cochlea. Hollow for reception of cochlear n.; forms medial wall of spiral canal.   **a**

23 *Base,* "basis modioli." Beginning of modiolus at base.   **a**

24 *Modiolar plate,* "lamina modioli." Upright end of bony spiral lamina.   **a**

25 *Spiral canal of modiolus,* "canalis spiralis modioli." Minute canal in axis wall near base of bony spiral lamina, for spiral ganglion.   **a**

26 *Longitudinal canals of modiolus,* "canales longitudinales modioli." Minute, centrally located bony canals for axons of cochlear part of vestibulocochlear n. from spiral ganglion.   **a**

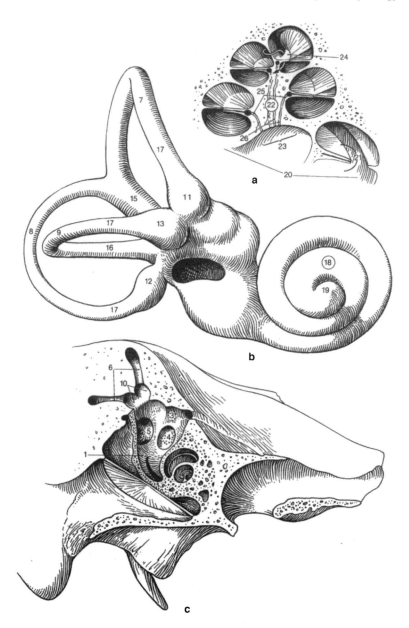

Fig. 1.55a–c (**a**) Cochlea, longitudinal section. (**b**) Cast of labyrinth. (**c**) Bony labyrinth, posterior wall.

(Fig. 1.56)

1 **Bony spiral lamina,** "lamina spiralis ossea." Two-layered bony lamella project-ing from modiolus into spiral cochlear canal; with cochlear duct, completely separates scala tympani from scala vestibuli.   **b**

2 *"Hamulus laminae spiralis."* Free, hook-like upper end of bony spiral lamina at apex of cochlea.   **b**

3 **"Helicotrema."** Connection between scala vestibuli and scala tympani at apex of cochlea; formed because bony spiral lamina and cochlear duct end before they reach apex.   **b**

4 **Secondary spiral lamina,** "lamina spiralis secundaria." Bony ridge in lower half of basal turn; projects from outer wall of spiral canal opposite bony spiral lamina. Lower part of basilar membrane is stretched between the two.   **b**

5 **Internal acoustic meatus,** "meatus acusticus internus." Begins on posterior wall of petrosal bone and contains vestibulocochlear n., facial n., and labyrin-thine a. and vein; approximately 1 cm long.   **a**

6 **Internal acoustic pore,** "porus acusticus internus." Entrance to internal acoustic meatus on posterior wall of petrosal bone above jugular foramen.   **a**

7 **Fundus of internal acoustic meatus,** "fundus meatus acustici interni." Floor of internal acoustic meatus; divided into several fields.   **a**

8 *Transverse crest,* "crista transversa." Divides fundus into upper and lower fields.   **a**

9 *Area of facial nerve,* "area nervi facialis." Contains origin of facial canal.   **a**

10 *Cochlear area,* "area cochleae." Larger field below transverse crest with forami-nous spiral tract.   **a**

11 *Foraminous spiral tract,* "tractus spiralis foraminosus." Perforated area corre-sponding to cochlear turns for passage of fibers from spiral ganglion to cochlear part of vestibulocochlear n.   **a**

12 *Superior vestibular area,* "area vestibularis superior." Lateral to facial canal for passage of utriculoampullary n. fibers.   **a**

13 *Inferior vestibular area,* "area vestibularis inferior." Lateral to facial canal for passage of utriculoampullary n. fibers.   **a**

14 *"Foramen singulare."* Small aperture behind inferior vestibular area for posterior branch of ampullary n.   **a**

15 **MIDDLE EAR,** "auris media." Consists of tympanic cavity, auditory tube, and cells of mastoid process.

16 **Tympanic cavity,** "cavitas tympanica." Medial to eardrum, obliquely situated, slitlike space, containing auditory ossicles; communicates at the top rear with air-containing mastoid process cells; at the bottom front, by way of auditory tube with nose–throat space.

17 **Tegmental wall,** "paries tegmentalis." Thin roof of tympanic cavity. Lies lateral to arcuate eminence of petrosal bone.   **c**

18 *Epitympanic recess,* "recessus epitympanicus." Dome of tympanic cavity, arching superiorly and laterally above margin of tympanic membrane.   **c**

19 *Cupular part,* "pars cupularis." Upper portion of epitympanic recess.   **c**

20 *Jugular wall,* "paries jugularis." Lower wall of tympanic cavity, facing jugular fossa.   **c**

21 *Styloid prominence,* "prominentia styloidea." Bulge in floor of tympanic cavity caused by styloid process.   **c**

22 **Labyrinthine wall,** "paries labyrinthicus." Medial wall of tympanic cavity.   **c**

23 *Oval window,* "fenestra vestibuli (fenestra ovalis)." Atrial window closed by base of stapes.   **c**

24 *Fossula of oval window,* "fossula fenestrae vestibuli." Small depression in medial wall of tympanic cavity between malleus and incus.   **c**

25 *Promontory,* "promontorium." Bulge caused by basal turn of cochlea.   **c**

26 *Promontory sulcus,* "sulcus promontorii." Branched grooves on promontory caused by tympanic plexus.   **c**

27 *Subiculum of promontory,* "subiculum promontorii." Small bony crest behind promontory and round window.   **c**

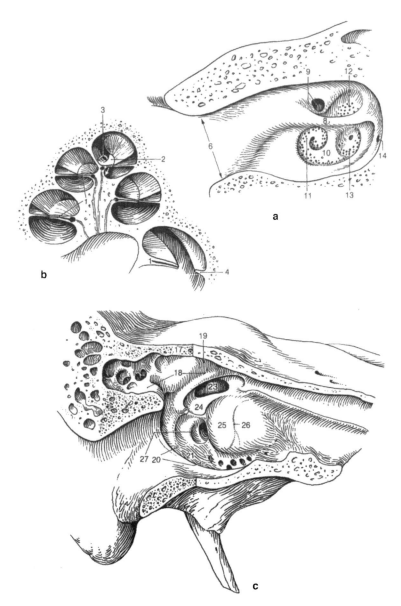

Fig. 1.56a–c (**a**) Internal acoustic meatus. (**b**) Section of cochlea. (**c**) Medial wall of tympanic cavity.

(Fig. 1.57)

1 *Tympanic sinus,* "sinus tympani." Deep groove behind promontory and round window. **d**

2 *Round window,* "fenestra cochleae rotunda." End of scala tympani, closed by secondary tympanic membrane. **d**

3 *Fossula of round window,* "fossula fenestrae cochleae." Groove leading to round window. **d**

4 *Crest of round window,* "crista fenestrae cochleae." Bony crest on edge of round window for attachment of secondary tympanic membrane. **d**

5 *Cochleariform process,* "processus cochleariformis." Spoon-shaped bony process above promontory at end of semicanal for tensor tympani muscle. With a loop of connective tissue it serves like a pulley for tensor m. of tympanum. **d**

6 **Secondary tympanic membrane,** "membrana tympani secundaria." Wall between scala tympani and tympanic cavity stretched across round window.

7 **["Adnexa mastoidea."],** Mastoid Process.

8 **Mastoid wall,** "paries mastoideus." Faces mastoid process. **d**

9 *Mastoid antrum,* "antrum mastoideum." Posterosuperior continuation of tympanic cavity. Mastoid air cells extend inferiorly from it. **d**

10 *"Aditus ad antrum."* Entrance to mastoid antrum from tympanic cavity. **d**

11 *Prominence of lateral semicircular canal,* "prominentia canalis semicircularis lateralis." Elevation above facial prominence due to lateral semicircular canal. **d**

12 *Prominence of facial canal,* "prominentia canalis facialis." Elevation between oval window and prominence of lateral semicircular canal due to facial canal. **d**

13 *Pyramidal eminence,* "eminentia pyramidalis." Bony cone at level of oval window, perforated at its apex. Tendon of stapedius m. passes through its apical opening. **d**

14 *Incudal fossa,* "fossa incudis." Small indentation for posterior ligament of incus in arch of aditus ad antrum. **d**

15 *Posterior sinus,* "sinus posterior." Small groove between incudal fossa and pyramidal eminence. **d**

16 *Opening of chorda tympani canal into tympanic cavity,* "apertura tympanica canaliculi chordae tympani." Near posterior edge of tympanic membrane at level of pyramidal eminence. **d**

17 *Mastoid air cells,* "cellulae mastoideae." Covered by flat or cuboidal epithelium, as in tympanic cavity. **d**

18 *Tympanic cells,* "cellulae tympanicae." Small depressions in floor of tympanic cavity. **d**

19 **Carotid wall,** "paries caroticus." Formed partly by carotid canal and partly by end of auditory tube. **d**

20 **Membranous wall,** "paries membranaceus." Formed principally by tympanic membrane. **b**

21 **Eardrum, tympanic membrane,** "membrana tympani." Stretched obliquely across end of external acoustic meatus; diameter, 9 to 11 mm. **ab**

22 **Shrapnell's membrane,** "pars flaccida Shrapnell's membrane." Small flaccid part of tympanic membrane above anterior and posterior mallear folds.   **ab**

23 **"Pars tensa."** Largest portion of tympanic membrane stretched across tympanic anulus.   **ab**

24 **Anterior mallear fold,** "plica mallearis anterior." On medial side of tympanic membrane. Runs anteriorly from base of handle of malleus; concave inferiorly.   **b**

25 **Posterior mallear fold,** "plica mallearis posterior." Runs posteriorly from base of handle of malleus on internal side of tympanic membrane; concave inferiorly.   **b**

26 **Mallear prominence,** "prominentia mallearis." Small elevation on outside of tympanic membrane caused by lateral process of malleus.   **a**

27 **Mallear stria,** "stria mallearis." Light-colored strip on outside of tympanic membrane caused by handle of malleus, as seen through semitransparent tympanic membrane.   **a**

28 **Umbo of tympanic membrane,** "umbo membranae tympani." At apex of handle of malleus, which draws tympanic membrane inward.   **a**

29 **Cutaneous layer,** "stratum cutaneum." Stratified squamous epithelium on outer side of tympanic membrane.   **c**

30 **Fibrocartilaginous ring,** "anulus fibrocartilagineus." Anchoring tissue of tympanic membrane in tympanic sulcus.   **c**

31 **Radiate layer,** "stratum radiatum." Group of external, radially oriented fibers of tympanic membrane.   **c**

32 **Circular layer,** "stratum circulare." Internally located fibers of tympanic membrane.   **c**

33 **Mucosal layer,** "stratum mucosum." Simple squamous epithelium of inner side of tympanic membrane.   **c**

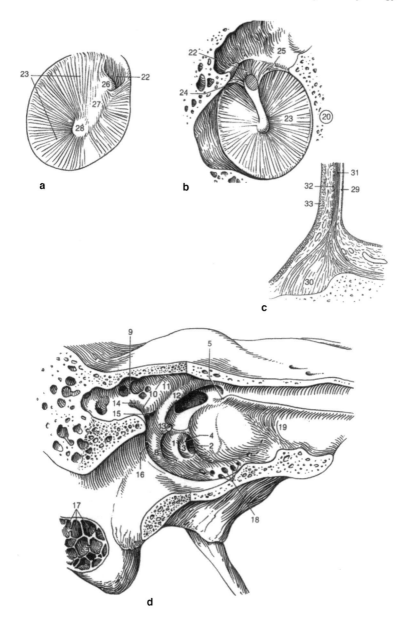

Fig. 1.57a–d   (**a**) Right eardrum, external view. (**b**) Lateral wall of tympanic cavity. (**c**) Attachment of eardrum. (**d**) Medial wall of tympanic cavity.

(Fig. 1.58)

1 **Auditory ossicles,** "ossicula auditus." Stapes, incus and malleus; transmit sound from tympanic membrane to inner ear.

2 **Stirrup,** "stapes." Base is inserted in oval window. **ab**

3 *Head of stapes,* "caput stapedis." Located opposite base and connected via lenticular process with long crus of incus. **ab**

4 *Anterior crus,* "crus anterius." Nearly straight crus of stapes. **ab**

5 *Posterior crus,* "crus posterius." Somewhat curved crus of stapes. **ab**

6 *Base of stapes,* "basis stapedis [ovalis]." Inserted into oval window. **ab**

7 **Anvil,** "incus." Located between head of malleus and stapes. **ad**

8 *Body of incus,* "corpus in cudis." Articulates with malleus via a saddle-shaped joint surface. **a**

9 *Long crus,* "crus longum." Runs downward almost vertically behind handle of malleus; bears lenticular process at its end. **a**

10 *Lenticular process,* "processus lenticularis." Minute piece of bone at end of long crus. Articulates with stapes. **a**

11 *Short crus,* "crus breve." Directed horizontally backward; attached by lig. in incudal fossa. **a**

12 **Hammer,** "malleus." Inserted between tympanic membrane and incus. **ac**

13 *Handle of malleus,* "manubrium mallei." Outer surface is attached to tympanic membrane up to lateral process. **a**

14 *Head of malleus,* "caput mallei." Bears convex articulating surface for body of incus. **a**

15 *Neck of malleus,* "collum mallei." Link between head and handle. **a**

16 *Lateral process,* "processus lateralis." Short process at end of handle, causing mallear prominence. **a**

17 *Anterior process,* "processus anterior." Elongated, slender process; extends into petrotympanic fissure in newborn, but atrophies in adult. **a**

18 **Articulations of auditory ossicles,** "articulationes ossiculorum auditus." Not true joints, but syndesmoses.

19 *Incudomallear articulation,* "articulatio incudomallearis." Connection between malleus and incus. Occasionally exhibits an articular cleft. **a**

20 *Incudostapedial articulation,* "articulatio incudostapedia." Connection between lenticular process of long crus of incus and stapes. **a**

21 *Tympanostapedial syndesmosis,* "syndesmosis tympanostapedia." Connective tissue attachment of base of stapes to oval window; wider anteriorly than posteriorly. **b**

22 **Ligaments of ossicles,** "ligg. ossiculorum auditus."

23 *Anterior ligament of malleus,* "lig. mallei anterius." Arises from anterior process of malleus; lies in anterior mallear fold and extends to petrotympanic fissure. **d**

24 *Superior ligament of malleus,* "lig. mallei superius." Runs from head of malleus to roof of epitympanic recess. **cd**

25 *Lateral ligament of malleus,* "lig. mallei laterale." Connects neck of malleus with upper margin of tympanic notch. **c**

26 *Superior ligament of incus,* "lig. incudis superius." Runs almost parallel to superior lig. of malleus; connects body of incus with roof of epitympanic recess.   **cd**

27 *Posterior ligament of incus,* "lig. incudis posterius." Runs from short crus of incus to lateral wall of tympanic cavity.   **cd**

28 *Stapedial membrane,* "membrana stapedis." Thin membrane between crura and base of stapes.   **b**

29 *Anular (annular) ligament of stapes,* "lig. anulare (annulare) stapedis." Ligamentous connection between base of stapes and margins of oval window; wider anteriorly than posteriorly.   **b**

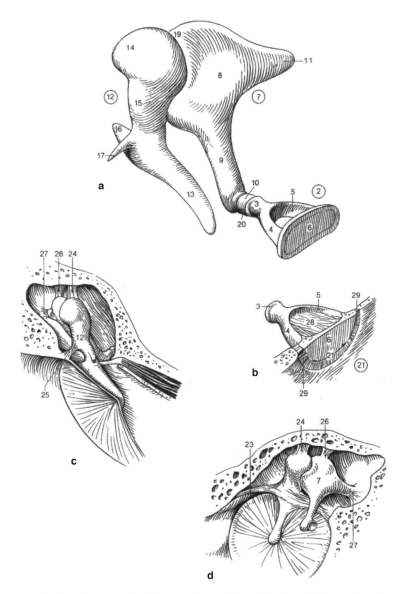

Fig. 1.58a–d (**a**) Auditory ossicles. (**b**) Base of stapes in oval window. (**c**) Tympanic cavity, posterior half. (**d**) Lateral wall of tympanic cavity.

(Fig. 1.59)

1 **Muscles of tympanic cavity,** "mm. ossiculorum auditus." Attached to auditory ossicles.

2 *Tensor muscle of tympanum,* "m. tensor tympani." Lies in semicanal for tensor m. of tympanum above auditory tube. Laterally its tendon winds around cochleariform process, at almost a right angle and is attached to base of handle of malleus.   **a**

3 *Stapedius muscle,* "m. stapedius." Arises in a bony canal on posterior wall of tympanic cavity; appears at apex of pyramidal eminence and attaches to head of stapes; by tilting stapes, reduces its vibrations.   **b**

4 **Mucosa of tympanic cavity,** "tunica mucosa cavi tympani." Composed of simple, flat to cuboidal epithelium and delicate lamina propria, rich in vessels.

5 **Posterior mallear fold,** "plica mallearis posterior." Extends from base of handle of malleus to posterosuperior portion of tympanic anulus. Contains posterior portion of chorda tympani.   **d**

6 **Anterior mallear fold,** "plica mallearis anterior." Extends from base of handle of malleus to anterosuperior portion of tympanic anulus. Contains anterior portion of chorda tympani, anterior process of malleus and anterior ligament of malleus.   **d**

7 **Fold of chorda tympani,** "plica chordae tympani." Between anterior and posterior mallear folds on neck of malleus.   **d**

8 **Anterior recess,** "recessus membranae tympani anterior." Mucosal pocket between anterior mallear fold and tympanic membrane.   **d**

9 **Superior recess,** Prussak's pouch, "recessus membranae tympani superior [Prussak's space]." Bounded laterally by Shrapnell's membrane and medially by head and neck of malleus and body of incus.   **d**

10 **Posterior recess,** "recessus membranae tympani posterior." Mucosal pocket between posterior mallear fold and tympanic membrane.   **d**

11 **Incudal fold,** "plica incudis." Mucosal fold between roof of epitympanic recess and head of incus; sometimes also extends from short crus of incus to posterior wall of tympanic cavity.   **d**

12 **Stapedial fold,** "plica stapedis." Mucosal fold between posterior wall of tympanic cavity and stapes; covers stapes and stapedius m.   **b**

13 **Auditory tube,** "tuba auditiva." Osteocartilaginous tube (eustachian tube) approximately 4 cm long, between middle ear and nasopharynx for ventilation of tympanic cavity.   **ac**

14 **Tympanic opening,** "ostium tympanicum tubae auditivae." In anterior wall of tympanic cavity, usually somewhat above floor.   **a**

15 **Osseous part,** "pars ossea tubae auditivae." Posterolateral upper bony portion, about one third of length of tube: lies under semicanal for tensor m. of tympanum; point of entry between carotid canal and spinous foramen.   **a**

16 *Isthmus,* "isthmus tubae auditivae." Narrowing of tube between cartilaginous and osseous portions.   **a**

17 *Air cells,* "cellulae pneumaticae." Small depressions in wall of bony portion of tube.   **a**

18 **Cartilaginous part,** "pars cartilaginea tubae auditivae." Located antero-medially; approximately 2.5 cm long.   **a**

19 *Cartilage of auditory tube,* "cartilago tubae auditivae." Hook shaped in cross section; decreases in height posterolaterally; consists of elastic cartilage only in angle between the two cartilaginous laminae.   **a**

20 *Medial lamina,* "lamina (cartilaginis) medialis." Rather wide plate.   **c**

21 **Lateral lamina,** "lamina (cartilaginis) lateralis." Low plated directed anterolaterally.   **c**

22 *Membranous lamina,* "lamina membranacea." Portion of wall of cartilaginous part.   **ac**

23 **Mucosa,** "tunica mucosa." Consists of a simple, ciliated epithelium. **c**

24 *Glands of tube,* "glandulae tubariae." Mucous glands, especially in cartilaginous part of tube.   **c**

25 **Pharyngeal orifice,** "ostium pharyngeum tubae auditivae." Funnel shaped or slitlike, located above levator elevation at level of inferior nasal meatus, 1 cm lateral and anterior to posterior pharyngeal wall.   **a**

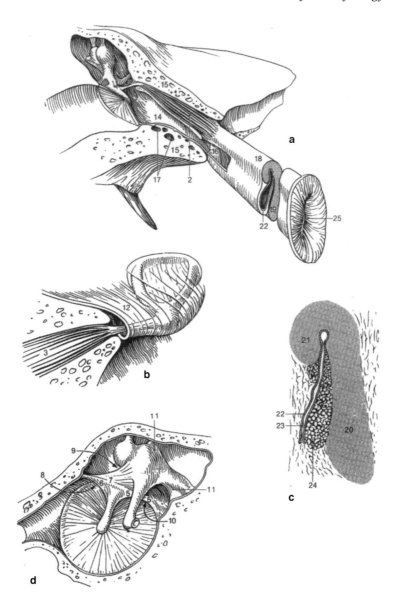

Fig. 1.59a–d (**a**) Auditory tube. (**b**) Stapedius muscle. (**c**) Auditory tube, cross section. (**d**) Lateral wall of tympanic cavity.

(Fig. 1.60)

1 **EXTERNAL EAR,** "auris externa." Comprises auricle and external acoustic meatus.

2 **External acoustic meatus,** "meatus acusticus externus." Flat, S-shaped osteocartilaginous external auditory canal, approximately 2.4 cm long and 6 mm in diameter.   **c**

3 **Opening of external acoustic meatus,** "porus acusticus externus."   **c**

4 **Cartilaginous external acoustic meatus,** "meatus acusticus externus cartilaginous." Lateral third of external acoustic meatus.   **c**

5 *Cartilage of acoustic meatus,* "cartilago meatus acustici." Connected with cartilage of auricle; not completely closed posterosuperiorly.   **d**

6 *"Incisurae cartilaginis meatus acustici."* Two slits in cartilage usually facing anteriorly and bridged by connective tissue.   **d**

7 **"Lamina tragic."** Lateral part of cartilaginous external acoustic meatus in front of opening of external acoustic meatus.   **d**

8 **Auricle,** "auricula."   **ab**

9 **Lobule,** "lobulus auriculae." Lower end of auricle, devoid of cartilage.   **abc**

10 **Auricular cartilage,** "cartilago auriculae." Basic framework of auricle composed of elastic cartilage.   **d**

11 **"Helix."** Outer curved margin of auricle.   **abcd**

12 *Crus of helix,* "curs helicis." Beginning of helix in concha of auricle.   **abd**

13 *Spine of helix,* "spina helicis," Small tubercle protruding anteriorly from crus.   **d**

14 *Tail of helix,* "cauda helicis." Posteroinferior terminal portion of auricular cartilage separated from antitragus by notch.   **d**

15 **"Anthelix."** Arched elevation in front of posterior portion of helix.   **abcd**

16 *Triangular fossa,* "fossa triangularis." Depression located anterosuperiorly, bounded by the two crura of anthelix.   **ad**

17 *Crura of anthelix,* "crura anthelicis." Two limbs of anthelix that enclose triangular fossa.   **ad**

18 **Scaphoid fossa,** "scapha." Posterior groove between helix and anthelix.   **ad**

19 **Concha of auricle,** "concha auriculae." Bounded by anthelix, antitragus, and tragus.   **a**

20 *"Cymba conchae."* Superior slit-like portion of concha between crura of helix and and thelix.   **a**

21 *Cavity of concha,* "cavum conchae." Main portion of concha below crus of helix and behind tragus.   **a**

22 **"Antitragus."** Small tubercle, continuation of anthelix, separated from tragus by intertragic notch.   **ad**

23 **"Tragus."** Low elevation in front of opening of external acoustic meatus.   **a**

24 **Anterior notch,** "incisura anterior (auris)." Between tragus (supratragic tubercle) and crus of helix.   **a**

25 **Intertragic notch,** "incisura intertragica." Fissure between tragus and antitragus.   **ad**

26 **Auricular of Darwin's tubercle,** "tuberculum auriculae [Darwin]." Occasionally occurring tubercle located posterosuperiorly on inner margin of auricle.   **a**

27 **Tip of auricle,** "apex auriculae." Occasionally occurring projection of external auricular margin in posterosuperior direction.   **b**

28 **Posterior auricular groove,** "sulcus auriculae posterior." Shallow indentation between antitragus and anthelix.   **a**

29 **Supratragic tubercle,** "tuberculum supratragicum." Occasionally occurring tubercle on upper end of tragus.   **a**

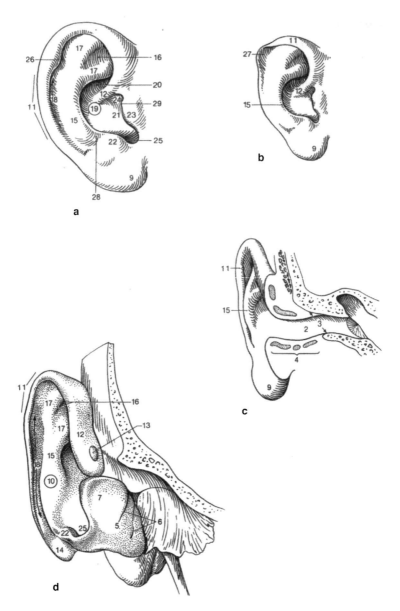

Fig. 1.60a–d (**a**) Auricle. (**b**) Auricle with a tip. (**c**) External acoustic meatus. (**d**) Auricular cartilage from front.

(Fig. 1.61)

1 **Isthmus of auricular cartilage,** "isthmus cartilaginis auris." Narrow connection between cartilaginous external acoustic meatus and lamina tragi of auricular cartilage.   **a**

2 **Terminal notch,** "incisura terminalis auris." Deep notch separating lamina tragi from auricular cartilage.   **a**

3 **Antitragohelicine fissure,** "fissura antitragohelicina." Located inferiorly between antitragus and helix, and, higher up, between anthelix and helix.   **a**

4 **Transverse anthelicine groove,** "sulcus anthelicis transverses." Visible from behind and medially; separates triangular and conchal eminences.   **a**

5 **Groove of curs of helix,** "sulcus cruris helicis." Shallow groove on back of auricular cartilage corresponding to anthelix on anterior side.   **a**

6 **Anthelicine fossa,** "fossa anthelicis." Depression on posterior surface or auricular cartilage corresponding to anthelix on anterior side.   **a**

7 **Eminence of concha,** "eminentia conchae." Bulge on posterior surface of auricular cartilage corresponding to cavity of concha.   **a**

8 **Eminence of scapha,** "eminentia scaphae." Curved bulge on posterior surface of auricular cartilage corresponding to scapha on anterior side.   **a**

9 **Eminence of triangular fossa,** "eminentia fossae triangular fossa."   **a**

10 **Auricular ligaments,** "ligg. auricularia." Attach articular cartilage to temporal bone.

11 **Anterior auricular ligament,** "lig. auriculare anterius." Extends from root of zygomatic arch to spine of helix.   **b**

12 **Superior auricular ligament,** "lig. auriculare superius." Runs from superior margin of external acoustic osseous meatus to spine of helix.   **b**

13 **Posterior auricular ligament,** "lig. auriculare posterius." Runs from conchal eminence to mastoid process.   **c**

14 **Auricular muscles,** "mm. auricularii."

15 **Larger muscle of helix,** "m. helicis major." Runs from spine of helix upward to helix.   **b**

16 **Smaller muscle of helix,** "m. helicis minor." Lies on crus of helix.   **b**

17 **Muscle of tragus,** "m. tragicus." Lies vertically on lamina tragi.   **b**

18 **Pyramidal muscle of auricle,** "m. pyramidalis auriculae." M. to spine of helix; occasionally present as an offshoot of m. of tragus.   **b**

19 **Muscle of antitragus,** "m. antitragicus." Fibers on antitragus that continue partly to tail of helix.   **b**

20 **Transverse muscle of auricle,** "m. transversus auricularis." On posterior surface of auricular cartilage between eminences of scapha and concha.   **c**

21 **Oblique muscle of auricle,** "m. obliquus auriculae." Fibers between eminences of concha and triangular fossa.   **c**

22 **Muscle of incisures of helix,** "m. incisurae helicis." Occasionally present caudal continuation of fibers of transverse m. of auricle.   **c**

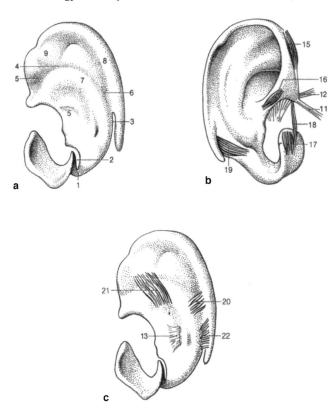

Fig. 1.61a–c (**a**) Auricular cartilage, medial view. (**b**) Auricular cartilage, lateral view. (**c**) Auicular cartilage, medial view.

Pathology of the Pinna and External Auditory Canal

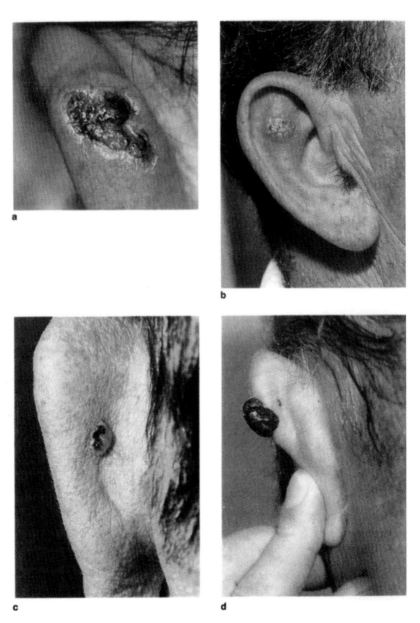

Fig. 1.62a–d   (**a**) Basal cell carcinoma of the left helix seen from behind. (**b**) Squamous cell carcinoma of the upper anthelix. (**c**) Pigmented basal cell carcinoma. (**d**) Nodular melanoma with small cutaneous metastases.

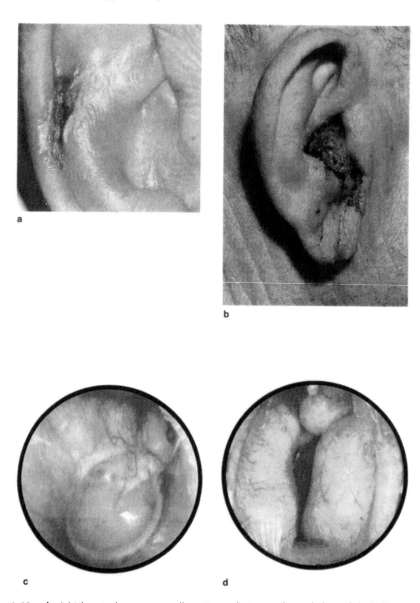

Fig. 1.63a–d (**a**) Ulcerated squamous cell carcinoma between the anthelix and the helix. (**b**) Middle ear carcinoma breaking through into the meatus. (**c**) Normal right tympanic membrane with mild reactive vascular injection. (**d**) Sessile meatal exostosis.

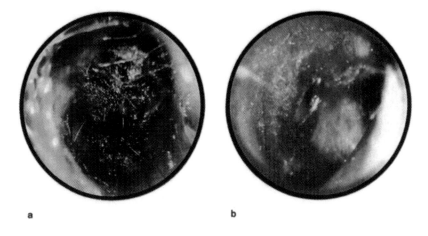

a   b

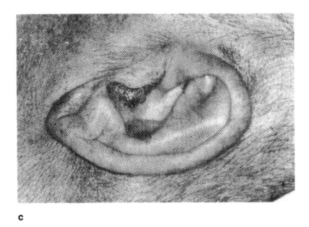

c

Fig. 1.64a–c (**a**) Keratosis obturans. (**b**) Right tympanic membrane perforation after slap to the ear. (**c**) Lateral basal skull fracture with cerebrospinal fluid (CSF) otorrhea: collection of CSF in the left concha (patient reclining).

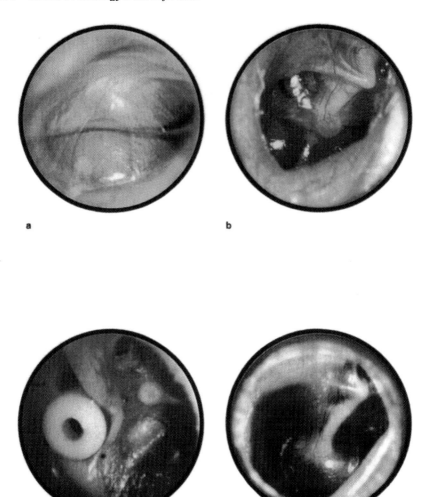

Fig. 1.65a–d (**a**) Serous middle ear effusion with fluid level. (**b**) Mucoid middle ear effusion with markedly retracted tympanic membrane. (**c**) Chronic middle ear effusion: aeration of the middle ear by a grommet. (**d**) Hemorrhagic middle ear effusion on the right with a "blue drum."

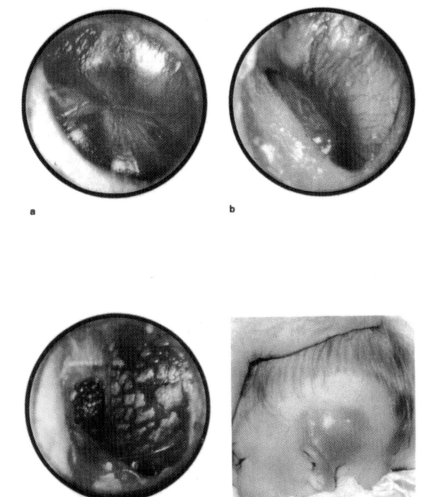

Fig. 1.66a–d (**a**) Early left-sided acute otitis media. (**b**) Left-sided acute otitis media with bulging of the posterosuperior quadrant of the tympanic membrane, and an exudate under pressure in the middle ear. (**c**) Hemorrhagic influenza otitis. (**d**) Mastoiditis with subperiosteal abscess.

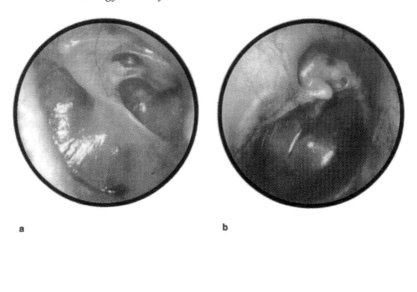

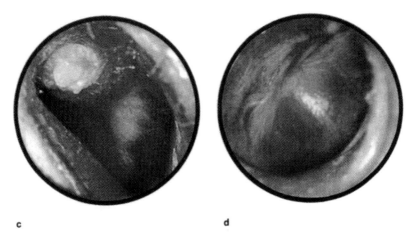

Fig. 1.67a–d (**a**) Retraction pocket in the posterosuperior quadrant with partial skeletonization of the long process of the incus and the head of the stapes (left ear). (**b**) Early cholesteatoma of the pars flaccid with invagination of the pars flaccid, in the presence of an effusion. The pars tensa is retracted. (**c**) Left-sided cholesteatoma of the pars flaccid. (**d**) Glomus tumor of the right arising from the hypotympanum.

2

Physical Acoustics

Table 2.1 Physical measurements of sound

Measurement	Unit	Physical Reference	Formula	Psychological Correlate
Frequency	cps (Hz)			Pitch
Intensity level	dB IL	10^{-16} watt/cm^2 10^{-12} watt/m^2 (SI)	$NdB = 10 \log Iql_r$	Loudness
Sound pressure level	dB SPL	0.0002 dyne/cm^2 20 µPa (SI)	$NdB = 20 \log P_0 P_R$	Loudness
Hearing level	dB HL	ANSI, 2010	$NdB = 20 \log P_0 P_R$	Loudness
Sensation level	dB SL	Hearing threshold of subject	$NdB = 20 \log P_0 P_R$	Loudness
Impedance	Ohm (Z)		$Z = \sqrt{R^2 + \left(2\pi f M \dfrac{S}{2\pi i}\right)^2}$	

Abbreviations: ANSI, American National Standards Institute; cps, cycles per second; dB, decibel; NdB, number decibels; dB IL, decibels intensity level.

Source: Martin, F.N. *Introduction to Audiology,* 4th ed. Needham Heights, MA: Allyn & Bacon, 1991. Reprinted by permission of Pearson Education, Inc., Upper Saddle River, NJ.

Table 2.2 Psychological measurements of sound

Measurement	Unit	Reference	Physical Correlate
Pitch	Mel	1000 mels (1000 Hz at 40 dB SL)	Frequency
Loudness	Sone	1 sone (1000 Hz at 40 dB SL)	Intensity
Loudness level	Phon	0 phon (corresponding to threshold at 1000 Hz)	Intensity
Quality			Spectrum

Source: Martin, F.N. *Introduction to Audiology,* 4th ed. Needham Heights, MA: Allyn & Bacon, 1991. Reprinted by permission of Pearson Education, Inc., Upper Saddle River, NJ.

Table 2.3 Units of acoustic measurement

Measurement	Unit CGS	Unit SI	Abbreviation CGS	Abbreviation SI	Equivalents
Length	Centimeter	Meter	cm	m	1 cm = 0.01 m 1 m = 100 cm
Mass	Gram	Kilogram	g	kg	1 g = 0.001 kg 1 kg = 1000 g
Area	Square centimeter	Square meter	cm^2	m^2	1 cm^2 = 0.0001 m^2 1 m = 10,000 cm^2
Work	Erg	Joule	e	J	1 e = 0.0000001 1 J = 10,000,000 e
Power	Ergs per second	Joules per second	e/sec	J/sec	1 e/sec = 0.0000001 J/sec 1 J/sec = 10,000,000 e/sec
	Watts	Watts	w	w	1 w = 1 J/sec 1 w = 10,000,000 e/sec
Force	Dyne	Newton	dyn	N	1 dyn = 0.00001 N 1 N = 100,000 dyn
Intensity	Watts per square centimeter	Watts per square meter	w/cm^2	w/m^2	1 w/cm^2 = 10,000 w/m^2 1 w/m^2 = 0.0001 w/cm^2
Pressure	Dynes per square centimeter	Newtons[a] per square meter Pascal	dyn/cm^2	N/m^2 Pa	1 dyn/cm^2 = 0.1 Pa 1 Pa = 10 dyn/cm^2 1 Pa = 1 N/m^2
Speed (velocity)	Centimeters per second	Meters per second	cm/sec	m/sec	1 cm/sec = 0.01 m/sec 1 m/sec = 100 cm/sec
Acceleration	Centimeters per square second	Meters per second squared	cm/sec^2	m/sec^2	1 cm/sec^2 = 0.01 m/sec^2 1 m/sec^2 = 100 cm/sec^2

[a]Related to but not strictly on the SI scale.

Source: Martin, F.N. Introduction to Audiology, 4th ed. Needham Heights, MA: Allyn & Bacon, 1991. Reprinted by permission of Pearson Education, Inc., Upper Saddle River, NJ.

Table 2.4   Earphone attenuation values—children

		Frequency (Hz)						
Earphone	*Measure*	*125*	*250*	*500*	*1000*	*2000*	*4000*	*8000*
Supra-aural	Mean	8.6	7.8	8.8	12.0	17.1	25.2	21.8
	SD	6.2	4.9	4.4	5.8	8.0	9.0	7.3
IE/3A	Mean	28.0	28.4	28.9	28.7	32.2	37.2	39.9
	SD	7.4	4.8	4.2	3.6	7.2	6.0	7.9
IE/3B	Mean	31.3	31.3	34.9	34.7	33.5	37.6	38.0
	SD	8.5	7.8	7.7	6.0	6.0	4.0	4.0
IE/3B minus IE/3A		3.3	2.9	6.0	6.0	1.3	0.4	−1.9

Note: Attenuation values (mean and standard deviations) for supra-aural and insert earphones using E-A-RLink 3A(IE/3A) and 3B (IE/3B) (E-A-R Corp., Portland, OR) earphones for children. (The attenuation differences for the IE/3B and IE/3A are shown at the bottom.)

Source: Wright, D.C. and Frank, T. (1992), "Attenuation values for a supra-aural earphone for children and insert earphone for children and adults," *Ear and Hearing*, 13(6): 456. Reprinted by permission.

Table 2.5   Earphone attenuation values—adults

	Frequency (Hz)								
Measure	*125*	*250*	*500*	*1000*	*2000*	*3150*	*4000*	*6300*	*8000*
Mean	28.2	30.0	33.8	35.7	34.8	38.2	37.6	39.1	42.4
SD	6.6	6.0	6.0	5.0	3.8	3.4	4.3	4.2	3.3

Note: Attenuation values (mean and standard deviations) for an insert earphone using E-A-RLink 3B for adults.

Source: Wright, D.C. and Frank, T. (1992), "Attenuation values for a supra-aural earphone for children and insert earphone for children and adults," *Ear and Hearing*, 13(6): 456. Reprinted by permission.

Table 2.6   Mean occlusion effect (in dB) for normal-hearing subjects

Study	Frequency (Hz)				
	250	*500*	*1000*	*2000*	*4000*
Elpern and Naunton (1963)	30.0	20.0	10.0		
Goldstein and Hayes (1965)	12.2	13.1	4.9	0.0	0.0
Hodgson and Tillman (1966)	22.0	19.0	7.0	0.0	0.0
Dirks and Swindeman (1967)	23.7	19.3	7.5	−0.6	0.0
Martin et al (1974)	20.0	15.0	5.0	0.0	0.0
Berger and Kerivian (1983)	20.3	21.6	7.5	−1.3	0.0
Mean	21.3	18.0	6.9	−0.3	0.0
Recommended occlusion effect values		**20.0**	**15.0**	**5.0**	

Source: Roeser, R.J., Valente, M., and Hosford-Dunn, H. (2007), *Audiology Diagnosis,* 2nd ed. New York: Thieme. Reprinted by permission.

Table 2.7   Mean interaural attenuation for insert earphones for pure-tone stimuli between 250 and 6000 hz (in dB)

Frequency Study	*250*	*500*	*1000*	*2000*	*3000*	*4000*	*6000*	*Mean*
Killion et al (1985)	95	85	70	75	80			81
Konig (1962)	95	90	83	75	80	82	70	82
Sklare and Denenberg (1987)	100	94+	81	71	69	77	75+	81+

Source: Roeser, R.J., Valente, M., and Hosford-Dunn, H. (2007), *Audiology Diagnosis,* 2nd ed. New York: Thieme. Reprinted by permission.

Table 2.8 Mean and ranges of interaural attenuation values for pure-tone air conduction signals using standard supra-aural earphones (in dB)

Study	Transducer		Frequency (Hz)								Mean
			250	500	1000	2000	3000	4000	6000	8000	
Chaiklin (1967)	TDH-39	Mean	51	59	69	61	68	70	65	57	62.5
		Range	44–58	54–65	57–66	55–72	56–72	61–85	56–76	51–69	
Coles and Priede (1970)	NR	Mean	61	63	63	63		68			63.6
		Range	50–80	45–80	40–80	45–75		50–85			
Killion et al (1985)	TDH-39	Mean	50	60	60	60	60	65			59.1
		Range	45–65	52–65	52–65	50–68	50–68	52–74			
Liden et al (1959)	NR	Mean	58	60	57	60		61		63	59.2
		Range	45–75	50–70	45–70	45–75		45–75		45–80	
Sklare and Denenberg (1987)	TDH-49	Mean	54	59	62	58	57	65	65		60.0
		Range	45–60	45–75	60–65	45–70	45–70	60–75	50–80		
Zwislocki (1950)	NR	Mean	45	50	55	60	–	65	–	–	55.0
	Overall Mean		55	59	61	60	62	66	65	60	

NR, not reported.
Source: Roeser, R.J., Valente, M., and Hosford-Dunn, H. (2007), *Audiology Diagnosis*, 2nd ed. New York: Thieme. Reprinted by permission.

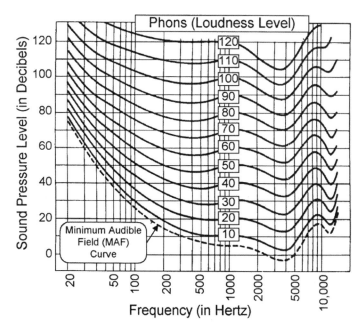

Fig. 2.1 Loudness-level or phon curves. [Based on data by Robinson and Dadson (1956) and ISO (1961).] The loudness level in phons is shown in the box at 1,000 Hz for each contour. The "0 phon line" corresponds to the minimum audibility field (MAF) curve. (From Gelfand, S. (2001), *Essentials of Audiology,* 2nd ed. New York: Thieme. Reprinted by permission.)

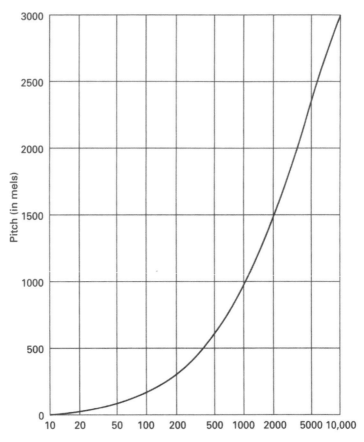

Fig. 2.2 Mel scale: relationship between pitch (in mels) and frequency (in Hz). (From Martin, F.N. *Introduction to Audiology,* 4th ed. Needham Heights, MA: Allyn & Bacon, 1991, page 52. Reprinted by permission.)

Table 2.9 Intensities of different speech sounds produced at conversational levels

Phoneme	Intensity (dB SPL)
C	65
E	61
I	58
1	58
ʃ	56
N	52
T	50
H	48
S	45
Θ	40

Source: Ross, M. and Giolas, T.D. (1978), *Auditory Management of Hearing-Impaired Children,* Austin, TX: PRO-ED. Reprinted by permission.

Table 2.10 Intensity levels of some familiar sounds

Sources (Measured at Operator/listener Distance from Source)	Aural Effect	Sound Level (dB)
Shotgun blast	Human ear pain threshold	140
Jet plane at takeoff		
Firecrackers, exploding		
Rock music (amplified)	Uncomfortably loud	120
Hockey game crowd		
Thunder, severe		
Pneumatic jackhammer		
Powered lawnmower	Extremely loud	100
Tractor, farm type		
Subway train (interior)		
Motorcycle		
Snowmobile		
Cocktail party (100 guests)		
Window air-conditioner	Moderately loud	80
Crowded restaurant		
Diesel-powered truck/tractor		
Singing birds	Quiet	60
Normal conversation		
Rustle of leaves	Very quiet	40
Faucet, dripping		
Light rainfall		
Whisper	Just audible	10

Source: Olishifski, J.B., and Harford, E.R., *Industrial Noise and Hearing Conservation,* 1975, page 2, National Safety Council, 625 North Michigan Ave., Chicago, IL 60611. Reprinted by permission.

Table 2.11   Sound levels generated by different instruments

Instrument	Average Sound Level (dBA)
Bass	80.5[1]
Cello	88.6[1]
Clarinet	85.3[1]
Drum rolls	106[2]
Drum set	93.5–94.6[1]
Flute	88.6–95.5[1]
Horn	90.2–98.6[1]
Marimba	91.3–95[1]
Oboe	88.3–93.5[1]
Piano played at moderate level	60–70[3]
Piano played loudly	92–95[4]
Piccolo	96–112[5]
Piccolo (near right ear)	102–118[5]
Sax	88.2–92[1]
Trombone	92.3–98[1]
Trumpet	97.6–98.5[1]
Tuba	87.9[1]
Viola	84.1–92.9[1]
Violin	85.5–87.8[1]

Data from: [1]Phillips and Mace, 2008; [2]Westmore and Eversden, 1981; [3]Sallows, 2001; [4]Hart, Geltman, Schupbach, and Santucci, 1987; [5]Chasin, 2006.

Source: Rawool, V. (2011), Hearing Conservation: In Occupational, Recreational, Educational, and Home Settings. New York: Thieme. Reprinted by permission.

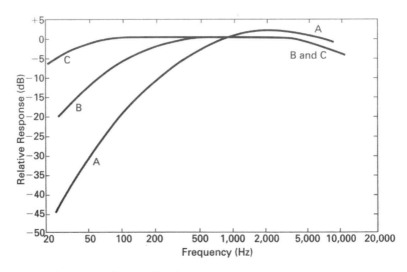

Fig. 2.3   Weighting curves for sound-level meters.

Table 2.12   Absorption coefficients for various materials

Material	Frequency (Hz)					
	125	*250*	*500*	*1000*	*2000*	*4000*
Ceilings						
Plaster or gypsum	0.14	0.10	0.06	0.05	0.04	0.03
Acoustic titles, ⅔ inch (suspended 16 inches from ceiling)	0.25	0.28	0.46	0.71	0.86	0.93
Acoustic titles, ½ inch (suspended 16 inches from ceiling)	0.52	0.37	0.50	0.69	0.79	0.78
Acoustic titles, ½ inch (cemented directly to ceiling)	0.10	0.22	0.61	0.56	0.74	0.72
High-absorbent panels, 1 inch (suspended 16 inches from ceiling)	0.58	0.88	0.75	0.99	1.00	0.96
Walls						
Brick	0.03	0.03	0.03	0.04	0.05	0.07
Concrete painted	0.10	0.05	0.06	0.07	0.09	0.08
Window glass	0.35	0.25	0.18	0.12	0.07	0.04
Marble	0.01	0.01	0.01	0.02	0.02	0.00
Plaster or concrete	0.12	0.09	0.07	0.05	0.05	0.04
Plywood	0.28	0.22	0.17	0.09	0.10	0.11
Concrete block (coarse)	0.36	0.44	0.31	0.29	0.39	0.25
Heavyweight drapery	0.14	0.35	0.55	0.72	0.70	0.65
Fiberglass wall treatment, 1 inch	0.08	0.32	0.99	0.76	0.34	0.12
Fiberglass wall treatment, 7 inches	0.86	0.99	0.99	0.99	0.99	0.99
Wood paneling on fiberglass blanket	0.40	0.99	0.80	0.50	0.40	0.30
Floors						
Wood parquet on concrete	0.04	0.04	0.07	0.60	0.06	0.07
Linoleum	0.02	0.03	0.03	0.03	0.03	0.02
Carpet on concrete	0.02	0.06	0.14	0.37	0.60	0.65
Carpet on foam rubber padding	0.08	0.24	0.57	0.69	0.71	0.73

Source: Valente, M., Hosford-Dunn, H., Roeser, R.J. (2008), *Audiology Treatment,* 2nd ed. New York: Thieme. Reprinted by permission.

Table 2.13 **Recommended unoccupied classroom noise levels to achieve optimum speech recognition for children with normal hearing and with hearing impairment**

Investigator/Year	Unoccupied Noise Level (dB(A))	Population
Niemoeller (1968)	30	Hearing impaired
Gengel (1971)	30	Hearing impaired
Ross (1978)	35	Hearing impaired
Knudsen and Harris (1978)	35	Normal hearing
Borrild (1978)	35	Normal hearing/hearing
	25	impaired
Fourcin et al (1980)	35	Hearing impaired
Bradley (1968)	30	Normal hearing
Finitzo-Hieber (1988)	35	Hearing impaired
Portuguese School Standard	35	Normal hearing/hearing impaired
German Performance/Design Standard (1989)	30	Normal hearing/hearing impaired
Swedish Board of Housing, Building, and Planning (1994)	30	Normal hearing/hearing impaired
Berg (1993)	35–40	Normal hearing
ASHA	30	Normal hearing/hearing impaired
Crandell et al (1995)	30–35	Normal hearing/hearing impaired
Crandell and Smaldino	30–35	Normal hearing/hearing impaired

Source: Adapted from Access Board. (1998). Retrieved from http://www.access-board.gov.

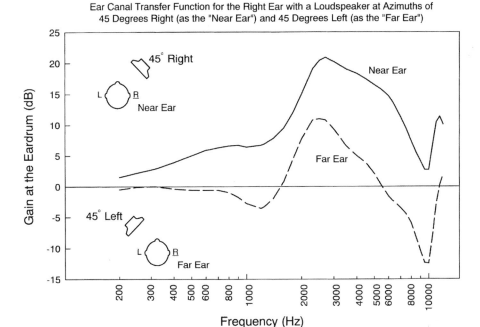

Fig. 2.4 Effect of azimuth: head-related transfer functions at the right ear when the loudspeaker is located at azimuths of 45 degrees to the right (a "near-ear" situation) versus 45 degrees to the left (a "far-ear" situation). (Based on data by Shaw (1974) and Shaw and Vaillancourt (1985).)

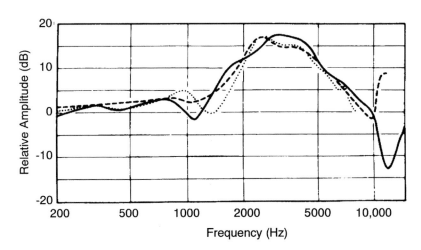

Fig. 2.5 Average head-related transfer functions (sound level at the eardrum compared with outside of the ear) for sounds presented from a loudspeaker directly in front of the subjects. *Dotted line,* data from Wiener and Ross (1946); *dashed line,* data from Shaw (1974); *solid line,* data from Mehrgardt and Mellert (1977). (From Mehrgardt, S. and Mellert, V., Transformation characteristics of the external human ear. J. Acoust. Soc. Am. 61, 1567 (1977). Reprinted by permission.)

Table 2.14 Ratios, logarithms, and outputs for determining number of decibels with intensity and pressure references

A Ratio	B Log	C Intensity outputs CGS (watt/m²)	SI (watt/cm²)	D dB IL[a]	E Equal amplitudes	F dB SPL[b]	G Pressure outputs CGS (dyne/cm²)	SI (µPa)
1:1	0	10^{-16}	10^{-12}	0	Threshold of Audibility	0	.0002	20.0 (2 × 10^1)
10:1	1	10^{-15}	10^{-11}	10		20	.002	200.0 (2 × 10^2)
100:1	2	10^{-14}	10^{-10}	20		40	.02	2,000.0 (2 × 10^3)
1,000:1	3	10^{-13}	10^{-9}	30		60	.2	20,000.0 (2 × 10^4)
10,000:1	4	10^{-12}	10^{-8}	40		80	2.0	200,000.0 (2 × 10^5)
100,000:1	5	10^{-11}	10^{-7}	50		100	20.0	2,000,000.0 (2 × 10^6)
1,000,000:1	6	10^{-10}	10^{-6}	60		120	200.0	20,000,000.0 (2 × 10^7)
10,000,000:1	7	10^{-9}	10^{-5}	70		140	2000.0	200,000,000.0 (2 × 10^8)
100,000,000:1	8	10^{-8}	10^{-4}	80	Threshold of pain			
1,000,000,000:1	9	10^{-7}	10^{-3}	90				
10,000,000,000:1	10	10^{-6}	10^{-2}	100				
100,000,000,000:1	11	10^{-5}	10^{-1}	110				
1,000,000,000,000:1	12	10^{-4}	10^{0}	120				
10,000,000,000,000:1	13	10^{-3}	10^{1}	130				
100,000,000,000,000:1	14	10^{-2}	10^{2}	140				

[a] The number of dB with an intensity reference ($I_R = 10^{-12}$ watt/m²) uses the formula: dB (IL) = 10 × log (I_O/I_R).

[b] The number of dB with a pressure reference ($P_R = 20$ µPa) uses the formula: dB (SPL) = 20 × log (P_O/P_R).

Source: Martin, F.N. Introduction to Audiology, 4th ed. Needham Heights, MA: Allyn & Bacon, 1991, page 30. Reprinted by permission of Pearson Education, Inc., Upper Saddle River, NJ.

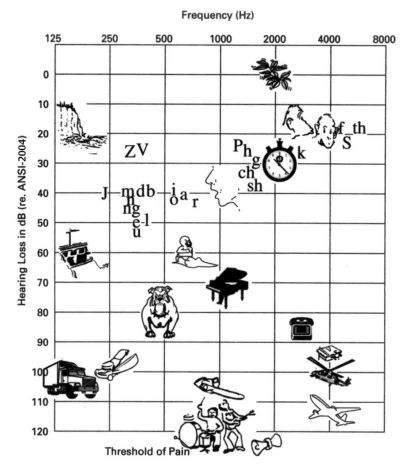

Fig. 2.6 Speech sounds and familiar sounds plotted on a standard audiogram form. Data for hearing loss is from American National Standards Institute, 1989. (From Northern, J. L., and Downs, M. P. (2002), *Hearing in Children*, 5th ed. Philadelphia: Lippincott Williams & Wilkins. Reprinted by permission.)

3

Audiometric Standards

Table 3.1 Minimum required frequencies and maximum hearing levels for pure-tone audiometers

Frequency (Hz)	Maximum Hearing Levels (dB HL)						
	Type 1[†§]		Type 2[†]		Type 3[†]		Type 4[‡]
	Air	Bone	Air	Bone	Air	Bone	Air
125	70	—	60	—	—	—	—
250	90	45	80	45	70	35	—
500	120	60	110	60	100	50	70
750	120	60	—	—	—	—	—
1000	120	70	110	70	100	60	70
1500	120	70	110	70	—	—	—
2000	120	70	110	70	100	60	70
3000	120	70	110	70	100	60	70
4000	120	60	110	60	100	50	70
6000	110	50	100	—	90	—	70
8000	100	—	90	—	80	—	—
Speech	100	60	60	55	—	—	—

[†]Sound field loudspeaker output within 250 to 6000 Hz is within 20 dB of the air tabled values for types 1, 2, and 3 for pure tones, warble tones, or speech.
[‡]Maximum HL is extended to 90 dB HL for type 4 if used for hearing conservation purposes.
[§]Maximum HL may be 10 dB less than tabled values for type 1 using circumaural or insert earphones.

Note: Maximum HL for type HF is 90 dB HL from 8000 to 11,200 Hz and 50 dB HL from 12,000 to 16,000 Hz; minimum HL is –20 dB HL at all frequencies above 8000 Hz.

Abbreviation: HF, high frequency.

Source: ANSI/ASA S3.6–2010 American National Standard Specification for Audiometers. Reprinted by permission.

Table 3.2 Reference equivalent threshold sound pressure levels (RETSPLs) for standard supraaural audiometric earphones expressed as the sound pressure levels (dB SPL in a 6-cc coupler, type NBA-9A) corresponding to 0 dB hearing level (HL)

Frequency (Hz)	125	250	500	750	1000	1500	2000	3000	4000	6000	8000	Speech
TDH-39 earphones	45.0	47.5	11.5	8.0	7.0	6.5	9.0	10.0	9.5	15.5	13.0	19.00
TDH-49 and -50 earphones	25.5	26.5	13.5	8.5	7.5	7.5	11.0	9.5	10.5	13.5	13.0	20.0

Source: Based on ANSI S3.6–2004.

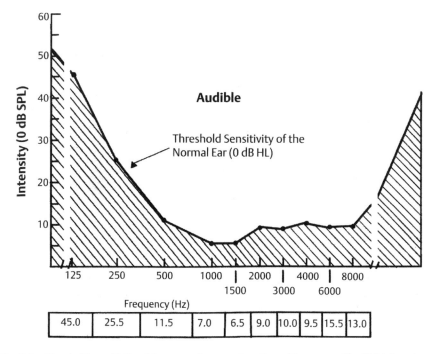

Fig. 3.1 Threshold sensitivity of the normal ear as a function of frequency. The 2004 American National Standards Institute reference equivalent threshold sound pressure levels (RETSPLs) shown at the bottom of the figure are required to reach 0 dB hearing level (HL) for a Telephonic Dynamic Headphones (TDH) 39 supra-aural earphone. (From Roeser, R.J. (2007), *Audiology Diagnosis*, 2nd ed. New York: Thieme. Reprinted by permission.)

Table 3.3 Reference equivalent threshold sound pressure levels (RETSPLs) for insert earphones corresponding to 0 dB hearing level (HL)

Frequency (Hz)	125	250	500	750	1000	1500	2000	3000	4000	6000	8000	Speech
dB SPL in occluded ear simulator	28.0	17.5	9.5	6.0	5.5	9.5	11.5	13.0	15.0	16.0	15.5	18.0
dB SPL in HA-2 coupler	26.0	14.0	5.5	2.0	0.0	2.0	3.0	3.5	5.5	2.0	0.0	12.5

Source: Based on ANSI S3.6–2004 RETSPLs for the HA-1 coupler, and the details about how the insert receiver is attached to the measurement device are provided in the standard.

Table 3.4 Bone-conduction vibrators as reference equivalent threshold force levels (RETFLs) in dB re: 1 μN, when measured on an artificial mastoid (mechanical coupler)

Frequency (Hz)	250	500	750	1000	1500	2000	3000	4000	6000	8000	Speech
Mastoid	67.0	58.0	48.5	42.5	36.5	31.0	30.0	35.5	40.0	40.0	55.0
Forehead	79.0	72.0	61.5	51.0	46.5	42.5	42.0	43.5	51.0	50.0	63.5

Source: Based on ANSI S3.6–2004.

Table 3.5 Minimum audible pressure (MAP) and minimum audible field (MAF): Summary of several investigations

Investigation	Test Conditions	Loudspeaker Azimuth[a]	Threshold Difference (MAP – MAF)	Subjects
Breakey and Davis (1949)	Earphone: unspecified (nonanechoic) field	0	3.4[b]	Normal hearing
Tillman, Johnson, and Olsen (1966)	Earphone: anechoic chamber	45	7.5	Normal hearing and sensorineural hearing loss
Dirks, Stream, and Wilson (1972)	Earphone: anechoic chamber	0	2.8	Young sophisticated listeners; hearing status unspecified
		30	5.6	
		60	7.0	
		90	6.6	
Tillman et al (1973)	Earphone: anechoic chamber	0	3.5	Normal hearing
		45	7.5	
	Earphone: sound-treated test booth	45	4.4	Normal hearing
Stream and Dirks (1974)[c]	Earphone: anechoic chamber	0	2.7[c]	Normal hearing
		30	5.6	
		60	7.1	
		90	6.7	

Breakey, M.R., and Davis, H. (1949), Comparisons of thresholds for speech: Words and sentence tests; receiver vs. field and monaural vs. binaural listening. *Laryngoscope.* 59:236–250.

Dirks, D.D., Stream, R.W., and Wilson, R.H. (1972), Speech audiometry: Earphone and sound field. *J. Speech Hear. Disord.* 37:162–176.

Stream, R.W., and Dirks, D.D. (1974), Effect of loudspeaker position on differences between earphone and free-field thresholds (MAP and MAF). *J. Speech Hear. Res.* 17:549–568.

Tillman, T., Johnson, R., and Olsen, W. (1966), Earphone versus sound field threshold sound pressure levels for spondee words. *J. Acoust. Soc. Am.* 39:125–133.

Tillman, T. W., Olsen, W.O., Killion, M.C., Block, M.G. (1973), MAP versus MAF for spondees: Nothing's really missing. Paper presented at the Convention of the American Speech and Hearing Association, October 12–15, Detroit.

[a] Reported in degrees relative to the midsagittal plane of the listener's head.
[b] Reported in decibels.
[c] Also reported binaural MAP and MAF data.

Source: Konkle, D.F., Rintelmann, W.F. (1983), *Principle of Speech Audiometry.* Austin, TX: PRO-ED. Reprinted by permission.

Table 3.6 One-third octave band maximum permissible ambient noise levels (MPANLs) for three test frequency ranges for ears covered with a supra aural or insert earphone and for ears not covered

Test Frequency Range One-Third Octave Band (Hz)	Ears Covered						Ears Not Covered		
	125–8000 Hz		250–8000 Hz		500–8000 Hz		125–8000 Hz	250–8000 Hz	500–8000 H
	TDH	Insert	TDH	Insert	TDH	Insert			
125	30.0*	54.0	34.0	62.0	44.0	73.0	24.0	30.0	39.0
250	20.0	48.0	20.0	48.0	30.0	59.0	16.0	16.0	25.0
500	16.0	45.0	16.0	45.0	16.0	45.0	11.0	11.0	11.0
800	19.0	44.0	19.0	44.0	19.0	44.0	10.0	10.0	10.0
1000	21.0	42.0	21.0	42.0	21.0	42.0	8.0	8.0	8.0
1600	25.0	43.0	25.0	43.0	25.0	43.0	9.0	9.0	9.0
2000	29.0	44.0	29.0	44.0	29.0	44.0	9.0	9.0	9.0
3150	33.0	46.0	33.0	46.0	33.0	46.0	8.0	8.0	8.0
4000	32.0	45.0	32.0	45.0	32.0	45.0	6.0	6.0	6.0
6300	32.0	48.0	32.0	48.0	32.0	48.0	8.0	8.0	8.0
8000	32.0	51.0	32.0	51.0	32.0	51.0	9.0	9.0	9.0

*Figures given are in decibels.

Note: Octave band MPANLs are 5 dB higher than each tabled level.

Source: ANSI/ASA S3.1–1999 (revised 2008) American National Standard Maximum Permissible Ambient Noise Levels for Audiometric Test Rooms. Reprinted by permission.

Table 3.7 Octave band maximum permissible ambient noise levels specified by Occupational Safety and Health Administration (OSHA) and ANSI S3.1–1999 (revised 2003) for ears covered for the test frequency range 500 to 8000 Hz

Octave Band (Hz)	OSHA (dB)	ANSI (dB)	Differences (dB)
125	—	49.0	—
250	—	35.0	—
500	40.0	21.0	19.0
1000	40.0	26.0	14.0
2000	47.0	34.0	13.0
4000	57.0	37.0	20.0
8000	62.0	37.0	25.0

Source: ANSI/ASA S3.1-1999 (revised 2008) American National Standard Maximum Permissible Ambient Noise Levels for Audiometric Test Rooms. Reprinted by permission.

Table 3.8 Monaural sound field RETSPLs reported in ANSI S3.6–2010, ASHA–1991, and the threshold differences

	Frequency (Hz)											
	125	250	500	750	1000	1500	2000	3000	4000	6000	8000	Speech
Monaural at 0 degree												
ANSI S3.6–2010	22.1	11.4	4.4	2.4	2.4	2.4	-1.3	-5.8	-5.4	-4.3	12.6	14.5
ASHA (1991)	32.0	16.0	9.5	7.5	5.5	4.5	2.5	0.05	1.5	7.5	13.0	16.5
Differences	-9.9	-4.6	-5.1	-5.1	-3.1	-2.1	-3.8	-5.85	-6.9	-11.8	-0.4	-2.0
Monaural at 45 degrees												
ANSI S3.6–2010	21.6	10.4	1.4	-1.1	-1.6	1.1	-4.3	-10.5	-9.4	-3.2	-7.1	12.5
ASHA (1991)	—	20.5	9.0	0.5	0.9	2.0	-0.5	-4.1	-3.1	3.8	—	12.5
Differences	—	-10.1	-7.6	-1.6	-2.5	-0.9	-3.8	-6.4	-6.3	-7.0	—	0.0
Monaural at 90 degrees												
ANSI S3.6–2010	21.1	9.4	-0.1	-2.6	-3.1	-2.6	-3.3	-8.3	-4.9	-5.2	4.1	11.0
ASHA (1991)	32.0	16.0	7.5	—	3.5	2.0	4.0	0.5	1.0	1.5	9.0	15.0
Differences	-10.9	-6.6	-7.6	—	-6.6	-4.6	-7.3	-8.8	-5.9	-6.7	-4.9	-4.0

Abbreviations: ANSI, American National Standards Institute; ASHA, American Speech-Language-Hearing Association; RETSPLs, reference equivalent threshold sound pressure levels.

Table 3.9   Audiometer inspection and listening checks: Example of an evaluation form

Speech and Hearing Clinic, Penn State University, 110 Moore Building, University Park, PA 16802

Audiometer Name/Model No: _____ Serial No: _____ Location: _____

Inspection Checks		Date and Tester Initials (If Inspection and Listening Check Are Okay Check Box; If Not Report Problem Immediately)										
Power Cord												
Earphone Cords												
Insert Earphone Tubing												
Bone Vibrator Cord												
Headband and Cushions												
Controls and Switches												
Listening Checks												
Frequency	Right											
	Left											
Attenuator Linearity	Right											
	Left											
Tone Switch, Hum, Static	Right											
	Left											
Crosstalk	Right											
	Left											
Known Threshold	Right											
	Left											
Acoustic Radiation												

© Tom Frank. Reprinted by permission.

Table 3.10 Calibration for earphone and bone vibrator output levels (ANSI S3.6–2004): Example of an evaluation form

Speech and Hearing Clinic, Penn State University, 110 Moore Building, University Park, PA 16802

Audiometer: _____ Serial No: _____ Channel: _____ Date: _____ Calibrated by: _____

Transducer Type	Frequency in Hertz (Hz)													
	125	250	500	750	1000	1500	2000	3000	4000	6000	8000	Speech
1. Right TDH 49/50, SPL*												
2. Left TDH 49/50, SPL*												
3. RETSPL + 70 dB HL	117.5	96.5	83.5	78.5	77.5	77.5	81.0	79.5	80.5	83.5	83.5	89.5
Rt TDH 49/50, Error (1–3)†												
Lt TDH 49/50, Error (1–3)†												
4. Right ER-3A, SPL‡												
5. Left ER-3A, SPL‡												
6. RETSPL + 70 dB HL	96.0	84.0	75.5	72.0	70.0	72.0	73.0	73.5	75.5	72.0	70.0	82.5
Right ER-3A. Error (4–6)†												
Left ER-3A, Error (4–6)†												
7. Bone Vib, Mastoid, FL§												
8. RETFL		67.0	58.0	48.5	42.5	36.5	31.0	30.0	35.5			
9. Hearing Level Setting		20	50	50	50	50	50	50	50			
Bone Vib, Error (7–(8+9))†												

*One-third octave band SPL in NBS 9A coupler with an HL setting of 70 dB.
†Error equals measured output level minus RETSPL/RETFL plus HL setting; tolerance is ± dB from 125–5000 Hz and ±5 dB at 6000 Hz and above.
‡One-third octave band SPL in HA-2 coupler with rigid tube attachment with a HL setting of 70 dB.
§Force level using B&K 4930 mechanical coupler.
© Tom Frank. Reprinted by permission.

141

Table 3.11 Calibration for attenuator linearity, frequency accuracy, tone switching, and on/off ratio: Example of an evaluation form

Speech and Hearing Clinic, Penn State University, 110 Moore Building, University Park, PA 16802

Audiometer: _____ Serial No.: _____ Channel: ____ Date: _____ Cal. by: _____

Attenuator Linearity				Frequency Accuracy				Tone Switching	
HL	*Output*	*Error**		*Freq.*	*Measured*	*Error†*		*Rise/Fall‡*	*Overshoot§*
120				125				/	
115				250				/	
110				500				/	
105				750				/	
100				1000				/	
95				1500				/	
90				2000				/	
85				3000				/	
80				4000				/	
75				6000				/	
70				8000				/	
65									

			On/Off Ratio‖			
60				*SA Phones TDH* _____		*Insert Phones* _____	
55			*Freq.*	*Right*	*Left*	*Right*	*Left*
50			125				
45			250				
40			500				
35			750				
30			1000				
25			1500				
20			2000				
15			3000				
10			4000				
5			6000				
0			8000				
Total							

*Error between 5-dB intervals is ≤1 dB, total error is ±2 dB from 125 to 5000 Hz and ±5 dB at 6000 Hz and above.

†Error is ±1% for type 1, ±2% for type 2, ±3% for types 3 to 5 of indicated frequency.

‡Error is <20 or >200 milliseconds.

§Error is >+1 dB.

‖SPL output with tone switch off must be ≥70 dB than with tone switch on.

© Tom Frank. Reprinted by permission.

Table 3.12 **American National Standards Institute (ANSI), International Organization for Standardization (ISO), and International Electrotechnical Commission (IEC) standards used for the calibration of audiometers and acoustic immittance instruments and other standards having application to audiology**

The following ANSI standards can be purchased from the Standards Secretariat, Acoustical Society of America, 35 Pinelawn Road, Suite 114E, Melville, NY 11747, or via the Internet (http://asastore.aip.org). ANSI standards referenced in this chapter are designated by an asterisk. The year in parentheses is the revision year.

S1.1–1994 (R2004) Acoustical Terminology
*S1.4–1983 (R2001) Specification for Sound Level Meters
S1.9–1996 (R2001) Instruments for the Measurement of Sound Intensity
*S1.11–2004 Specification for Octave-Band and Fractional-Octave-Band Analog and Digital Filters
S1.13–2005 Measurement of Sound Pressure Levels in Air
*S1.40–1984 (R2001) Specification for Acoustic Calibrators
S1.42–2001 Design Response of Weighting Networks for Acoustical Measurements
S1.43–1997 (R2002) Specifications for Integrating-Averaging Sound Level Meters
*S3.1–1999 (R2003) Maximum Permissible Ambient Noise Levels for Audiometric Test Rooms
S3.2–1989 (R1999) Method for Measuring the Intelligibility of Speech Over Communication Systems
S3.4–2005 Procedure for the Computation of Loudness of Noise
S3.5–1997 (R2002) Methods for Calculation of Speech Intelligibility Index
*S3.6–2004 Specification for Audiometers
*S3.7–1995 (R2003) Method for Coupler Calibration of Earphones
*S3.13–1987 (R2002) Mechanical Coupler for Measurement of Bone Vibrators
S3.20–1995 (R2003) Bioacoustical Terminology
S3.21–2004 Method of Manual Pure-Tone Threshold Audiometry
*S3.25–1989 (R2003) Occluded Ear Simulator
*S3.39–1987 (R2002) Specifications for Instruments to Measure Aural Acoustic Impedance and Admittance (Aural Acoustic Immittance)
The following ISO standards can be purchased from the Central Secretariat, International Organization for Standardization (ISO), 1 rue de Varembe, Case Postale 56, CH-1211 Geneva 20, Switzerland, or via the Internet (http://asastore.aip.org/shop.do?cID=11). ISO standards referenced in this chapter are designated by an asterisk.
ISO 389–1:1998 Acoustics—Reference zero for the calibration of audiometric equipment. Part 1: Reference equivalent threshold sound pressure levels for pure tones and supra-aural earphones
*ISO 389–2:1994 Acoustics—Reference zero for the calibration of audiometric equipment. Part 2: Reference equivalent threshold sound pressure levels for pure tones and insert earphones
*ISO 389–3:1994 Acoustics—Reference zero for the calibration of audiometric equipment. Part 3: Reference equivalent threshold force levels for pure tones and bone vibrators
*ISO 389–4:1994 Acoustics—Reference zero for the calibration of audiometric equipment. Part 4: Reference levels for narrow band masking noise
ISO/TR 389–5:1998 Acoustics—Reference zero for the calibration of audiometric equipment. Part 5: Reference equivalent threshold sound pressure levels for pure tones in the frequency range 8 kHz to 16 kHz
*ISO 389–7:1996 Acoustics—Reference zero for the calibration of audiometric equipment. Part 7: Reference threshold of hearing under free-field and diffuse-field listening conditions

(continued on next page)

Table 3.12 *(Continued)*

ISO 389–8:2004 Acoustics—Reference zero for the calibration of audiometric equipment. Part 8: Reference equivalent threshold sound pressure levels for pure tones and circum-aural earphones

The following IEC standards can be purchased from the International Electrotechnical Commission (IEC) Central Office, 1 rue de Varembe, CP-131 Geneva 20, Switzerland, or via the Internet (http://www.iec.ch/searchpub/cur_fut.htm (key word: electroacoustics)). IEC standards referenced in this chapter are designated by an asterisk.

IEC 60318–1 (1998–07) Electroacoustics—Simulators of human head and ear. Part 1: Ear simulator for the calibration of supra-aural earphones

*IEC 60318–2 (1998–08) Electroacoustics—Simulators of human head and ear. Part 2: An interim acoustic coupler for the calibration of audiometric earphones in the extended high-frequency range

*IEC 60318–3 (1998–08) Electroacoustics—Simulators of human head and ear. Part 3: Acoustic coupler for the calibration of supra-aural earphones used in audiometry

*IEC 60373 (1990–01) Mechanical coupler for measurements on bone vibrators

IEC 60645 (2001–06) Electroacoustics—Audiological equipment. Part 1: Pure-tone audiometers

*IEC 60645 (2004–11) Electroacoustics—Audiological equipment. Part 5: Instruments for the measurement of aural acoustic impedance/admittance

*IEC 60711 (1981–01) Occluded-ear simulator for the measurement of earphones coupled to the ear by ear inserts

Table 3.13 Standards for classroom acoustics

American Academy of Audiology. (2008) *Remote Microphone Hearing Assistance Technologies for Children and Youth from Birth to 21 Years.* www.audiology.org/resources/documentlibrary/documents/hatguideline.pdf

American National Standards Institute. (2002) *Acoustical Performance Criteria, Design Requirements, and Guidelines for Schools* (ANSI/ASA S12.6–2002). New York: American National Standards Institute.

American National Standards Institute. (2009) *American National Standard Acoustical Performance Criteria, Design Requirements, and Guidelines for Schools, Part 2: Relocatable Classroom Factors* (ANSI/ASA S12.60–2009). New York: American National Standards Institute

American National Standards Institute. (2010) *American National Standard Acoustical Performance Criteria, Design Requirements, and Guidelines for Schools, Part 1: Permanent Schools* (ANSI/ASA S12.60–2010). New York: American National Standards Institute

American Speech-Language-Hearing Association Working Group on Classroom Acoustics. (2005) *Guidelines for Addressing Acoustics in Educational Settings.* Asha.org/docs/html/gl2005–00023.html#sec1.1.

Eargle J. (2003) *Loudspeaker Handbook.* New York. Springer

4

Audiological Procedures/Materials

General

Table 4.1 Objectives of audiological assessment

Audiological assessment for children from birth to 5 years of age is designed to serve the following purposes:
- to determine the status of the auditory mechanism
- to identify the type, degree, and configuration of hearing loss for each ear
- to characterize associated disability and potentially handicapping conditions
- to access the ability to use auditory information in a meaningful way
- to identify individual risk factors and the need for surveillance of late-onset or progressive hearing loss
- to access candidacy for sensory devices
- to refer for additional evaluation and intervention services when indicated
- to provide culturally and linguistically sensitive counseling for families/caregivers
- to communicate findings and recommendations, with parental consent, to other professionals
- to consider the need for additional assessments and/or screenings (i.e., speech-language, cognitive, behavioral)

Source: American Speech-Language-Hearing Association. (2004). Guidelines for the audiologic assessment of children from birth to 5 years of age. http://www.asha.org/members/deskref-journals/deskref/default. Reprinted by permission.

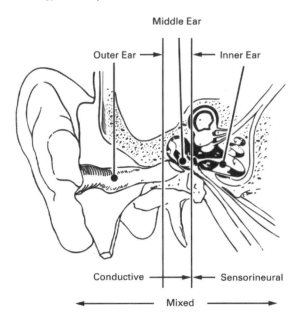

Fig. 4.1 Classification of hearing loss type by anatomic site. (From Roeser, R.J. In: Roeser, R.J. and Downs, M.P. (1994), *Auditory Disorders in School Children*, 3rd ed., page 31. New York: Thieme. Reprinted by permission.)

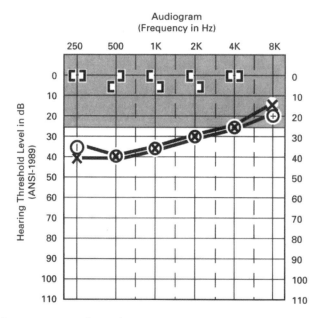

Fig. 4.2 Audiogram type—conductive hearing loss. (From Roeser, R.J. In: Roeser, R.J. and Downs, M.P. (1994), *Auditory Disorders in School Children*, 3rd ed., page 31. New York: Thieme. Reprinted by permission.)

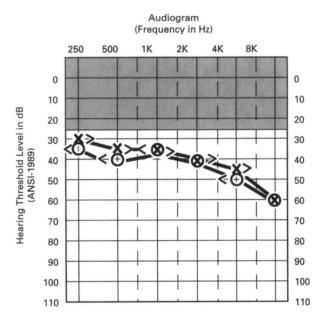

Fig. 4.3   Audiogram type—sensorineural hearing loss. (From Roeser, R.J. In: Roeser, R.J. and Downs, M.P. (1994), *Auditory Disorders in School Children*, 3rd ed., page 32. New York: Thieme. Reprinted by permission.)

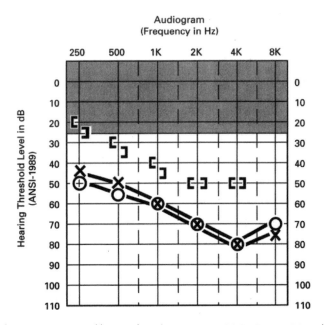

Fig. 4.4   Audiogram type—mixed hearing loss. (From Roeser, R.J. In: Roeser, R.J. and Downs, M.P. (1994), *Auditory Disorders in School Children*, 3rd ed., page 32. New York: Thieme. Reprinted by permission.)

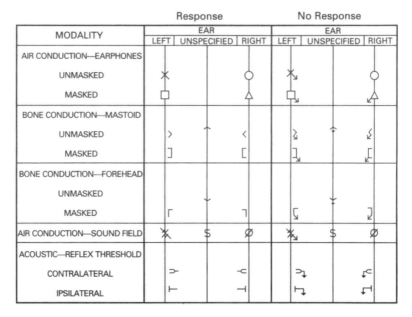

Fig. 4.5 Audiometric symbols. The symbols recommended in this guideline were taken directly from those specified in appropriate standards (ANSI S3.21–1978, R-1986; ANSI S3.39–1987), with two exceptions. (Color coding might still be considered if it is felt that it would further clarify results.) (From American Speech and Hearing Association, Committee on Audiometric Evaluation. Guidelines for audiometric symbols. *Asha* 1990;32(Suppl):25–30. Reprinted by permission.)

Table 4.2 Masking guidelines

A. PURE-TONE AIR-CONDUCTION TESTING
   I. When to mask:
      Basic rule—Use masking when the air-conduction threshold of the test ear exceeds the bone-conduction threshold of the nontest ear by 40 dB or more.
      Corollary—Because bone-conduction thresholds will not significantly exceed air-conduction thresholds, it follows that masking is needed when the air-conduction threshold of the test ear exceeds the air-conduction of the nontest ear by 40 dB or more.
   II. How to mask:
      Basic rule—When the need for masking is indicated, introduce masking noise into the nontest (masked) ear at an effective level 10 to 15 dB above its air-conduction threshold. It is necessary to find a plateau.
B. PURE-TONE BONE-CONDUCTION TESTING
   I. When to mask:
      Basic rule—Use masking when the air-conduction threshold of the test ear and the bone-conduction threshold of the same ear differ by more than 10 dB. That is, mask when there is an air–bone gap of more than 10 dB.

Table 4.2 (*Continued*)

II. How to mask:

Basic rule—When the need for masking is indicated, introduce masking noise into the nontest ear via air conduction. The initial effective level should equal the air-conduction threshold of this ear plus 10 to 15 dB plus the occlusion effect[a] for the frequency being tested when the nontest ear is normal or has a sensorineural hearing loss. It is necessary to find a plateau.

C. SPEECH RECOGNITION THRESHOLD TESTING

I. When to mask:

Basic rule—Use masking when the speech recognition threshold of the test ear exceeds the best bone-conduction threshold in the speech range (500, 1,000 and 2,000 Hz) in the nontest ear by 45 dB or more.

Corollary—Because bone-conduction thresholds will not significantly exceed air-conduction thresholds, it follows that masking is needed when the speech recognition threshold in the test ear exceeds the speech recognition threshold of the nontest ear by 45 dB or more.

II. How to mask:

Effective masking for the speech recognition threshold, when indicated, equals the presentation level of the signal in the test ear minus 35 dB plus the average air-bone gap in the speech frequencies of the nontest (masked) ear if one exists. It is necessary to find a plateau.

D. WORD/SPEECH RECOGNITION TESTING

I. When to mask:

Basic rule—Use masking when the presentation level of the signal in the test ear exceeds the best bone-conduction threshold in the speech range (500, 1,000, and 2,000 Hz) in the nontest ear by 35 dB or more.

Corollary—Because bone-conduction thresholds will not significantly exceed air-conduction thresholds, it follows that masking is needed when the presentation level of the signal in the test ear exceeds the speech recognition threshold of the nontest ear by 35 dB or more.

II. How to mask:

Effective masking for word/speech recognition testing, when indicated, equals the presentation level of the signal in the test ear minus 25 dB plus the average air-bone gap in the speech frequencies in the nontest (masked) ear if one exists. Since testing is at a fixed intensity, it is not necessary to change the level of masking.

Note: For additional information see Goldstein, B.A., and Newman, C.W., Clinical masking: a decision-making process. In Katz, J. (ed.), *Handbook of Clinical Audiology,* 4th ed., Baltimore: Williams & Wilkins, 1994.

[a]The occlusion effect is 20–30 dB at 250 Hz, 15–20 dB at 500 Hz, and 5–10 dB at 1,000 Hz.

Source: Roeser, R.J., Valente, M., and Hosford-Dunn, H (2007), *Audiology Diagnosis,* 2nd ed. New York: Thieme. Reprinted by permission.

Table 4.3 Summary of masking rules

| Test | When Should Masking Be Done? | | How Much Masking Is Needed? | |
	Supra-Aural Earphones	Insert Earphones	Supra-Aural Earphones	Insert Earphones
Pure-Tone AC	When the AC threshold of the TE exceeds the threshold of the NTE BC by 40 dB or more	When the AC threshold of the TE exceeds the threshold of the NTE BC by 50 dB or more	Threshold of the NTE + CF + the safety factor (10 to 15 dB)	Threshold of the NTE + CF + the safety factor (10 to 15 dB)
Pure-Tone BC	When the AC and BC thresholds differ by more than 10 dB in the same ear	When the AC and BC thresholds differ by more than 10 dB in the same ear	Threshold of the NTE + CF + the safety factor (10 to 15 dB) + occlusion effect if needed	Threshold of the NTE + CF + the safety factor (10 to 15 dB) + occlusion effect if needed
SRT	When the PL in the TE exceeds the best BC thresholds in the speech frequencies in the NTE by 45 dB or more	When the PL in the TE exceeds the best BC thresholds in the speech frequencies in the NTE by 55 dB or more	PL in the TE minus 35 dB + the average ABG in the speech frequencies	PL in the TE minus 45 dB + the averages ABG in the speech frequencies
WRS	When the PL in the TE exceeds the best BC thresholds in the speech frequencies in the NTE by 35 dB or more	When the PL in the TE exceeds the best BC thresholds in the speech frequencies in the NTE by 45 dB or more	PL in the TE minus 25 dB + the average ABG in the speech frequencies	PL in the TE minus 35 dB + the average ABG in the speech frequencies

Abbreviations: ABG, air–bone gap; AC, air conduction; BC, bone conduction; CF, carrier frequency; NTE, nontest ear; PL, presentation level; SRT, speech-reception threshold; TE, test ear; WRS, word/speech recognition score.

Source: Roeser, R.J. and Clark, J. Clinical masking. In: Roeser, R.J., Valente, M., and Hosford-Dunn, H. (eds.) (2007), *Audiology Diagnosis*, 2nd ed., pp. 261–287. New York: Thieme. Reprinted by permission.

Table 4.4   Central masking effect for pure-tone air-conduction and bone-conduction stimuli between 500 and 4,000 Hz presented at 20 to 80 dB HL

	Pure-Tone Air Conduction				Pure-Tone (Mastoid) Bone Conduction			
dB	*500*	*1,000*	*4,000*	*Mean*	*500*	*1,000*	*4,000*	*Mean*
20	0.2	1.2	0.6	0.7	0.5	0.9	0.6	0.7
40	1.8	3.0	2.2	2.3	2.9	4.5	1.6	3.0
60	3.6	4.5	3.1	3.7	5.0	5.9	2.1	4.3
80	7.2	8.8	6.2	7.4	7.8	10.6	7.3	8.6
Mean				3.5				4.2

Abbreviation: HL, hearing level.
Source: Dirks, D. and Malmquist, C. (1964). Changes in bone conducted thresholds produced by masking in the non-test ear. Journal of Speech and Hearing Research, 50, 271–278. Reprinted by permission of ASHA.

Table 4.5   Communication difficulty as a function of degree of hearing loss

Level of Hearing Loss Based on Better Ear Pure-Tone Average (500, 1,000, 2,000 Hz)	Degree of Hearing Loss	Effects of Hearing Loss
26 to 40	Mild	Child has difficulty understanding soft-spoken speech; needs preferential seating and may benefit from speech-reading training; good candidate for a hearing aid.
41 to 55	Moderate	Child demonstrates an understanding of speech at 3 to 5 feet; requires amplification, preferential seating, speech-reading training, and speech therapy.
56 to 70	Moderate to severe	Speech must be loud for auditory reception; child has difficulty in group and classroom discussion; may require special classes for hearing impaired, plus all of the above needs.
71 to 90	Severe	Loud speech may be understood at 1 foot from ear; child may distinguish vowels but not consonants; requires classroom for hearing impaired and mainstreaming at a later date.
91+	Profound	Child does not rely on audition as primary modality for communication; may work well with total communication approach; may eventually be mainstreamed at higher grade levels.

Source: Goodman, A. (1965), Reference zero levels for pure tone audiometers, *Asha* 7:262–263. Reprinted by permission.

Table 4.6   A plethora of hearing loss labels (hearing level in dB; ANSI–1969)

	Davis (1970)	Goodman (1965)	Northern and Downs (1978)	O'Neill and Oyer (1973)	Rintelmann and Bess (1977)	Sweitzer (1977) Children	Sweitzer (1977) Adults
Slight	25–40			27–40			
Mild	40–55	27–40	15–30		25–40	21–35	27–40
Moderate		41–55	31–50	41–55	40–65	36–55	41–55
Moderately severe		56–70				56–70	56–70
Marked	55–70			56–70			
Severe	70–90	71–90	51–80	71–90	65–95	71–90	71–90
Profound		91+	81–100		95+	91+	91+
Extreme	90+			91+			
Anacusis (or total hearing loss)			101+				

Source: Clark, J.G. *Audiology for the School Speech-Language Clinician.* Springfield, IL: Charles C. Thomas, 1980. Reprinted by permission.

4 Audiological Procedures/Materials • 153

Term	Description	Audiometric Configuration
Flat	There is little or no change in thresholds (+ or − 20 dB) across frequencies	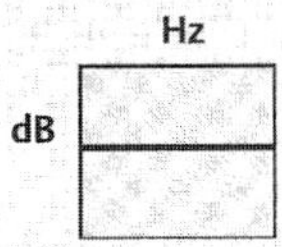
Sloping	As frequency increases, the degree of hearing loss increases	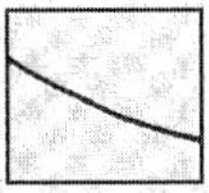
Rising	As frequency increases, the degree of hearing loss decreases	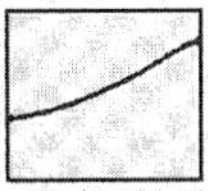
Precipitous	There is a very sharp increase in the hearing loss between octaves	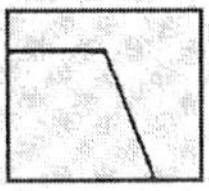
Scoop or trough shape	The greatest hearing loss is present in the midfrequencies, and hearing sensitivity is better in the low and high frequencies	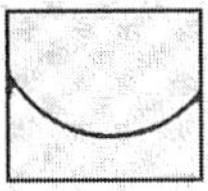
Inverted scoop or trough shape	The greatest hearing loss is in the low and high frequencies, and hearing sensitivity is better in the midfrequencies	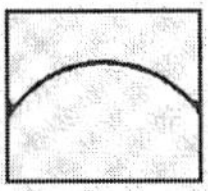
High frequency	The hearing loss is limited to the frequencies above the speech range (2000–3000 Hz)	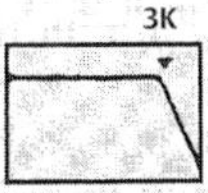
Fragmentary	Thresholds are recorded only for low frequencies, and they are in the severe-to-profound range	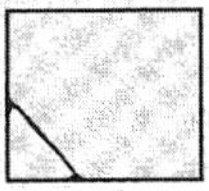
4000 to 6000 Hz notch	Hearing is within normal limits through 3000 Hz, and there is a sharp drop in the 4000 to 6000 Hz range, with improved thresholds at 8000 Hz	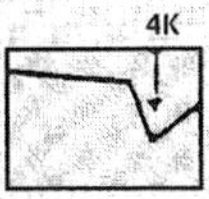

Fig. 4.6 Common terms used to describe pure-tone audiograms. (From Roeser, R.J., Valente, M., Hosford-Dunn, H. (2007), *Audiology Diagnosis,* 2nd ed. New York: Thieme. Reprinted by permission.)

Duele

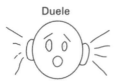

Fig. 4.7 Pictorial representations for assessing loudness levels: Uncomfortably Loud (Duele), Too Strong (Muy Fuerte), a Little Strong (un Poco Fuerte, Is Comfortable (Es Correcto), and Too Soft (Muy Suave).

Muy Fuerte

Un Poco Fuerte

Es Correcto

Muy Suave

Table 4.7 Description of hearing loss by degree of loss

Average threshold level (dB)[a]	Suggested description
−10 to 15[b]	Normal hearing
16 to 25[b]	Slight hearing loss
26 to 40	Mild hearing loss
41 to 55	Moderate hearing loss
56 to 70	Moderately severe hearing loss
71 to 90	Severe hearing loss
91 +	Profound hearing loss

[a]Average threshold level (ANSI–1989) for 0.5,1, and 2 kHz.
[b]Modified by Clark (1981); Goodman recommended normal hearing from −10 to 25 dB.
Sources: Roeser, R.J. In: Roeser, R.J. and Downs, M.P. (1994), *Auditory Disorders in School Children*, 3rd ed. New York: Thieme. Reprinted by permission. Modified from Goodman, A. (1965), Reference zero levels for pure-tone audiometer. *Asha* 7:262–263.

Table 4.8 Summary of tuning-fork tests

Test	Purpose	Placement of Fork	Normal Hearing	Conductive Loss	Sensorineural Loss
Schwabach	Compare patient's BC to normal	Mastoid process	Normal Schwabach: patient hears tone for as long as examiner	Normal or prolonged Schwabach: patient hears tone as long as, or longer, than examiner	Diminished Schwabach: patient hears tone for shorter time than examiner
Rinne	Compare patient's AC to BC	Alternately mastoid process and at ear opening	Positive Rinne: louder at ear	Negative Rinne: louder behind ear	Positive Rinne: louder at ear
Bing	Determine presence or absence of occlusion effect	Mastoid process	Positive Bing: tone sounds louder with ear opening occluded	Negative Bing: tone does not sound louder with ear opening occluded	Positive Bing: tone sounds louder with ear opening occluded
Weber	Determine conductive versus sensorineural loss (in unilateral losses)	Midline of head	Tone heard equally in both ears	Tone louder in poorer ear	Tone louder in better ear

Abbreviations: AC, air conduction; BC, bone conduction.

Source: Martin, F.N., *Introduction to Audiology*, 4th ed. Needham Heights, MA: Allyn & Bacon, 1991. Reprinted by permission of Pearson Educations, Inc., Upper Saddle River, NJ.

Table 4.9   Tests for pseudohypoacusis

Procedure	Hearing Loss for Test Is Applicable	Type of Test
Basic audiometry	Unilateral/bilateral	Qualitative
Test–retest threshold reliability	Unilateral/bilateral	Qualitative
SRT/PTA agreement	Unilateral/bilateral	Qualitative
Speech threshold/PTA agreement	Unilateral	Qualitative
Failure to demonstrate shadow curve		
Tests for pseudohypoacusis		
Stenger (minimum contralateral interference level) test	Unilateral	Quantitative
Doerfler-Stewart test*	Unilateral/bilateral	Qualitative
Lombard reflex*	Unilateral/bilateral	Qualitative
Delayed auditory feedback*	Unilateral/bilateral	Qualitative
Swinging story/varying intensity story test (VIST)	Unilateral/bilateral	Qualitative
Immittance measures	Unilateral/bilateral	Quantitative
Otoacoustic emissions	Unilateral/bilateral	Quantitative
Auditory evoked potentials		
Electrocochleography	Unilateral/bilateral	Quantitative
ABR	Unilateral/bilateral	Quantitative
Middle latency response	Unilateral/bilateral	Quantitative
Late latency response	Unilateral/bilateral	Quantitative

*Historical tests not routinely used in daily audiological practice.

Abbreviations: ABR, auditory brainstem response; PTA, pure-tone average; SRT, speech recognition threshold.

Source: Adapted from *Diagnostic Audiology* (p. 43), by R. J. Roeser, 1986, Austin, TX: PRO-ED. Copyright 1986 by PRO-ED, Inc. Adapted by permission.

Table 4.10   Causes of audiometric changes

The following factors have been demonstrated to influence audiometric measurements. Not all of these factors are of concern in the industrial hearing conservation program. The list is presented to illustrate the potential complexity of audiometry.

Physical variables
  Improper placement of earphones
  Ambient noise levels in test room
  Equipment variables, such as accuracy of attenuator steps, type of earphone cushions, hum, noise, etc.
Physiological variables
  Age and sex
  Pathology of the auditory organs
  General health of subject
  Temporary threshold shift
  Tinnitus and other head noises
Psychological variables
  Motivation of subject
  Momentary fluctuations of attention
  Attitude toward the test situation
  Personality attributes
  Intellectual factors
  Comprehension of instructions
  Experience in test taking of any sort
  Response conditions
  Type of response required of subject, e.g., button pressing, finger raising, verbal response, etc.
Methodological variables
  Testing technique used
  Time interval between successive tests
  Instructions to subjects
  Order of presentation of frequencies

Source: Adapted from *Guide for Conservation of Hearing in Noise*, published by the Committee on Conservation of Hearing of the American Academy of Ophthalmology and Otolaryngology.

Table 4.11   Guidelines for hearing screening from birth through 65+ years

Age	Test Type	Opportunity to Screen	Referral Criteria
Birth to 4	OAE screen[1] ABR screen	• All newborns not screened in hospital • Any child who presents with Parental concern Speech delay Language delay Behavioral problems Social problems School performance problems	• Those with high-risk criteria[1] not already screened • Those with failing OAE or ABR screen • Those with 3 months of continuous bilateral otitis media with effusion
4 to 18	Audiometric screen at 20 HL at 1,000, 2,000, and 4,000 Hz[2]	• School hearing screening • Any child who presents with Parental concern Speech delay Language delay Behavioral problems Social problems School performance problems Excessive noise exposure	• Rescreen those who fail at any frequency in either ear immediately • Rescreen those who fail within 1 to 2 weeks • Refer those who fail screen upon second visit
18 to 65	Audiometric screen at 25 dB HL at 500, 1,000, 2,000, and 4,000 Hz	• Periodic health assessment • Parent/family complaint • Poor or declining socialization of work habits • Excessive noise exposure	• Rescreen those who fail at any frequency in either ear immediately • Rescreen those who fail within 1 to 2 weeks • Refer those who fail screen upon second visit
65+	Audiometric screen at 25 dB or 40 dB HL at 500, 1,000, 2,000, and 4,000 Hz (audioscope); Hearing Handicap Index	• Periodic health assessment • Parent/family complaint • Poor or declining socialization of work habits • Excessive noise exposure • Note that OSHA necessitates threshold testing (not screening)	• Counsel those failing 25 dB screen that they have a problem • Refer those failing 40 dB screen at any frequency except 4,000 Hz • Refer those failing Hearing Handicap Index

Abbreviations: ABR, auditory brainstem response; HL, hearing level; OAE, otoacoustic emissions; OSHA, Occupational Safety and Health Administration.

[1] Joint Committee on Infant Hearing. (1991). 1990 position statement. ASHA Supplementum, 5, 3–6
[2] American Speech-Language-Hearing Association, Panel on Audiologic Assessment. (1996). Guidelines for audiologic screening. Rockville, MD: Author.

Table 4.12   Summary of the major components of hearing impairment screening protocols throughout the age range recommended by ASHA (1997) guidelines

Population (Testing Method)	Frequencies Tested (Hz)	Screening Level (dB HL)	Pass Criteria
Newborn–6 months			ABR at ≤ 35 dB nHL, or TEOAE or DPOAE, in both ears
7 months–2 years (Visual Reinforcement Audiometry)		30	Respond at all frequencies in both ears
7 months–2 years (Conditioned Play Audiometry)	1,000, 2,000, and 4,000	20	
3–5 years (Conditioned Play Audiometry)		20	Respond to at least two of three presentations at all frequencies in both ears
5–18 years		20	Respond at all frequencies in both ears
Adults		25	

Abbreviations: ABR, auditory brainstem response; DPOAE, distortion product otoacoustic emissions; nHL, normalized hearing level; TEOAE, transient evoked otoacoustic emissions.
Source: Gelfand, S.A. (2001), *Essentials of Audiology,* 2nd ed. New York: Thieme. Reprinted by permission.

Table 4.13 Calculation of sensitivity, specificity, predictive value, and efficiency

Test Outcome	Retrocochlear Site (Retrocochlear Disorder Present)	Cochlear Site (Cochlear Disorder Present)	Total
Positive for retrocochlear disorder	A True positive (hit rate)	B False positive (miss rate)	Number positive (A + B)
Negative for retrocochlear disorder	C False negative (false alarm)	D True negative (correct negative)	Number negative (C + D)
Total	Number with retrocochlear disorder (A + C)	Number with cochlear disorder (B + D)	Total
	Sensitivity	= True positive (A)/ Total number with retrocochlear disorder (A + C)	
	Specificity	= True negative (D)/ Total number with cochlear disorder (B + D)	
	Predictive value (positive result)	= True positive (A)/ Total number positive (A + B)	
	Predictive value (negative result)	= True negative (D)/ Total number negative (C + D)	
	Efficiency	= True positive + true negative/ Total number of patients (A + B + C + D)	

1. *Sensitivity.* The sensitivity of a test is its accuracy in correctly identifying disordered subjects; in the case of audiological tests, sensitivity is the ability to identify a retrocochlear disorder. Sensitivity is calculated by dividing the true-positive results by the total number of patients.
2. *Specificity.* The specificity of a test is its accuracy in correctly rejecting patients without retrocochlear disorder; that is, these patients would be classified as having a cochlear site of lesion. Specificity is calculated by dividing true-negative results by the total number of patients.
   Sensitivity and specificity are generally related inversely. As one increases, the other decreases.
3. *Predictive value.* The predictive value (PV) of a test is related to the number of false-negative results and the number of false-positive results. PV is influenced by the prevalence of the disorder. The PV+ is calculated by dividing the true-positive findings by the total number of positive tests, whereas PV– is calculated by dividing the true-negative findings by the total number of negative tests.
4. *Efficiency.* Efficiency specifies a test's overall accuracy. Efficiency is calculated by dividing the true-positive plus the true-negative findings by the total number of patients.

Table 4.14 Summary of etiologies resulting in unilateral hearing loss

Study	No. of Patients	Pathology	Percentage
Kinney (1953)	310	Meningitis Measles Mumps	
Tieri et al (1988)	280	Mumps	23
Everberg (1960)	122	Congenital: heredity Other etiologies: Chicken pox Cogan's syndrome Congenital cholesteatoma Cytomegalovirus Embolism External ear deformities Herpes zoster oticus Hyperbilirubinemia Hypertension Intraventricular hemorrhage Labyrinth membrane rupture Low birth weight Meniere's disease Multiple sclerosis Neoplasms Otitis media Perilymph fistula Persistent pulmonary Post-otologic surgical Sludging of blood Syphilis Thrombosis Trauma Vascular pathologies Viral labyrinthitis	75

Source: Valente, M., *Strategies for Selecting and Verifying Hearing Aid Fittings*, 2nd ed. New York: Thieme. Reprinted by permission.

Table 4.15   Spanish instructions

A. *Pure-tone testing* (raising a hand):
USTED VA A ESCUCHAR UNOS SONIDOS. POR FAVOR LEVANTE SU MANO CUANDO OIGA EL SONIDO. NO IMPORTA SI EL SONIDO ES FUERTE O SUAVE. LEVANTE SU MANO AUNQUE EL SONIDO ESTE BIEN SUAVECITO O SUENE BIEN LEJOS. BAJE LA MANO TAN PRONTO DEJE DE OIR EL SONIDO. HA ENTENDIDO?

B. *Pure-tone testing* (pushing a button):
USTED VA A ESCUCHAR UNOS SONIDOS. POR FAVOR APRIETE EL BOTON CUANDO OIGA EL SONIDO. NO IMPORTA SI EL SONIDO ES FUERTE O SUAVE. APRIETE EL BOTON AUNQUE EL SONIDO ESTE BIEN SUAVECITO O SUENE BIEN LEJOS. DEJE DE APRETAR EL BOTON CUANDO YA NO OYE EL SONIDO. HA ENTENDIDO?

C. *Speech thresholds:*
POR FAVOR REPITA LAS PALABRAS QUE VOY A DECIR. DESPUES, LAS PALABRAS VAN A SER DICHAS MAS SIJAVEMEMTE GRADIJALMENTE. NECESITO SABER A QUE NIVEL USTED YA NO ME PUEDE ENTENDER. TRATE DE ADIVINAR LA PALABRA SI NO ME ENTIENDE. ESCUCHE ATENTAMENTE.

D. *Word recognition:*
USTED VA A ESCUCH AR UNA GRABACION A UN NIVEL MAS O MENOS COMODO. POR FAVOR REPITA LA ULTIMA PALABRA QUE USTED OIGA. POR EJEMPLO, USTED OIRA: "D1GA LA PALABRA AGUA." USTED REPITE "AGUA." HA ENTENDIDO?

E. *Masking:*
VOY A PONERLE UN RUIDO ES ESTE OIDO (POINT TO EAR WHERE MASKING WILL BE INTRODUCED). SONARA COMO UN VIENTO O CUANDO SE LE SALE EL AIRE A UNA LLANTA. NO LE PONGA ATENCION A ESTE RUIDO. IGNORELO POR COMPLETO. QUIERO QUE SOLAMENTE LEVANTE LA MANO [O APRIETE EL BOTON (or push the button)] CUANDO OIGA EL SONIDO, NO IMPORTA CUAN FUERTE EL RUIDO SE PONGA EN ESTE OIDO. HA ENTENDIDO?

F. *Immittance:*
VOY A PONER UN TAPONCITO EN ESTE OIDO (POINT TO EAR). VA A SENTIR AIRE O UN POQUITO DE PRESION EN EL OIDO, PARECIDO A CUANDO ESTA EN UN ELEVADOR O EN UN AVION. TAMBIEN VA A OIR UNOS SONIDOS FUERTES. NO TIENE QUE LEVANTAR LA MANO. NO SE MUEVA, NI HABLE. NI SE RIA. ESTE EXAMEN ES SENCILLO Y NO DUELE. LOS RESULTADOS ME DIRAN SI TIENE ALGUN PROBLEMA EN LA PARTE EXTERNA O MEDIA DEL OIDO, O NO.

G. *Uncomfortable loudness level (ULL):*
LE VOY A HABLAR. MI VOZ SE PONDRA GRADUALMENTE MAS Y MAS FUERTE. NECESITO QUE USTED LEVANTE LA MANO CUANDO MI VOZ SE PONE TAN FUERTE QUE USTED NO LA PUEDE TOLERAR O SOPORTAR. ES MUY IMPORTANTE QUE USTED LEVANTE LA MANO CUANDO EL VOLUMEN DE MI VOZ ES MUY INCOMODO PARA USTED Y *NO* CUANDO SOLAMENTE SE PONE FUERTE.

H. *Real-ear measurement:*
SIENTESE EN FRENTE DE ESTA BOCINA. LE VOY A PONER ESTE TUBITO PLASTICO EN EL OIDO. QUIZA LE DE COSQUILLA. NO LE DEBE DE DOLER PERO SI LE MOLESTA. POR FAVOR DIGAME. DESPUES LE PONDRE EL AUDIFONO. ESTA COMPUTADORA ME VA A DEJAR TOMAR MEDIDAS EXACTAS DE COMO EL SONIDO AMPLIFICADO A TRAVES DE SU AUDIFONO REACCIONA DENTRO DEL CANAL AUDITIVO. UNA VEZ ESTAS MEDIDAS SON OBTENIDAS, YO PODRE HACER MODIFICACIONES NECESARIAS PARA QUE USTED PUEDA OIR MEJOR
O SENCILLAMENTE VERIFICAR QUE TODO ESTA BIEN. USTED NO NECESITA HACER NADA. SIENTESE TRANQUILO Y RELAJESE.

Table 4.15   *(Continued)*

I. *ABR—Instructions to parents of children being tested*[a]

Por favor dé le la medicina al niño. Ahora voy a limpiar la piel y después esperaremos 20–30 minutos para que el niño se duerma. Cuándo esté dormido, voy a poner estos platillos (o electrodos) en la piel y tambien voy a poner los audifonos. El ninño va a oir algunos sonidos fuertes y bajitos. Los platillos (o electrodos) registran la respuesta del nervio del oido a los sonidos y así podemos decir si el niño puede oir bien o si no oye bien.

J. *ABR—Instructions to adult patient*[a]

Por favor sientese (o acuestese) aqui. Ahora voy a limpiar la piel y voy a poner estos platillos (o electrodos), los platillos (o electrodos) registran la respuesta del nervio del oído a varios sonidos fuertes y bajitos. Usted no tiene que hacer nada, no mas cierre los ojos y sientese (o acuestese) muy quieto y relajado sin moverse lo mas que pueda. Este examen dura 30–45 minutos.

Abbreviation: ABR, auditory brainstem response.

[a]Jameson, S.D., M.A., CCC-A, Callier Center/University of Texas at Dallas.

Source: Briseida Northrup, M.S., CCA-A, Callier Center/University of Texas at Dallas. Reprinted by permission.

Infants and Children

Table 4.16 Chronology of development in the human auditory system*

Gestation weeks	Event
3	Otic placode
3	Otic pit
3	Otic vesicle
4	Fold I of the otic vesicle
4	Auditory dendrites grow toward cochlea
4	Acousticovestibular ganglia begin to separate
5	Auditory nerve fibers reach brainstem
5	Periotic cartilaginous matrix forms
6	Cochlear nucleus and superior olive can be identified
8	Medial geniculate can be identified
8–9	Central nucleus of inferior colliculus can be identified
8–9	Calbindin present in auditory ganglion cells
8–9	Three turns present in the cochlea
9	Auditory dendrites penetrate the cochlear epithelium
10	Tectoral membrane can be identified
10	Hair cell differentiation begins
11	Perilymphatic spaces can be identified
11	Ciliogenesis on the hair cells
11	Brachium of the inferior colliculus can be identified
12	Acetylcholinesterase fibers in the internal capsule
12	Afferent synapses seen on the hair cells
15	Tunnel of Corti begins to open
16	Perilymphatic spaces reach the apex
16–20	Ossification of the periotic capsule begins
20	Outer hair cells present in the apex of the cochlea
20	Onset of myelination in the auditory nerve and auditory striae
20	Estimated onset of function in the cochlea
21	Tunnel of Corti present in all turns of the cochlea
20–24	Acetylcholinesterase fibers seen in the cortical subplate
24	Onset of myelination in the brachium of the inferior colliculus
25	Ossification of the periotic capsule is complete
24–28	Acetylcholinesterase fibers seen in the cortical plate
28	Columns of acetylcholinesterase in the cortex
30	Gross morphological maturity of the cochlea
35	Threshold sensitivity of the click brainstem evoked auditory potential (CBEAP) is adult-like
36–40	Large fibers in the lateral lemniscus and trapezoid body myelinate
40–44	Onset of myelination in the auditory radiations

*Other chronologies of human auditory system development are available in Rubel, E.W., Ontogeny of structure and function in the vertebrate auditory system. In Jacobson, M. (ed.), *Development of Sensory Systems.* New York: Springer-Verlag, 1978: 135–237; and Anson, B.J. and Davies, J., Developmental anatomy of the ear. In: Paparella, M.M. and Shumrick, D.A. (eds.), *Otolaryngology, Vol. I.* Philadelphia: WB Saunders, 1980:3–25.

Source: Willard, F. (1990), Analysis of the development of the human auditory system. *Seminars in Hearing* 11(2):108. New York: Thieme. Reprinted by permission.

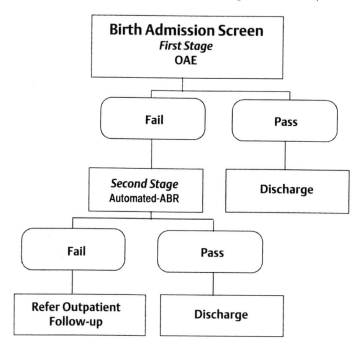

Fig. 4.8 Flow chart illustrating the two-stage screening protocol (otoacoustic emissions [OAE] followed by auditory brainstem response [ABR]) endorsed by the National Institutes of Health at the 1993 consensus meeting. (From Roeser, R.J., Valente, M., Hosford-Dunn, H. (2007), *Audiology Diagnosis,* 2nd ed. New York: Thieme. Reprinted by permission.)

Table 4.17 Hearing loss risk indicators for neonates from birth to 28 days of age

Risk indicators based on the JCIH (2000) position statement
- Neonatal condition requiring care in the neonatal intensive care unit for ≥ 48 hours
- Familial history of permanent sensorineural hearing loss in childhood
- Infections during pregnancy (e.g., rubella, cytomegalovirus, herpes, toxoplasmosis)
- Craniofacial anomalies, including pinna and ear canal abnormalities
- Stigmata (or other findings) associated with syndromes involving sensorineural and/or conductive hearing impairments

Risk indicators included in JCIH (1994) but omitted from JCIH (2000)
- Low birth weight (< 1,500 g or < 3.3 pounds)
- Hyperbilirubinemia requiring transfusion
- Ototoxic medications (aminoglycoside antibiotics or others) in multiple courses or combined with loop diuretics
- Bacterial meningitis
- Low Apgar scores[a] (0–4 at 1 minute, or 0–6 at 5 minutes)
- Mechanical ventilation for ≥ 5 days

[a]Many earlier listings referred to asphyxia and/or anoxia.

Source: Gelfand, S.A. (2001), *Essentials of Audiology,* 2nd ed. New York: Thieme. Reprinted by permission.

Table 4.18 Hearing loss risk indicators for rescreening infants from 29 days to 2 years of age

Risk indicators based on the JCIH (2000) position statement
- Concern about hearing, speech, language, or developmental delay by parent or caregiver
- Infections during pregnancy (e.g., syphilis, toxoplasmosis, rubella, cytomegalovirus, herpes)
- Postnatal infections (including bacterial meningitis) associated with sensorineural hearing loss
- Neonatal conditions such as hyperbilirubinemia requiring transfusion, persistent pulmonary hypertension of the newborn with mechanical ventilation, and those requiring extracorporeal membrane oxygenation
- Familial history of permanent sensorineural hearing loss in childhood
- Syndromes associated with progressive hearing loss (e.g., neurofibromatosis, Usher syndrome, osteopetrosis)
- Neurodegenerative disorders (e.g., Hunter syndrome) or sensorimotor neuropathies (e.g., Charcot-Marie-Tooth syndrome, Friedreich's ataxia)
- Stigmata (or other findings) associated with syndromes that involve sensorineural or conductive hearing impairments, or eustachian tube dysfunction
- Head trauma
- Persistent or recurrent otitis media with effusion lasting ≥ 3 months

Risk indicator included in JCIH (1994) but omitted from JCIH (2000)
- Ototoxic medications (aminoglycoside antibiotics or others) in multiple courses or combined with loop diuretics

Source: Gelfand, S.A. (2001), *Essentials of Audiology,* 2nd ed. New York: Thieme. Reprinted by permission.

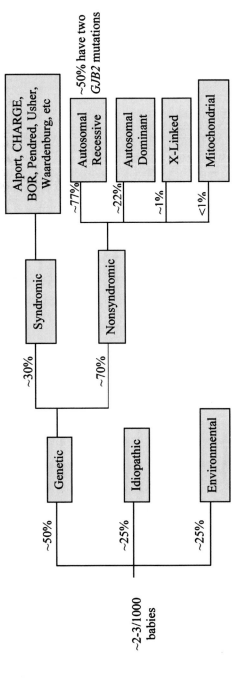

Fig. 4.9 Breakdown of etiologies of hearing loss. CHARGE, a syndrome of associated defects, including coloboma, heart anomaly, atresia choanae, retardation, and genital and ear anomalies; BOR, branchio-oto-renal syndrome. (From Madell, J.R. and Flexer, C. (2008) *Pediatric Audiology.* New York: Thieme. Reprinted by permission.)

Table 4.19 Middle ear abnormalities of congenital origin

Chromosomal Defects	
Syndrome	*Middle Ear Defect*
Turner syndrome (gonadal aplasia)	Middle ear hypoplasia, stapes malformation
Goldenhar syndrome	Malformed or absent ossicles Oval window hypoplasia
Patau syndrome (trisomy 17–15)	Small tympanic membrane, thickened manubrium, distorted IS joint
Down syndrome (trisomy 21)	Deformed stapes
Trisomy 22	Nonpneumatized middle ear, absence of stapes and oval window; bony closure of round window niche

Familial (Inherited) Disorders		
Syndrome	*Pattern of Inheritance*	*Middle Ear Defect*
Achondroplasia	Autosomal dominant	Fusion of ossicles, undeveloped ossicular mass
Apert syndrome	Autosomal dominant	Fixation of footplate
Atresia auris congenital	Autosomal dominant	Absence or fusion of ossicles Abnormal IS or MI joint
Klippel-Feil syndrome	Autosomal recessive	Stapes footplate fistula
Pierre Robin syndrome	Autosomal dominant	Thick stapes and footplate Absence of middle ear
Cleidocranial dysostosis	Autosomal dominant	Small ossicles, absence of manubrium and long process of uncus, stapes fixation
Mobius syndrome	Autosomal	Undeveloped ossicular mass
Crouzon syndrome	Autosomal dominant	Absence of TM, malleus fixation/deformation, stapes fixation, narrow middle ear, narrow round window niche
Duane syndrome	Autosomal/X-linked	Ossicular fusion, disarticulation
Hurler disease	Autosomal recessive	Absence of IM joint, deformed stapes, fibrous invasion of middle and inner ear
Letterer-Siwe disease	Autosomal recessive	Bony destruction of canal and middle ear structures
Teacher-Collins syndrome	Autosomal dominant	Ossicles deformed, absence of stapes/tensor tympani muscle

Table 4.19 (*Continued*)

Congenital Syndromes with Associated Middle Ear Defects

Syndrome	Pattern of Inheritance	Middle Ear Defect
Fanconi syndrome	Autosomal recessive	Stapes fixation
Mohr syndrome	Autosomal recessive	Absence of IS joint
Osteitis deformans (Padgett)	Autosomal dominant	Abnormal stapes ossification
Osteopetrosis	Autosomal	Abnormal ossicles, small middle ear space
Otopalatal digital syndrome	Autosomal recessive	Immature ossicles, fixed stapes, absence of oval window

Abbreviations: IM, incudo-malleus; IS, Incudo-stapedial; MI, Malleo-incudal; TM, tympanic membrane.

Source: Martin, F.N. and Clark, J.G., *Hearing Care for Children,* 1st ed, 1996. Reprinted by permission of Pearson Education, Inc., Upper Saddle River, NJ.

Table 4.20   A summary of tests used in pediatric assessments

Test	Expected Infant/ Child Response	Cognitive Age Range	Benefit	Challenges
Behavioral Observation Audiometry (BOA)	Change in sucking in response to auditory stimulus; other behavioral changes are not accepted because they usually indicate supra-threshold responses	Birth–6 months	Enables the audiologist to obtain valuable behavioral responses in infants; part of the cross-check principle. Testing can be conducted in sound field, with earphones, bone oscillator, hearing aids, or cochlear implants. Enables accurate fitting of technology because minimal response levels (MRLs) can be obtained.	Requires careful observation of infant sucking on the part of the audiologist. Cannot be used with infants who do not suck, e.g., infants who use feeding tubes. Testing can be performed only when the infant is in a calm, awake, or light sleep state. BOA has not been generally accepted in the audiology community because audiologists typically have not been trained to use a sucking response paradigm.
Visual Reinforcement Audiometry (VRA)	Conditioned head turn to a visual reinforcer, usually a lighted animated toy	5–36 months	Enables the audiologist to obtain valuable behavioral responses in infants and young children; part of the cross-check principle.	Because responses are conditioned, more responses can be obtained in one test session. Testing can be conducted in sound field, with earphones, bone oscillator, hearing aids, or cochlear implants. Enables accurate fitting of technology because MRL can be obtained. The state of the infant or child is less problematic because the child can be more easily involved in the task. Some children will not accept earphones, so obtaining individual ear information can be challenging.
Conditioned Play Audiometry (CPA)	Child performs a motor act in response to hearing a sound (e.g., the listen-and-drop task)	30 months to 5 years	Accurate responses can be obtained at threshold level. Testing can be conducted in sound field, with earphones, bone oscillator, hearing aids, or cochlear implants.	Keeping the child entertained and involved long enough to obtain all the necessary information can be challenging.

Test			Description	Requirements/Limitations
Immittance	None	All	Provides information about middle ear functioning and about intactness of the auditory system reflex arc.	The child must sit still, not speaking or moving during the test battery.
Transient Otoacoustic Emissions (TOAE)	None	All	Measures outer hair cell function. Presence of emissions indicates no greater than a mild hearing loss. Contributes to evaluation of the overall function of the auditory system.	The infant or child must sit still, not speaking during testing. Cannot rule out mild hearing loss.
Distortion Product Otoacoustic Emissions (DPOAE)	None	All	Measures outer hair cell function. Presence of emissions indicates no greater than moderate hearing loss. Contributes to evaluation of the overall function of the auditory system.	The infant or child must sit still, not speaking during testing. Cannot rule out moderate hearing loss.
Auditory Brainstem Response (ABR) Testing	None	All	Tonal ABR provides frequency specific threshold information. Click ABR provides information about the intactness of the auditory pathways, including measures contributing to the diagnosis of auditory neuropathy.	The infant or child must be asleep, sedated, or very still for the duration of testing. ABR testing is not a direct measure of hearing and is not a substitute for behavioral audiological testing.

Source: Madell, J.R. and Flexer, C. (2008), *Pediatric Audiology*. New York: Thieme. Reprinted by permission.

Table 4.21 Functional auditory assessment tools for infants and young children

Measurement Tool	Authors	Age Range	Purpose
Auditory Behavior in Everyday Life (ABEL) (2002)	Purdy et al, 2002	2–12 years	Twenty-four-item questionnaire with three subscales (aural-oral, auditory awareness, social/conversational skills) that evaluates auditory behavior in everyday life
Children's Home Inventory for Listening Difficulties (CHILD) (2000)	Anderson and Smaldino, 1998, 2000	3–12 years	Parent and self-report versions that assess listening skills in 15 natural situations
Children's Outcome Worksheet (COW) (2003)	Williams, 2003	4–12 years	Teacher, parent, and child rating scales of classroom and home listening situations with amplification device; to specify five situations where improved hearing is desired
Early Listening Function (ELF) (2000)	Anderson, 1989, 2000	5 months to 3 years	Parent observational rating scale of structured listening activities conducted over time to record distance learning
Functional Auditory Performance Indicators (FAPI) (2003)	Stredler-Brown and Johnson, 2001–2003	Infants through school-age children	Parent or interventionist assessment of functional auditory skills over time
Infant-Toddler Meaningful Auditory Integration Scale (IT-MAIS) (1997)	Robbins, Renshaw, and Berry, 1991	Infant-toddler and older child versions	Structured parent interview scale designed to assess spontaneous auditory behaviors in everyday listening situations
Listening Inventories for Education (LIFE.) (1998)	Anderson and Smaldino, 1998, 2000	6 years and above	Student and teacher rating scales designed to assess listening difficulty in the classroom

Little Ears (2003)	Kuhn-Inacker et al, 2003	Birth and up	Questionnaire for the parent with 35 questions, based on the child's age, that assess auditory development
Meaningful Auditory Integration Scale (MAIS) (1991)	McKonkey Robbins et al, 1991	3 to 4 years and up	Parental interview with 10 questions that evaluate the child's meaningful use of sound in everyday situations, attachment with hearing instrument, ability to alert to sound, ability to attach meaning to sound
Parent's Evaluation of Aural/Oral Performance of Children (PEACH) (2000)	Ching, Hill, and Psarros, 2006	Preschool to 7 years	Interview with parent with 15 questions targeting the child's everyday environment; includes scoring for five subscales (use, quiet, noise, telephone, environment)
Preschool Screening Instrument For Targeting Educational Risk (Preschool SIFTER) (1996)	Anderson and Matkin, 1996	3 to 6 years	Questionnaire with 15 items completed by the teacher that identifies children at risk for educational failure; has five subscales (academics, attention, communication, class participation, behavior)
Screening Inventory for Targeting Educational Risk (SIFTER) (1989)	Anderson, 1989, 2000	6 years through secondary school	Teacher questionnaire designed to target academic risk behaviors in children with hearing problems; has five subscales (academics, attention, communication, class participation, behavior)
Teacher's Evaluation of Aural/Oral Performance of Children (TEACH) (2000)	Ching, Hill, and Psarros, 2006	Preschool to 7 years	Interview with teacher having 13 questions targeting the child's everyday environment; includes scoring for five subscales (use, quiet, noise, telephone, environment)

Source: Cole, E.B. and Flexer, C. *Children with Hearing Loss: Developing Listening and Talking, Birth to Six* (pp. 157–158). Copyright © 2007 Plural Publishing, Inc. All rights reserved. Used by permission.

Table 4.22 Number and prevalence (%) of school-age children (*N* = 1218) exhibiting minimal sensorineural hearing loss, conductive hearing loss, and other hearing loss (e.g., mixed) as a function of grade, race, and sex

Hearing Loss Category	Grade			Race			Sex	
	3 (%)	6 (%)	9 (%)	Black (%)	White (%)	Other (%)	Male (%)	Female (%)
Bilateral sensorineural hearing loss	5 (0.88)	3 (0.86)	4 (1.32)	5 (0.93)	7 (1.07)	0 (0)	3 (0.53)	9 (1.38)
High-frequency hearing loss	6 (1.06)	5 (1.43)	6 (1.98)	5 (0.93)	12 (1.83)	0 (0)	11 (1.95)	6 (0.92)
Unilateral sensorineural hearing loss	23 (4.07)	5 (1.43)	9 (2.97)	20 (3.72)	16 (2.45)	1 (3.85)	12 (2.12)	25 (3.85)
Conductive hearings loss	28 (4.96)	9 (2.57)	4 (2.57)	9 (1.68)	31 (4.74)	1 (3.85)	21 (3.72)	20 (3.08)
Other	18 (3.19)	2 (0.66)	2 (0.66)	13 (2.42)	17 (2.60)	0 (0)	10 (1.77)	20 (3.08)

Source: Bess, F.H. and Gravel, J.S. (2006), *Foundations of Pediatric Audiology.* Plural Publishing, Inc. Copyright Fred H. Bess. Reprinted by permission.

Table 4.23 High-risk factors for deafness: Mnemonic ABC TORCH DEFG

Asphyxia
Bacterial meningitis
Congenital perinatal infections
Toxoplasmosis
Other bacterial infections (i.e., syphilis)
Rubella virus
Cytomegalovirus
Herpes simplex virus
Defects of the head and neck
Elevated bilirubin
Family history
Gram birthweight less than 1500 g (3.3 lbs)

Table 4.24 Exogenous causes of prelingual deafness

Preconception and prenatal causes
  Rubella
  Cytomegalovirus
  Ototoxic and other drugs, maternal alcoholism
  Hypoxia (and its possible causes: high altitude, general anesthetic, severe hemorrhage)
  Syphilis
  Toxemia, diabetes, other severe systemic maternal illness
  Parental irradiation
  Toxoplasmosis
Perinatal causes
  Hypoxia
  Traumatic delivery
  Maternal infection
  Ototoxic drugs
  Premature delivery
Neonatal and postnatal causes
  Hypoxia
  Infection
  Ototoxic drugs
  Erythroblastosis fetalis
  Infantile measles or mumps
  Otitis media (acute, chronic, serous)
  Noise-induced
  Meningitis
  Encephalitis

Source: Northern, J.L. and Downs, M.P. (2002), *Hearing in Children,* 5th ed. Philadelphia: Lippincott Williams & Wilkins. Reprinted by permission.

Table 4.25 Summary of audiologic evaluation procedures for infants and young children

Test	Technique	Developmental Age Range	Advantages	Disadvantages
Behavioral observation audiometry	Conditioning: none; reinforcement: none	0–6 months	No specialized equipment needed; can be used with children who cannot be conditioned	Rapid habituation; only sensitive to patients with severe to profound hearing losses; not sensitive to unilateral hearing loss; large inter- and intrasubject variability
Conditioned orienting response/visual reinforcement audiometry	Conditioning: head turn; reinforcement: lighted/animated toy and social	6–30 months	Can present stimuli through speakers, earphones, or bone oscillator; less inter- and intrasubject variability; can obtain minimal response levels close to thresholds; sensitive to even mild hearing losses	Some infants cannot be conditioned until about 12 months of age; many infants will not tolerate earphones or will not turn their heads when wearing earphones; specialized equipment is required
Tangible reinforcement operant conditioning audiometry (TROCA)	Conditioning: press button/lever; reinforcement: candy, cereal, small toys, etc.	30 months–4 years	Accurate thresholds can be obtained reliably; stimuli can be presented through speakers, earphones, or bone oscillators	May require numerous sessions; patient habituates when satiated by reinforcer; reinforcers may not be appropriate/safe
Conditioned play audiometry	Conditioning: play activity; reinforcement: play activity and social; may also use visual reinforcement	30 months–4 years	Accurate thresholds can be reliably obtained; can be accomplished with traditional equipment; stimuli can be presented through speakers, earphones, or the bone oscillator	May have to change activities many times to keep child's interest; child may need to be reconditioned when activities change

Source: Roeser, R.J., Valente, M., Hosford-Dunn, H. (2007), *Audiology Diagnosis*, 2nd ed. New York: Thieme. Reprinted by permission.

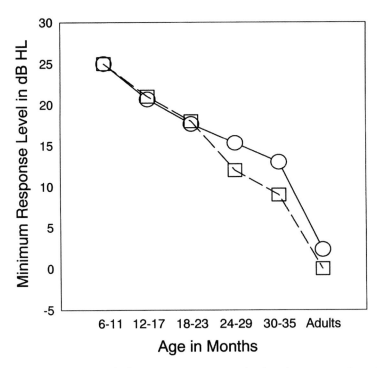

Fig. 4.10   The improvement of infants' minimum response levels with maturation from 6 to 35 months of age using visual reinforcement audiometry and adult thresholds for comparison. Based on data by Matkin (1977). (From Gelfand, S.A. (2001), *Essentials of Audiology,* 2nd ed. New York: Thieme. Reprinted by permission.)

Table 4.26 Auditory skill development sequence

Auditory Skills	Child Behaviors	Stimulation Skills
1. Attending/detection	Child attends to environmental sounds and voices. Child attends to distinct speech sounds.	Use auditory clues, show child sources of sound and reinforce child's responses to sound.
2. Recognizing	Child recognizes objects and events from their sounds.	Point out sounds and reinforce child's recognition of sound sources. Allow sound to be child's first source of information.
3. Locating	Child locates sound sources in space.	Create localization opportunities and reinforce all child's attempts to localize.
4. Distances and levels	Child locates sound sources at increased distances and above and below.	Create opportunities for child to hear sounds above and below and at distances; reinforce child's responses.
5. Environmental discrimination, identification, and comprehension	Child discriminates, identifies, and comprehends environmental sounds.	Repeatedly stimulate the child with environmental sounds and reinforce child's discrimination, identification, and comprehension of sounds.
6. Vocal discrimination, identification, and comprehension	Child discriminates, identifies, and comprehends gross vocal sounds, words, and phrases.	Provide opportunities for child to discriminate, identify, and comprehend onomatopoeic sounds, words, and phrases.
7. Speech discrimination, identification, and comprehension	Child discriminates, identifies, and comprehends fine speech sounds: vowels, then consonants.	Provide stimulation of vowel, then consonant sounds in meaningful words. Create opportunities for child to demonstrate discrimination, identification, and comprehension of these words.

Source: Schow, R.L. and Nerbonne, M.A., *Introduction to Aural Rehabilitation*, 2nd ed. © 1991. Reprinted by permission of Pearson Education, Inc., Upper Saddle River, NJ.

Table 4.27 Children's picture spondaic word list

cupcake	toothbrush	popcorn	flashlight
airplane	bathtub	fire	bluebird
baseball	ice	mailman	toothpaste
cowboy	shoelace	snowman	reindeer
hotdog	football	sailboat	seesaw

Sources: Based on Frank, T. (1980). Clinical significance of the relative intelligibility of pictorially represented spondee words. *Ear and Hearing, 1,* 46–49. Baltimore: Lippincott Williams & Wilkins; and American Speech-Language-Hearing Association (ASHA). (1988). Guidelines for determining threshold level for speech. *ASHA, 30,* 85–89. Reprinted by permission.

Table 4.28 Multisyllabic lexical neighborhood test (MLNT; Kirk, Pisoni, and Osberger, 1995)

List 1 (Easy Words)	List 1 (Hard Words)	List 2 (Easy Words)	List 2 (Hard Words)
children	butter	water	puppy
animal	lion	banana	pickle
monkey	money	glasses	button
finger	jelly	airplane	summer
pocket	yellow	window	bottom
apple	purple	tiger	finish
morning	hello	cookie	bunny
sugar	carry	again	belly
alright	corner	another	couple
about	heaven	almost	under
because	measles	broken	naughty
crazy	ocean	china	really

Source: Indiana University; David B. Pisoni and Karen Kirk. Reprinted by permission. (Test recording available from Auditec of St. Louis.)

Table 4.29   Word intelligibility by picture identification (WIPI) test word lists

List 1	List 2	List 3	List 4
school	broom	moon	spoon
ball	bowl	bell	bow
smoke	coat	coke	goat
floor	door	corn	horn
fox	socks	box	block
hat	flag	bag	black
pan	fan	can	man
bread	red	thread	bed
neck	desk	nest	dress
stair	bear	chair	pear
eye	pie	fly	tie
knee	tea	key	bee
street	meat	feet	teeth
wing	string	spring	ring
mouse	clown	crown	mouth
shirt	church	dirt	skirt
gun	thumb	sun	gum
bus	rug	cup	bug
train	cake	snake	plane
arm	barn	car	star
chick	stick	dish	fish
crib	ship	bib	lip
wheel	seal	queen	green
straw	dog	saw	frog
pail	nail	ail	tail

Source: Ross, M. and Lerman, J. (1971). *Word Intelligibility by Picture Identification (WIPI).* St. Louis: Auditec. Reprinted by permission.

Table 4.30   Northwestern University Children's Perception of Speech (NU-CHIPS) test word lists (alphabetical order)

ball	horse
bear	house
bike	juice
bird	light
boat	man
bus	meat
cake	milk
clock	mouth
coat	nose
comb	purse
cup	school
dog	shirt
door	shoe
dress	sink
duck	smile
food	snake
foot	soap
frog	spoon
girl	teeth
gum	tongue
gun	train
hair	tree
ham	truck
hand	watch
head	witch

Source: Elliott, L. and Katz, D. (1980). Northwestern University Children's Perception Speech (NU-CHIPS). St. Louis: Auditec. Reprinted by permission.

Table 4.31 Features of auditory skill assessments

Test	Ages	Scoring*	Stimuli/Features Assessed	Skills Assessed	Response Set	Comments
Early Speech Perception Test (ESP) (Moog and Geers, 1990)	2 years through teens	CR	Syllable number; spondees differing in consonant and vowel content; vowels	Discrimination; identification	Closed	Toys available for use by young children
Test of Auditory Comprehension (TAC) (Trammel, 1976)	4–12 years	STD-HI	Environmental sounds; nonverbal human sounds; words, phrases, sentences, short stories	Discrimination; identification; memory for two and four critical elements; sequencing; recalling details; listening in noise	Closed	Out of print, but widely used in programs for children with hearing loss; normative data from children with cochlear implants not available
Auditory Perception Test for the Hearing Impaired (APT-HI) (Allen and Serwatka, 1994)	5 years through teens	CR	Syllables; pitch; vowels; consonant difference in words; sentences	Auditory awareness; discrimination; identification; comprehension of questions	Closed; open set for comprehension	
Test of the Auditory Perceptual Skill–Revised (TAPS-R) (Gardner, 1996)	4–13 years	STD-NL	Words and numbers; words differing in vowel or consonant content; sentences	Memory; discrimination; comprehension	Open	

Test	Age	Scoring	Stimuli	Skills	Format	Notes
The Listening Test (Barrett, Hui)	6–12 years	STD-NL	Paragraphs	Getting the main idea; remembering details; applying conceptual vocabulary; inferring answers; story comprehension	Open; concepts section supplies pictures for topic	
Speech Perception Instructional Curriculum and Evaluation (SPICE) – Rating form (Moog, Biedenstein, and Davidson, 1995)	3–12 years	CR	Syllables; words; sentences; questions	Detection; suprasegmental discrimination; vowel and consonant discrimination; identification of words and sentences; comprehension	Ranging from closed to open set	This is a rating form for placement on the Developmental Approach to Successful Listening (DASL) curriculum and for documenting progress
Developmental Approach to Successful Listening II (DASL-II) – Placement test (Stout and Windle, 1992)	3–18 years	CR	Syllables; words; sentences	Detection; suprasegmental discrimination; vowel and consonant discrimination; identification of words and sentences; comprehension	Ranging from closed to open set	This is a rating form for placement on the DASL curriculum and for documenting progress

*Scoring categories: CR, criterion reference; STD-HI, standardized with children with hearing impairment; STD-NL, standardized with children with normal hearing.

Source: Roeser, R.J. In: Roeser, R.J., and Downs, M.P. (2004), *Auditory Disorders in School Children*, 4th ed. New York: Thieme. Reprinted by permission.

Table 4.32   Behaviors of children that are associated with hearing loss

1. Frequently asks to have things repeated
2. Turns one side of head toward speaker
3. Talks too loudly or too softly
4. Shows strain in trying to hear
5. Watches and concentrates on teacher's lips
6. Is inattentive in classroom discussion
7. Makes frequent mistakes in following directions
8. Makes unusual mistakes in taking dictation
9. Tends to isolate self
10. Tends to be passive
11. Is tense
12. Tires easily
13. Has a speech problem
14. Is not working up to apparent capacity
15. Has academic failure following severe illness

Physical symptoms may include:
1. Mouth breathing
2. Draining ears
3. Earaches
4. Dizziness
5. Reports of ringing, buzzing, or roaring in ears

Table 4.33 (S)TORCH complex—associated clinical manifestations

Disease	Primary Symptoms	Prevalence of Hearing Loss (%)	Type and Degree of Hearing Loss
Syphilis	Enlarged liver and spleen, snuffles, rash, hearing loss	35	Severe to profound bilateral SNHL; configuration and degree varies
Toxoplasmosis	Chorioretinitis, hydrocephalus, intracranial calcifications, hearing loss	17	Moderate to severe bilateral SNHL; may be progressive
Rubella	Heart and kidney defects, eye anomalies, mental retardation, hearing loss	20–30	Profound bilateral SNHL—"cookie-bite" audiogram is common; may be progressive
Cytomegalovirus	Mental retardation, visual defects, hearing loss	17	Mild to profound bilateral SNHL; may be progressive
Herpes simplex	Enlarged liver, rash, visual abnormalities, psychomotor retardation, encephalitis, hearing loss	10	Moderate to severe unilateral or bilateral SNHL

Abbreviation: SNHL, sensorineural hearing loss.

Source: Bess, F.H. and Humes, L. E. *Audiology—The Fundamentals.* Baltimore: Lippincott Williams & Wilkins, 1990:87. Reprinted by permission.

Table 4.34 Establishing effective communication with hearing-impaired children: Methods for parents

Objectives	Method
Establish an effective communication setting	1. Keep background noises at a minimum when communicating with child.
	2. Allow child freedom to explore and play. Child must have chance to explore objects and learn what they are and do if he is to understand communication about them.
	3. Serve as a "communication consultant." Place child near you so you can frequently communicate with him.
	4. Use interactive turn-taking. Encourage child to "take turns" in a variety of activities and situations.
	5. Get down on child's level, as close to him as possible. Speech is most intelligible 3 to 4 feet from child.
	6. Occasionally provide *ad concham* stimulation (talk directly into child's ear).
	7. Maintain eye contact and direct conversation to child.
Establish effective nonverbal communication	1. Use interesting, varied facial expressions.
	2. Use varied intonation and rhythm patterns.
	3.
	4. Use natural gestures.
	Touch child in stimulating way while vocalizing.

Table 4.34 (*Continued*)

Objectives	Method
Establish effective verbal communication	1. Regard child's cry as communicative and respond accordingly.
	2. Imitate and expand child's babbling and vocal play. Imitate and expand child's motions and add vocalizations. Introduce a few new babbling sounds each week for the child to hear.
	3. Identify and respond to child's verbal and nonverbal intents (vocalizing, pointing, tugging, stretching, looking, playing) with simple language.
	4. Use conversational turn-taking (wait expectantly for a response, signal the child to take a turn, use prods, chains, questions, etc., to keep conversation going).
	5. Talk about obvious objects and events. Talk about child's meaningful daily activities and emotional experiences.
	6. Talk about fun topics that interest child. Take advantage of child's curiosity.
	7. Use short, simple sentences and expressions rather than long, complicated ones.
	8. Communicate to child in ways he can understand (match child's communication level).
	9. When child is ready, encourage a more mature communication level.

Source: Schow, R.L. and Nerbonne, M.A., *Introduction to Aural Rehabilitation*, 2nd ed. © 1991. Reprinted by permission of Pearson Education, Inc., Upper Saddle River, NJ.

Table 4.35   Handicapping effects of hearing loss in children

Average Hearing Level 500–2,000 Hz	Description	Possible Condition	What Can Be Heard Without Amplification	Handicapping Effects (If Not Treated in First Year of Life)	Probable Needs
0–15 dB	Normal Range	Conductive hearing losses	All speech sounds	None	None
15–25 dB	Slight hearing loss	Conductive hearing losses, some sensorineural hearing losses	Vowel sounds heard clearly; may miss unvoiced consonant sounds	Mild auditory dysfunction in language learning	Consideration of need for hearing aid; speechreading, auditory training, speech therapy, preferential seating
25–30 dB	Mild hearing Loss	Conductive or sensorineural hearing loss	Only some of speech sounds, the more loudly voiced sounds	Auditory learning dysfunction, mild language retardation, mild speech problems, inattention	Hearing aid, speechreading, auditory training, speech therapy
30–50 dB	Moderate hearing loss	Conductive hearing loss from chronic middle-ear disorders; sensorineural hearing losses	Almost no speech sounds at normal conversational level	Speech problems, language retardation, learning, dysfunction, inattention	All of the above, plus consideration of special classroom situation
50–70 dB	Severe hearing loss	Sensorineural or mixed losses due to a combination of middle-ear disease and sensorineural involvement	No speech sounds at normal conversational level	Severe speech problems, language retardation, learning dysfunction, inattention	All of the above, probable assignment to special classes
70+ dB	Profound hearing loss	Sensorineural or mixed losses due to a combination of middle-ear disease and sensorineural involvement	No speech or other sounds	Severe speech problems, language retardation, learning dysfunction, inattention	All of the above, probable assignment to special classes

Source: Northern, J.L. and Downs, M.P. (2002), Hearing in Children, 5th ed. Philadelphia: Lippincott Williams & Wilkins. Reprinted by permission.

Table 4.36 Expected auditory responses to various sounds for normal-hearing infants

	Stimulus			
Age	*Noisemakers (dB SPL)*	*Warbled Pure Tone (dB HL)*	*Speech[a] (dB HL)*	*Expected Response*
Birth–6 weeks	50–10	78 (SD = 6)	40–60	Eye widening, eye blink, stirring or arousal from sleep, startle
6 weeks–4 months	50–60	70 (SD = 10)	47 (SD = 2)	Eye widening, eye shift, eye blink, quieting; beginning rudimentary head turn by 4 months
4–7 months	40–50	51 (SD = 9)	21 (SD = 8)	Head turn on lateral plane toward sound; listening attitude
7–9 months	30–40	45 (SD = 15)	15 (SD = 7)	Direct localization of sounds to side, indirectly below ear level
9–13 months	25–35	38 (SD = 8)	8 (SD = 7)	Direct localization of sounds to side, directly below ear level, indirectly above ear level
13–16 months	25–30	32 (SD = 10)	5 (SD = 5)	Direct localization of sound on side, above, and below
16–21 months	25	25 (SD = 10)	5 (SD = 1)	Direct localization of sound on side, above, and below
21–24 months	25	26 (SD = 10)	3 (SD = 2)	Direct localization of sound on side, above, and below

Abbreviation: SD, standard deviation.

[a]Adapted from Northern, J.L. and Downs, M.P. (1984), *Hearing in Children*, 3rd ed. Baltimore: Williams & Wilkins.

Source: Bess, F.H. and Humes, L. E. *Audiology—The Fundamentals.* Baltimore: Lippincott Williams & Wilkins, 1990:87. Reprinted by permission.

Table 4.37 Comparison of several recommended screening guidelines

Source	Test Frequencies	Intensity Level (ANSI–1989)	Pass-Fail Criteria
American Speech and Hearing Association Committee on Identification Audiometry (1975)[a]	1,000, 2,000, and 4,000 Hz	20 dB at 1,000 and 2,000 Hz 25 dB at 4,000 Hz	Fail to respond to any frequency in either ear
American Speech-Language-Hearing Association (1985)[b]	1,000, 2,000, and 4,000 Hz	20 dB	Fail to respond to one tone in either ear
Anderson[c]	1,000, 2,000, and 4,000 Hz	20 dB	Fail to respond to any one signal in any ear
Downs[d]	1,000, 2,000, 4,000, and 6,000 or 8,000 Hz	15 dB	Fail to respond to either 1,000 or 2,000 Hz or to both 4,000 and 6,000–8,000 Hz in either ear
National Conference on Identification Audiometry[e]	1,000, 2,000, 4,000, and 6,000 Hz	20 dB at 1,000, 2,000, and 6,000 Hz 30 dB at 4,000 Hz	Fail to hear any signals at these levels in either ear
Northern and Downs[f]	1,000, 2,000, 3,000, and/or 4,000 and 6,000 Hz	25 dB	Fail to respond to one tone at 1,000 or 2,000 Hz; or fail to respond to two of three tones at 3,000, 4,000, and 6,000 Hz
State of Illinois Department of Public Health[g]	500, 1,000, 2,000, and 4,000 Hz	25 or 35 dB	Fail to respond to one tone at 35 dB in either ear or respond to any two tones at 25 dB in the same ear

[a]American Speech and Hearing Association (ASHA) Committee on Audiometric Evaluation Guidelines for Identification Audiometry. *Asha* 17 (1975), 94–99.
[b]American Speech-Language-Hearing Association (ASHA), Guidelines for screening hearing impairment and middle ear disorders. *Asha* 32: (Suppl) 2, (1990), 17–24.
[c]Anderson C.V., Conversation of hearing. In: Katz J. (ed.) *Handbook of Clinical Audiology*, 2nd ed. Baltimore: Williams & Wilkins, 1978.
[d]Downs, M.P., Auditory screening. *Otolaryngol. Clin. North Am.* 11 (1968), 611–629.
[e]Darley, F.L., Identification audiometry for school-age children: basic procedures, J. *Speech Hear. Dis.* Suppl 9,1962, 26–34.
[f]Northern, J.L. and Downs M.P., *Hearing in Children*, 4th ed. Baltimore: Williams & Wilkins, 1991.
[g]*A Manual for Audiometrists.* Springfield, IL: Illinois Department of Public Health, 1974.

Table 4.38 Helping families encourage infant communication

Techniques that support both auditory and visual communication
- Understand that daily routines such a feeding, changing, and comforting are effective situations for encouraging infant communication development.
- Watch closely for communication "signals" such as points, gestures, gazes, and facial expressions and respond to them.
- Think about what the infant's signal is meant to convey and give the words/signs for that person, object, or action.
- Talk/sign to the infant about what is happening.
- Use lots of facial expression when communication and be certain that your expression matches your words/signs.
- Use natural gestures in combination with words and signs.
- Use reciprocal, or "back and forth" communication, pausing where the infant's turn should be and encouraging the infant to take a turn.

Techniques that support early listening and speech
- Encourage the infant to wear his or her hearing aids or cochlear implant during all waking hours.
- Point out interesting or meaningful sounds and show what is making the sound.
- Be certain that sounds are loud enough to be heard (30 to 50 dB above threshold) and vary them to maintain interest.
- Get close when you talk. This provides a more audible signal and minimizes interference from other noises in the room.
- Remember that infants like listening to speech. Make your voice as interesting as possible by using lots of intonation (up or down inflection) when talking.
- Encourage vocalization and use of voice for communication. Show how happy and excited you are when the infant vocalizes in return.
- Respond to all vocalizations as if they were communication.
- Using vowels and consonants, focus on specific speech sounds by associating them with activities such as sucking or toy movement.

Techniques that support early visual communication
- Pay attention to hand movements and respond positively to this "manual babbling" in the same way you might respond to vocalization.
- Pay close attention to what the infant is looking at and provide the sign. Make the sign close to the object or bring the object into the infant's attention before signing. You may need to wait patiently or touch the child's shoulder.
- Make signs easy to see by positioning yourself at the infant's eye level.

Source: Roeser, R.J. In Roeser, R.J. and Downs, M.P. (2004), *Auditory Disorders in School Children*, 4th ed. New York: Thieme. Reprinted by permission.

Table 4.39 Expanding cochlear implant candidacy criteria

Year of FDA Approval	1985*	1990*	1995*	1997*	1998*	2000**
Age at implantation	≥ 18 years	≥ 2 years	≥ 2 years	≥ 18 months	≥ 18 months	≥ 1 year
Onset of Hearing Loss	Postlinguistic	Adults: postlinguistic Children: no stated requirement	Adults: pre-, peri-, and postlinguistic Children: no stated requirement	Adults: pre-, peri-, and postlinguistic Children: no stated requirement	Adults: pre-, peri-, and postlinguistic Children: no stated requirement	Adults: pre-, peri-, and postlinguistic Children: no stated requirement
Degree of Sensorineural Hearing Loss	Profound (no statement re: bilateral)	Adults: profound (no statement re: bilateral) Children: profound, bilaterally	Postlinguistic adults: moderate to profound for low frequencies and profound (≥ 90 dB HL) for mid- to high speech frequencies, bilaterally Pre- or perilinguistic adults: profound Children: profound, bilaterally	Postlinguistic adults: moderate to profound for low frequencies and profound (≥ 90 dB HL) for mid- to high speech frequencies, bilaterally Pre- or perilinguistic adults: profound Children: profound, bilaterally	Postlinguistic adults: moderate to profound for low frequencies and profound (≥ 90 dB HL) for mid- to high speech frequencies, bilaterally Pre- or perilinguistic adults: profound Children: profound, bilaterally	Adults: moderate to profound for low frequencies and profound (≥ 90 dB HL) for mid- to high speech frequencies, bilaterally Infants (12 to 24 months): profound, bilaterally Children (≥ 2 years): severe to profound, bilaterally
Limited Benefit from Amplification	Little or no benefit from a hearing aid	Little or no benefit from a hearing aid	Postlinguistic: ≤ 30% open-set sentence recognition, best-aided condition	Postlinguistic: ≤ 30% open-set sentence recognition, best-aided condition	Postlinguistic: ≤ 40% open-set sentence recognition, best-aided condition	≤ 50% aided open-set sentence recognition in the ear to be implanted (≤ 60% best-aided condition)

Adults	No stated speech perception requirement[1]	No stated speech perception requirement[1]	Pre- or perilinguistic: no stated speech perception requirement[2]	Pre- or perilinguistic: no stated speech perception requirement[2]	Pre- or perilinguistic: no stated speech perception requirement[2]
Limited Benefit from Amplification	Not candidates	Failure to improve on age-appropriate closed-set word identification tasks after a recommended minimum 6-month hearing aid or vibrotactile device	Failure to improve on age-appropriate closed-set word identification tasks after a recommended minimum 6-month hearing aid or vibrotactile device	Failure to improve on age-appropriate closed-set word identification tasks after a recommended minimum 6-month hearing aid or vibrotactile device	
Children				Older children: < 20% aided open-set speech recognition as measured by MLNT/LNT (after a required minimum 3- to 6-month trial) Younger children: lack of progress in the development of simple auditory skills with appropriate amplification (after a required minimum 3- to 6-month trial) and intensive aural rehabilitation	Older Children: ≤ 30% aided open-set speech recognition as measured by MLNT/LNT Younger children: lack of progress in auditory skill development with appropriate amplification and intervention over a 3- to 6-month period, desirably quantified by a measure such as the MAIS or ESP test

Abbreviations: ESP, Early Speech Perception (Moog and Geers, 1990); LNT, Lexical Neighborhood Test (Iler-Kirk et al., 1995); MAIS, Meaningful Auditory Integration Scale (Robbins, Renshaw, and Berry, 1991); MLNT, Multisyllabic Lexical Neighborhood Test (Iler-Kirk, Pisoni, and Osberger, 1995).

*Nucleus® 24.

**Nucleus® 24 Contour™ to Current System.

[1]Typically, zero or close to zero aided speech perception.

[2]Typically, would fall within the same range as postlinguistic.

Source: Cochlear Americas (Centennial, CO). Reprinted by permission.

Table 4.40 Education laws for children with hearing loss

Education Laws	Coverage	Relevant Federal Agency	Web Resources
IDEA Public Law 108–446	Primary federal law addressing the educational needs of children with disabilities. Requires that states and local school districts provide free and appropriate early intervention and educational services that address the child's specific needs.	Department of Education	www.ed.gov/legislation/ covers children 3 to 21 years of age. http://ww2.ed.gov/legislation/FedRegister/finrule/2006–3/081406a.pdf. www.ed.gov/policy/speced/guid/idea/modelform-iep.pdf
Part B	Focuses on school-based services and covers children 3 to 21 years of age.	Department of Education	www.nectac.org/idea/idea.asp
Part C	Addresses EI services for children up to 3 years of age. Provides grants to states to develop early intervention programs for young children who have a diagnosed condition that could impact on the child's development	Department of Education	
NCLB, 2001	By focusing on academic achievement, the law's intent is to hold schools accountable for ensuring that all students—including those with disabilities—meet specific standards. IDEA focuses on access to the child's educational program, whereas NCLB provides a mechanism for monitoring the quality and impact of services provided under IDEA.	Department of Education	www.ed.gov/policy/elsec/guid/edpicks.jhtml?src=fp www.whitehouse.gov/news/releases/2002/01/20020108.html
Section 504 of the Rehabilitation Act	For children who do not qualify for special education services under IDEA, Section 504 can be utilized to provide related services such as FM systems or captioning. See General Access on other Sec 504 elements.	Relevant Federal Agency	www.usdoj.gov/crt/ada/cguide.htm#anchor65610 www.section508.gov/index.cfm?FuseAction=Content&ID=15
ADA, Title II (public schools) and Title III (private schools)	Can be applied in similar fashion to Section 504. Private schools and higher education institutions are required to make their programs communications accessible.	Access Board (guidelines) Department of Justice (enforcement)	See General Access

Abbreviations: ADA, Americans with Disabilities Act; EI, early intervention; FM, frequency modulation; IDEA, Individuals with Disabilities Education Act; NCLB, No Child Left Behind Act.

Source: Madell, J.R. and Flexer, C. (2008), *Pediatric Audiology.* New York: Thieme. Reprinted by permission.

Table 4.41   Model letter to teachers for children who fail pure-tone hearing screening

Student's Name:_____

Dear:_____

The above-named child, who is enrolled in your class, was tested and found to have a hearing impairment. With the parent's permission we are sending you this letter providing you with suggestions for helping a hearing-impaired child succeed in a class with normally hearing children.

1. *Preferential seating.* Seat the child close to where you usually stand to give instruction. Check to make sure that the lighting is such that the child can see your face while you are talking. It is also helpful if you do not give important instructions while you are walking about the room or when your back is toward the child. When other children recite, allow the child to turn around to that he or she can see the child reciting. The child's face should be toward the speaker.
2. *Talking to the child.* Secure the child's attention before you begin to speak. Then talk naturally in your normal tone of voice. Shouting is not helpful. If the child does not understand something, repeat what you just said. If he or she still seems uncertain, then rephrase what you said using different words.
3. *Special hints.* If the child has trouble during spelling tests, try using the words in a sentence. Many words look alike to the lip-reader. When the child makes other mistakes, make sure he or she has understood the question or direction (by having the child repeat) before you correct the error. When giving homework assignments or important directions, have the child write the assignment so you can make sure he or she understands what to do.

   Children with a hearing loss who need to see the speaker's face often cannot take notes and listen at the same time. You may wish to allow a "buddy" to take notes for the child using carbon paper. Special assignments requiring the child to watch a television program may also be difficult, as the child cannot always see the speaker's face. Providing notes for the child to study at home would be helpful in this situation. During reading class you should make sure that the child knows the meaning of the words and does not simply "call" words that he or she does not understand. In a reading circle these children will have difficulty keeping their places because they cannot see and understand the other children as well as they do the teacher. Another problem area for some hearing-impaired children is hearing the various bells used to signal the end of class, fire drills, etc. Assign these children a "buddy" to tap them on the shoulder to alert them to the bell.
4. *Parents can be helpful.* Because children with a hearing loss can follow instructions better if they are already prepared for the vocabulary in the new lesson, it is often most helpful if teachers allow interested parents to bring the child's textbooks home. Using the teacher's recommendations, the parent can individually introduce the child to the vocabulary in the next lesson.
5. *The hearing aid.* Even if the child wears a hearing aid, he or she still needs to watch the face of the speaker to understand what is being said. A child with a hearing aid should wear it constantly while at school except for swimming class. Encourage the parents to provide the child with an extra battery so that the battery can be replaced if it goes out while the child is in school. We have enclosed additional information regarding hearing aid use and maintenance that you may wish to refer to for further assistance.

Your understanding of this child can be an important contribution to his or her success in school. If you have questions or comments concerning this letter, please feel free to call me.

Yours very truly,

_____ MS, COC/A
Clinical Audiologist

Source: Diagnostic Audiology, by R. J. Roeser, 1986, Austin, TX: PRO-ED. Copyright 1986 by PRO-ED, Inc. Reprinted by permission.

Table 4.42   Summary of communication approaches and philosophies

Approach/Philosophy	Definition
A-O approach (now called AVEd by many professionals)	This approach has spoken language as a desired outcome. Active listening, enhanced by the use of hearing aids or cochlear implants, is accompanied by speech reading to receive instructional and conversational information (Clark, 2006). The use of natural gestures is acceptable; sign language is not used. Children with hearing loss may be grouped together in auditory-oral classrooms for specialized oral instruction, at least in preschool and kindergarten, with mainstreaming being a goal. Family members will need to learn how to manage auditory technology, and how to provide an enriched spoken language environment for their child.
AVT approach (also called "unisensory" and "acoupedic")	This is primarily an early intervention therapeutic approach in which technology (hearing aids or cochlear implants) is paired with specific techniques and strategies that teach children to listen and understand spoken language. The 10 principles of auditory-verbal practice focus on parent coaching to foster cognition, speaking, reading, and learning through the auditory modality. Visual cues (lipreading and sign language) are not used or taught during therapy so that the child can develop the auditory system through directed listening practice. The foremost goals of AVT are to guide parents and caregivers as the primary facilitators for helping their children develop intelligible spoken language through listening, and to advocate for their children's inclusion in regular schools. AVT uses one-on-one teaching of parent or caregiver and child, focusing on strong family involvement; children are mainstreamed from the beginning (Estabrooks, 2006). However, some children will require additional auditory support after entering the mainstream. Parents are key partners in AVT.
BiBi	A person who achieves fluency in ASL and English (or another language) is bilingual. Using this approach, ASL is often taught as the first language and English is taught as a second language to develop literacy skills. English may be taught by using a sign system or through print; spoken English is not featured. The child will need to be in an ASL self-contained classroom, or require an ASL interpreter if placed in a general education classroom. Family members will also need to learn ASL and the English-based sign system to communicate with their child.

Table 4.42 (*Continued*)

Approach/Philosophy	Definition
Cued speech	A supplement to spoken English, cued speech is intended to make important features of spoken language fully visible, since approximately 60% of the phonemes are not visible through speech reading. This system enhances speech reading by employing phonemically based gestures to distinguish between similar visual speech patterns. The goal of cued speech is the reception and expression of spoken communication. Family members will need to learn cued speech to communicate with their child. Children are expected to be able to drop the use of cues once their oral language skills are firmly established.
Sign-supported speech and language	Signs are used occasionally to support spoken language development. Signs function as a bridge to enhance the meaning of oral communication. The signs also can serve to enhance understanding in certain challenging situations such as noisy environments or when a hearing device is not in use. Family members will need to learn sign language in addition to oral communication techniques to communicate with their child.
Simultaneous communication	This is the concurrent use of signs and speech. To provide language using two modalities simultaneously, a sign system, rather than a signed language, is used. This visual representation of the oral language is accomplished using manual symbols and signs. If not in a self-contained classroom that uses sign language, the child will require a sign language interpreter. Family members will need to learn both sign language and oral communication techniques to communicate with their child.
TC (also called a multi-sensory approach)	Introduced in the 1960s, this philosophy aims to make use of several strategies or modes of communication including sign, speech, auditory, written, and other visual aids. First developed by Roy Holcomb, the choice of modalities depends on the particular needs and abilities of the child, and professes to provide whatever is needed to foster communicative success. Children will need to be placed in a TC classroom, or have an interpreter if in general education classrooms. Family members also will need to learn sign language and other prescribed techniques to communicate with their child.

Abbreviations: AVEd, Auditory–Verbal Education; A-O, Auditory-Oral; ASL, American Sign Language; AVT, Auditory Verbal Therapy; BiBi, Bilingual Bimodal; TC, Total Communication.

Note: This table was developed with Arlene Stredler Brown.

Source: Madell, J.R. and Flexer, C. (2008), *Pediatric Audiology*. New York: Thieme. Reprinted by permission.

Speech Audiometry

Table 4.43 Speech perception test measures: Hierarchical listing

I. Detection
  A. Two-alternative, forced-choice detection. The speech element occurs in one interval while silence occurs in the other interval. The student must indicate in which interval the speech stimulus occurred.
  B. Open-set detection. The student must indicate when the speech stimulus is heard.
II. Discrimination (same versus different)
  A. Presentation of two stimuli. The stimuli are the same/different in one or more specified dimensions (frequency, intensity, duration, etc.). The student states whether the two stimuli are the same/different.
  B. AXB paradigm. A and B are two different stimuli. The student must state whether X is the same as A or B. X is presented second and is one presentation away from each of the reference stimuli.
  C. ABX paradigm. The task is the same as the previous task, but while X is one presentation away from the B stimulus, it is two presentations away from the A stimulus. This increases the load on short-term memory.
  D. Oddball detection in a three-interval, forced-choice procedure. Two of the stimuli are identical and one differs. The position of the oddball varies randomly across presentations. The student needs to indicate which of the three stimuli was the oddball.
III. Identification
  A. Closed-set (forced-choice) identification. There are a minimum of two choices. The student is required to identify which of the items was spoken.
  B. Open-set recognition. The student repeats what he or she has heard.
IV. Comprehension
  A. Word associations. These include responding with a synonym or stating the category in which the word belongs.
  B. Yes/No questions.
  C. WH questions (Where, What, Who, When, Why, How).
  D. Open-ended questions.
  E. Answer questions in response to a connected discourse recording.

Note: The above list does not detail specialized test procedures, such as sound-symbol relations, auditory synthesis/analysis, sequencing, memory span, and processing speed, which can also be assessed in hierarchical fashion.
Source: Medwetsky, L., Educational audiology. In: Kate, J. (ed.), *Handbook of Clinical Audiology*, 4th ed., 1994, page 507. Baltimore: Lippincott Williams & Wilkins. Reprinted by permission.

Table 4.44 Hierarchy of speech perception measures

Code	Test	Author	Recommended Age	Stimuli	Presentation Format	Response	Norms
Awareness							
SDT	Speech detection threshold	ASHA (1988)	Birth to 3 years	Monosyllabic words	Live voice	Behavioral change	Northern and Downs (1991)
Discrimination							
ADT	Auditory Discrimination Test	Wepman (1973)	5–8 years	Monosyllabic word pairs	Live voice	Respond verbally, same/different	Yes
Identification							
SRT	Speech recognition threshold	ASHA (1988)	3 years–adult	Spondees	Tape or CD[1,6]	Repeat the word or point to pictures	ANSI (2004)
Goldman-Fristoe Woodcock (GFW)	GFW Diagnostic Auditory Discrimination Test	Goldman et al (1974)	3 years–adult	Monosyllabic words presented in quiet	Tape[4]	Point to one of two pictures	Included in manual, based on age
WIPI	Word Intelligibility by Picture Identification	Ross and Lerman (1970; rev. 2004)	4–6 years	Four equivalent lists of 25 monosyllabic words each	Tape or CD[1]	Point to one of six pictures	Papso and Blood (1989), Sanderson-Leepa and Rintelmann (1976)
NU-CHIPS	Northwestern University Children's Perception of Speech	Elliott and Katz (1980)	3–5 years	50 monosyllabic words	Tape or CD[1]	Point to one of four pictures	Included in manual

(continued on next page)

Table 4.44 (Continued)

Code	Test	Author	Recommended Age	Stimuli	Presentation Format	Response	Norms
PSI	Pediatric Speech Intelligibility Test	Jerger and Jerger (1982)	3–6 years	20 monosyllabic words and two sentence formats in two lists of 10 sentences each	Tape or CD[1]	Point to one of five pictures	Jerger and Jerger (1982)
TAC	Test of Auditory Comprehension	Trammel (1981)	4–17 years	Environmental sounds, words, stereotypic messages arranged in 10 subtests	Tape[2]	Point to one of three pictures	Included in manual, based on PTA and age
PBK	Phonetically balanced kindergarten word lists	Haskins (1949)	6–12 years	50 monosyllabic words	Tape or CD[1]	Repeat the words	Sanderson-Leepa and Rintelmann (1976)
BKB SIN	Bamford-Kowal-Bench Speech in Noise	Etymotic Research (2005)	5–14 years	Sentences	CD[7]	Repeat the sentence	Included in manual
HINT-C	Hearing in Noise Test for Children	Nilsson et al (1996)	6–12 years	Sentences	CD[5]	Repeat the sentence	Included in manual
HINT	Hearing in Noise Test	Nilsson et al (1994)	13 years and up	Sentences	CD[5]	Repeat the sentence	Included in manual
Quick SIN	Quick Speech in Noise	Etymotic Research (2001)	12 years and up	Sentences	CD[7]	Repeat the sentence	Included in manual

Abbreviation	Name	Reference	Age	Material	Format	Task	Source
PAL PB 50	Psychoacoustics Laboratory phonetically balanced 50-word lists	Eagan (1948)	12 years and up	Monosyllabic words	Tape or CD[1]	Repeat the words	Yellin et al (1989)
CID W-22	Central Institute for the Deaf W-22	Hirsh et al (1952)	12 years and up	Monosyllabic words	Tape or CD[1]	Repeat the words	Yellin et al (1989)
NU-6	Northwestern University 6	Tillman and Carhart (1966)	12 years and up	Monosyllabic words	Tape or CD[1]	Repeat the words	Dubno et al (1995)
SPIN	Revised Speech Perception in Noise	Bilger et al (1984)	12 years and up	High- and low-predictability sentences	Tape[3]	Repeat the final word of the sentence	Included in manual
SSI	Synthetic Sentence Identification	Speaks and Jerger (1965)	12 years and up	Sentences that do not convey meaning	Tape or CD[1,6]	Identify the sentence from a list of ten	Jerger (1973)

Abbreviations: ANSI, American National Standards Institute; ASHA, American Speech-Language-Hearing Association; CD, compact disc; PTA, pure-tone average.

[1]Available from Auditec of St. Louis, 2515 South Big Bend Boulevard, St. Louis, MO 63143; 314-781-8890, http://www/auditec.com.

[2]Portions are available from Forewords Publications, Box 82289, Portland, OR; 503-653-2614; http://www.foreworks.com/fore.html.

[3]Available from University of Illinois, Department of Speech and Hearing Science, 901 South Sixth Street, Champaign, IL 61820; 217-333-2230.

[4]Available from American Guidance Service, 4201 Woodland Road, Circle Pines, MN 55014-1796; 800-328-2560.

[5]Available from Bio-logic Systems Corp, One Bio-logic Plaza, Mundelein, IL 60060; 800-272-8075; www.blsc.com/hearing/hint.html.

[6]Comparable materials in Spanish and French are available from Auditec of St. Louis, 2515 South Big Bend Boulevard, St. Louis, MO 63143; 314-781-8890; http://www/auditec.com.

[7]Available from: Etymotic Research, Inc., 61 Martin Lane, Elk Grove Village, IL 60007; www.etymotic.com.

Source: Roeser, R.J., Valente, M., Hosford-Dunn, H (2007), *Audiology Diagnosis*, 2nd ed. New York: Thieme. Reprinted by permission.

Table 4.45 Diagnostic significance of speech audiometry*

Hearing Status	SRT	WRS (NU-6 Lists)	SRS (SSI)	PBmax vs. SSImax	PI Function	UCL for Speech
Normal hearing	SRT ± 10 dB = PTA	88% or higher on 25-word list presented at 30 dB above SRT	100% at MCR of 0 dB	PBmax = SSImax	No decline > 20% in performance as intensity is increased	UCL – SRT > 100 dB
Conductive hearing loss	SRT ± 10 dB = PTA	88% or higher on 25-word list presented at 30 dB above SRT	100% at MCR of 0 dB	PBmax = SSImax	No decline > 20% in performance as intensity is increased	UCL – SRT > 100 dB
Cochlear hearing loss	SRT ± 10 dB = PTA	Reduced re: that expected for PTA	Flat: Reduced by same degree as WRS sloping: reduced by same degree as WRS	Flat: PBmax = SSImax Rising: PBmax – SSImax = 2% Sloping 2 kHz: PBmax = SSImax Sloping 1 kHz: PBmax – SSImax = –12% Sloping 0.5 kHz: PBmax – SSImax = –20%	No decline > 20% in performance as intensity is increased	UCL – SRT < 100 dB Recruitment

Retrocochlear hearing loss	SRT ± 10 dB = PTA	Disproportionately low re: that expected for PTA	Eighth nerve: rollover-decline in PI function > 20% on affected side Central: rollover can be present on side opposite lesion	Eighth nerve: PBmax = SSImax Central: PBmax − SSImax > 2% in the side opposite the lesion	Eighth nerve: rollover-decline in PI function > 20% on affected side Central: rollover can be present on side opposite lesion	UCL − SRT < 100 dB Derecruitment
Presbycusis	SRT ± 10 dB = PTA	Disproportionately low re: that expected for PTA	Reduced usually more than PBmax	PBmax − SSImax > 10%	Rollover: decline in PI function > 20%	UCL − SRT < 100 dB

Abbreviations: MCR, message-to-competition ratio; NU-6, Northwestern University 6; PBmax, highest score on phonetically balanced word list; PI, performance intensity; PTA, pure-tone average; SRS, sentence recognition score; SRT, speech recognition threshold; SSImax, highest score on Synthetic Sentence Identification in the ipsilateral competing condition at 0 dB message-to-competition ratio; UCL, uncomfortable loudness level; WRS, word recognition score.

*Classifications based on Thornton and Raffin (1978), Dubno et al (1995), Jerger and Jerger (1971), Jerger and Hayes (1977), and Jerger et al (1978).

Source: Roeser, R.J., Valente, M., Hosford-Dunn, H. (2007), *Audiology Diagnosis,* 2nd ed. New York: Thieme. Reprinted by permission.

Table 4.46 Comparison of test instruments to assess speech recognition in the communication system

Test	Signal	Masker	Procedure	Items	Test	Results
NST	Male voice, CVs or VCs with carrier phrase	Edited cafeteria noise	Fixed level; closed set	91 items organized into 11 subsets of 7 to 9 syllables	1 set unaided and aided (182 syllables)	Percent correct; auditory feature matrix
NU-6 and CID W-22	CVCs with carrier phrase	Optional, not standardized	Fixed level; open set	50 items, phonemically balanced word lists	1 list unaided and 1 list aided (100 words)	Percent correct
SPIN	Male voice, last word in sentence	12-talker babble	Fixed level; can vary SNR	50 sentences per list; both low- and high-probability lists	1 list unaided and aided (100 key words)	Percent correct
SSI	Male voice, synthetic sentences	Male voice, single talker	Fixed level varying SNR; closed set	10 sentences per list	3 lists unaided and four lists aided (70 sentences)	PI functions in noise
SIN	Female voice, IEEE sentences	4-talker babble	4 SNR (0, +5, +10, +15)	5 sentences with 5 key words per test condition	1 set unaided and aided (200 key words)	PI functions in noise
Quick SIN	Female voice, IEEE sentences	4-talker babble	6 SNR (0, +5, +10, +15, +20, +25)	1 sentence with 5 key words per test condition	1 set unaided and aided (60 key words)	SNR loss (re: normal hearing)
HINT	Male voice, revised Bamford-Kowel-Bench sentences	Noise matched to long-term average spectrum of signal	Adaptive for Reception Threshold for Sentences with masker fixed at 65 dBA	10 phonemically balanced sentences per list; SNR	2 lists unaided and aided (40 sentences)	SNR for 50% correct in noise
CST	Female voice, continuous speech	6-talker babble	Fixed-level presentation	25 key words in 10 sentences per passage	2 passages unaided and aided (100 key words)	Percent correct (RAU)

Abbreviations: CID, Central Institute for the Deaf; CST, Connected Speech Test; CV, consonant-vowel; CVC, consonant-vowel-consonant; dBA, decibel average; HINT, Hearing in Noise Test; IEEE, Institute of Electrical and Electronics Engineers; NST, nonsense syllable test; NU, Northwestern University; PI, performance intensity; Quick SIN, quick speech-in-noise test; RAU, rationalized arcsine unit; SIN, speech-in-noise test; SNR, signal-to-noise ratio; SPIN, Speech Perception in Noise; SSI, Synthetic Sentence Identification; VC, vowel-consonant.

Source: Valente, M., Hosford-Dunn, H., Roeser, R.J. (2008), *Audiology Treatment*, 2nd ed. New York: Thieme. Reprinted by permission.

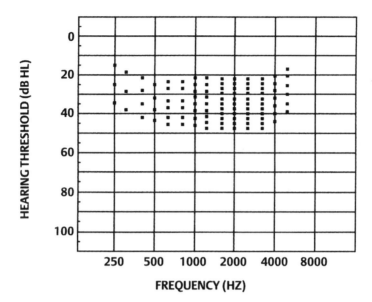

Fig. 4.11 Count-the-dot audiogram. HL, hearing level. (Adapted from Mueller, H.G., and Killion, M.C. (1990). An easy method for calculating the articulation index. Ear and Hearing, 43, 14–17. Baltimore: Lippincott Williams & Wilkins. Reprinted by permission.)

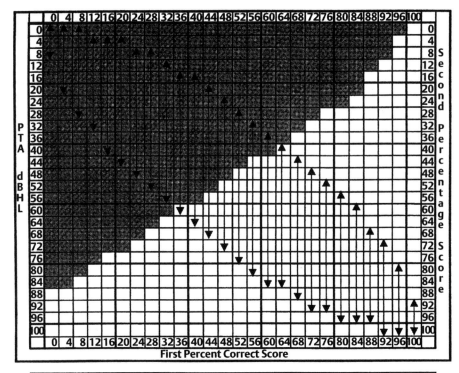

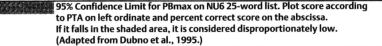

95% Confidence Limit for PBmax on NU6 25-word list. Plot score according to PTA on left ordinate and percent correct score on the abscissa. If it falls in the shaded area, it is considered disproportionately low. (Adapted from Dubno et al., 1995.)

95% Critical differences for 25-word list. Plot first and second score according to the abscissa and right ordinate. If it falls within the arrow, the two scores are not significantly different. (Adapted from Thornton & Raffin, 1978.)

Fig. 4.12 Speech Recognition Interpretation (SPRINT) chart for 25-word NU-6 lists. HL, hearing level; PTA, pure-tone average. (Copyright Linda M. Thibodeau. Reprinted by permission.)

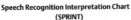

Speech Recognition Interpretation Chart
(SPRINT)

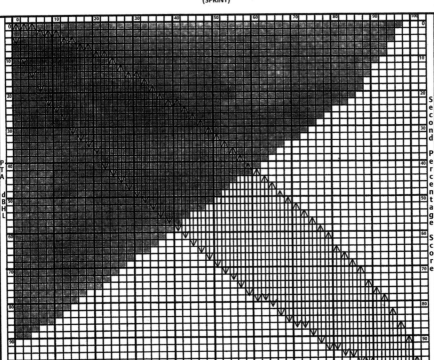

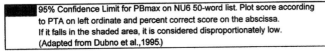

95% Confidence Limit for PBmax on NU6 50-word list. Plot score according to PTA on left ordinate and percent correct score on the abscissa. If it falls in the shaded area, it is considered disproportionately low. (Adapted from Dubno et al., 1995.)

95% Critical differences for 50-word list. Plot first and second score according to the abscissa and right ordinate. If it falls within the arrow, the two scores are not significantly different. (Adapted from Thornton & Raffin, 1978.)

Fig. 4.13 Speech Recognition Interpretation (SPRINT) chart for 50-word NU-6 lists. HL, hearing level; PTA, pure-tone average. (Copyright Linda M. Thibodeau. Reprinted by permission.)

Table 4.47 Auditec Northwestern University/NU-6 binaural fusion speech test: Normative data for adult subjects*

Test	Left Ear— Low Frequency; Right Ear— High Frequency	Right Ear— Low Frequency; Left Ear— High Frequency	Left Ear— Both Bands	Right Ear— Both Bands
Form A mean	81.5	83.2	77.8	76.9
SD	8.9	7.5	9.8	9.9
Range	66–92	66–94	58–92	48–88

Abbreviation: SD, standard deviation.

*Wilson, L. and Mueller, H.G. (1984), Performance of normal hearing individuals on Auditec filtered speech tests. *Asha* (abstract).

Source: Mueller, H.G. and Bright, K.E. Monosyllabic procedures in central testing. In: Kate, J. (ed.), *Handbook of Clinical Audiology*, 4th ed., 1994, page 227. Baltimore: Lippincott Williams & Wilkins. Reprinted by permission.

Table 4.48 Auditec NU-6 filtered-speech tests: Normative data for adult subjects*

Test		List 1	List 2	List 3	List 4
500 Hz	Mean	46.1	49.9	40.6	43.9
(Form A)	SD	13.3	12.0	12.1	10.5
	Range	26–76	20–66	8–64	8–64
750 Hz	Mean	78.4	75.2	74.0	79.3
(Form B)	SD	10.2	12.0	13.2	11.9
	Range	64–100	50–94	48–94	52–94
1,000 Hz	Mean	89.3	91.5	93.3	91.0
(Form C)	SD	7.1	5.8	5.0	6.4
	Range	68–100	76–100	80–100	76–100

Abbreviation: SD, standard deviation.

*Wilson, L. and Mueller, H.G. (1984), Performance of normal hearing individuals on Auditec filtered speech tests. *Asha* (abstract).

Source: Mueller, H.G. and Bright, K.E. Monosyllabic procedures in central testing. In: Kate, J. (ed.), *Handbook of Clinical Audiology*, 4th ed., 1994, page 224. Baltimore: Lippincott Williams & Wilkins. Reprinted by permission.

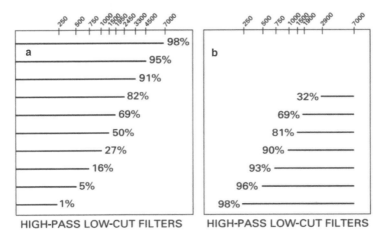

Fig. 4.14a,b Maximum discrimination for syllable articulation for high-pass filter conditions as related to the cutoff frequency. The discrimination scores were derived from the curves of French and Steinberg (1947) at an orthotelephonic gain of +10 dB (75 dB SPL). ([a] From French, N.R., and Steinberg, J.C., (1947) Factors governing the intelligibility of speech sounds. *J. Acoust. Soc. Am.* 19:90–119. [b] From Goetzinger C.P., Word discrimination testing. In: J. Katz (ed.), *Handbook of Clinical Audiology*, 2nd ed. Baltimore: Williams & Wilkins, 1978.)

Table 4.49 Speech intelligibility/recognition test materials, procedures, and guidelines

Type of Stimuli	Investigator (Year)	Task	Name	Items per List	Alternate Forms	Commercial Recordings Available for Purchase
Monosyllables						
Open-set	Fry and Kerridge (1939)	Word or phoneme recognition	Word Tests for Deaf People	25	5	No
	Egan (1948)	Word recognition	PAL PB-50	50	20	Yes
	Hirsh et al (1952)	Word recognition	CID-W-22	50	4	Yes
	Lehiste and Peterson (1959)	Word recognition	CNC Lists	50	10	No
	Fry (1961)	Word recognition or phoneme recognition	Fry Lists	35	10	Yes
	Tillman and Carhart (1966)	Word recognition	NU-6	50	4	Yes
	Boothroyd (1968)	Word recognition or phoneme recognition	Short Isophonemic Word Lists	10	15	No
	Beykirch and Gaeth (1978)	Number, letter, word recognition	Speech Discrimination Scale	8 numbers/16 letters and words	—	No
Closed-set	Fairbanks (1958)	Initial consonant identification	Rhyme Test	50	5	No
	House et al (1965)	Initial and final consonants identification	Modified Rhyme Test	50	6	No
	Griffiths (1967)	Initial and final consonants identification	Rhyming Minimal Contrast	50	5	No
	Kruel et al (1968)	Initial and final consonants identification in filtered noise	Modified Rhyme Test	50	6	Yes
	Schultz and Schubert (1969)	Initial and final consonants identification	Multiple Choice Discrimination Test (MCDT)	50	4	Yes (CID W-22)

	Task	Test	Items		
Pederson and Studebaker (1972)	Initial and final consonants/vowel identification	Oklahoma University Closed Response Speech Test	80/64	5	No
Owens and Schubert (1977)	Initial and final consonants identification	California Consonant Test	100	2	Yes
McPherson and Pang-Ching (1979)	Initial and final consonants identification	Distinctive Feature Discrimination Test	50	4	No
Wilson and Antablin (1980)	Word/picture identification	Picture Identification Task	50	4	Yes
Sentences					
Open-set					
Fry and Kerridge (1939)	Repeat sentences	Sentence Tests for Deaf People	25 sentences/100 words	5	No
McFarlan (1945)	Repeat sentences	Nonsense Sentences			No
Silverman and Hirsh (1955)	Repeat sentences	CID Everyday Sentences	10 sentences/50 key words	10	Yes
Kalikow et al (1977)	Repeat last word in sentence	Speech Perception in Noise Test (SPIN)	50	8	No[a]
Fry (1961)	Repeat sentences	Fry Revised Sentences	25 sentences/100 words	10	Yes
Closed-set					
Bilger (1984)	Repeat last word in sentence	Revised SPIN Test	50	8	No[a]
Speaks and Jerger (1965)	Identify sentence from printed list	Synthetic Sentence Identification (SSI)	10	24	Yes
Closed-set					
Berger(1969)	Select key word among five choices	KSU Speech Discrimination	13	8	Yes
Sergeant et al (1981)	Identify three individual words	Naval Submarine Medical Research Laboratory Tri-Test of Intelligibility	150	3	No[a]

(continued on next page)

Table 4.49 (Continued)

Type of Stimuli	Investigator (Year)	Task	Name	Items per List	Alternate Forms	Commercial Recordings Available for Purchase
Nonsense syllable						
Open-set	Edgerton and Danhauer (1979)	Bisyllable or phoneme recognition	NST	25	2	Yes
Closed-set	Resnick (1976)	Initial and final consonants identification	CUNY NST	7 or 9	7	Yes
	Feeney and Franks (1982)	Middle consonant identification	Distinctive Feature Difference	13	1	No

Source: Hearing Assessment, by W.F. Rintelmann, 1991, Austin, TX: PRO-ED. Copyright 1991 by PRO-ED, Inc. Reprinted by permission.
[a]Contact authors for information regarding availability of tape recordings.

Table 4.50 Speech intelligibility/recognition test materials: Summary for children

Test Name	Investigator	Material	Number of Lists	Items per List	Response Format	Response Task	Age Range	Commercially Available?
Children's lists								
1. PBK-50	Haskins (1949)	Monosyllables	4	50	Open-set	Verbal	6–9 years	No
2. Discrimination by Identification of Pictures (DIP)	Siegenthaler and Haspiel (1966)	Monosyllables	3	48	Closed-set (2-picture matrix)	Psychomotor	2 years, 10 months–8 years, 3 months	Yes
3. Word Intelligibility by Picture Identification (WIPI)	Ross and Lerman (1970)	Monosyllables	4	25	Closed-set (6-picture matrix)	Psychomotor	3–6 years	Yes
4. Goldman-Fristoe-Woodstock Test of Auditory Discrimination (GFW)	Goldman, Fristoe, and Woodcock (1970)	Monosyllables	1	30	Closed-set (4-picture matrix)	Psychomotor	≥ 4 years	Yes
5. Sound Effects Recognition Test (SERT)	Finitzo-Hieber et al (1980)	Environmental sounds	3	10	Closed-set (4-picture matrix)	Psychomotor	≥ 3 years	Yes
6. Spondee Recognition Test	Erber (1974)	Spondees	1	25	Closed-set	Written	8–16 years	No
7. WIPI Sentences	Weber and Redell (1976)	Sentences	4		Closed-set (6-picture matrix)	Psychomotor	3–6 years	No
8. Five Sound Test	Ling (1978)	Vowels /u/, /a/, /i/, /ʃ/, /s/	1	5	Open-set	Psychomotor	Infants/children	No
9. Perception of Words and Word Patterns	Erber and Witt (1977)	Monosyllables, spondees, and trochees	3	10	Closed-set	Psychomotor and verbal	9–13 years	No

(continued on next page)

Table 4.50 (Continued)

Test Name	Investigator	Material	Number of Lists	Items per List	Response Format	Response Task	Age Range	Commercially Available?
10. Children's Perception of Speech (CHIPS)	Katz and Elliott (1978)	Monosyllables	4[a]	50	Closed-set	Psychomotor	≥ 3 years	No
11. Synthetic Sentence Identification of Children (SSIC)	Wilson (1978)	Synthetic sentences	10[a]	1.0	Closed-set	Verbal	≥ 7 years	No
12. BKB Sentences	Bench, Koval, and Bamford (1979)	Sentences	21 / 11	16 / 16	Open-set	Verbal	8–15 years	No
13. Auditory Numbers Test (ANT)	Erber (1980)	Numbers	1	5	Closed-set	Psychomotor	3–8 years	No
14. Pediatric Speech Intelligibility Test	Jerger et al (1980)	Monosyllables and sentences	1 / 2	20 / 10	Closed-set	Verbal	3–10 years	No

[a]Source: *Principles of Speech Audiometry*, by D.F. Kindle and W.F. Rintelmann, 1983, Austin, TX: PRO-ED. Copyright 1983 by PRO-ED, Inc. Reprinted by permission.

Table 4.51 Speech reception threshold (SRT) procedures: Guidelines

Investigator	Method	Initial Trial				Threshold Search				Threshold Criterion
		Starting Level	Words per Level	Step Size (dB)	Termination	Starting Level	Words per Level	Step Size (dB)	Termination	
Hudgins et al (1947) PAL No. 9	Descending					<24 dB above expected threshold	6	4	Administer at least 2 lists; if thresholds within 4 dB terminate tests; if not, continue	Count words correct and consult table for dB equivalent Subtract from starting point, and average for 2 lists
Hirsh et al (1952)	Descending					<33 dB above expected threshold	3	3	Not stated	Subtract number of words correct from starting level and add 1.5 dB for 50% criterion
Newby (1958)	Descending and bracketing	15 to 20 dB above estimated threshold	3–4	5		Bracketing around level at which words were missed	1–2		Not stated	Level at which about half of spondees missed
Jerger et al (1959)	Descending and bracketing	20 to 30 dB above estimated threshold	2–3	10	Level at which 2 consecutive words were missed	Bracketing around level at which words were missed	4	2	Not stated	Lowest level at which 2 out of 4 words are repeated correctly, or level at which 3 out of 4 are correct if next lower level yields only 1 out of 4 correct

(continued on next page)

Table 4.51 (Continued)

Investigator	Method	Initial Trial				Threshold Search				
		Starting Level	Words per Level	Step Size (dB)	Termination	Starting Level	Words per Level	Step Size (dB)	Termination	Threshold Criterion
Chaiklin (1959)	Descending		5	5	Level at which 1 word was missed	5 to 6 dB above level at which word is missed in initial descent	3–6	2	When 4 words are missed at each of 3 consecutive levels	Lowest level at which 3 out of possible 6 words are repeated correctly (threshold search repeated 3 times)
Chaiklin and Ventry (1964)	Descending	25 dB above 2-frequency pure-tone average	1	5	Level at which 1 word was missed	10 dB above level at which in initial descent	3–6	5	When 4 words are missed at 2 consecutive levels	Lowest level at which 3 out of 6 possible words are repeated correctly
Chaiklin and Ventry (1964)	Descending	25 dB above 2-frequency pure-tone average	1	5	Level at which 1 word was missed	5 to 6 dB above level at which word is missed in initial descent	2–4	2	When 3 words are missed at 3 consecutive levels, or no words are repeated correctly at 2 consecutive levels	Lowest level at which 2 out of 4 possible words are repeated correctly

Chaiklin, Font, and Dixon (1967)	Ascending	−10 dB HL	1	10	Level at which 1 word was repeated correctly	Decrease 20 dB below level at which 1 word is repeated correctly	3–6	5	Level at which 3 out of possible 6 words are repeated correctly	Lowest level at which 3 out of 6 possible words are repeated correctly
Hopkinson (1972)	Descending and bracketing	20 dB above 1,000-Hz threshold	1	2	Level at which words missed		Varies	159	Not stated	2 dB above lowest level at which any word is repeated
Tillman and Olsen (1973)	Descending	30 to 40 dB above expected threshold	1–2	10	Level at which 2 consecutive words are missed	10 dB above level at which 2 words are missed in initial descent	2	2	If less than 5 of 6 words are repeated correctly in first 3 steps, increase level 4 to 6 dB and begin new descent; terminate when 5 of 6 consecutive words are missed	Subtract number of words repeated correctly from starting level, and add 1 dB for 50% criterion

(continued on next page)

Table 4.51 (Continued)

Investigator	Method	Initial Trial				Threshold Search				
		Starting Level	Words per Level	Step Size (dB)	Termination	Starting Level	Words per Level	Step Size (dB)	Termination	Threshold Criterion
Wilson, Morgan, and Dirks (1973)	Descending	30 to 40 dB above expected threshold	1–2	10	Level at which 2 words are missed	10 dB above level at which 2 words are missed	2 or 5	2 or 5	If less than 5 of 6 words in first 3 steps (2 dB/ step) or less than all 5 words (5 dB/ step) are repeated correctly, increase level 4 to 10 dB and begin new descent; terminate when 5 of 6 words (2 dB/ step) or all 5 words (5 dB/ step) are missed	Subtract number of words repeated correctly from starting level, and add 1 dB (2 dB/ step) or 2 dB (5 dB/ step) for 50% criterion

Study	Approach	Starting level								
Martin and Stauffer (1975)	Descending	50 dB HL unless incorrect response, then increase in 20-dB steps	1–2	10	Same procedure as used in Tillman and Olsen	16 dB above level at which 2 words are missed in initial descent	2	Same procedure and criteria as used in Tillman and Olsen	2	Same procedure and criteria as used in Tillman and Olsen
ASHA (1977)	Ascending	–10 dB HL	1	10	Level at which 1 word is repeated correctly	15 dB below level at which 1 word is repeated correctly in initial ascent	4	Level at which at least 3 words are repeated correctly; repeat again, beginning 10 dB below level at which at least 3 words are repeated correctly; repeat above process a third time	5	Lowest level at which of words are repeated correctly in minimum of 2 ascending series
ASHA (1988)	Descending	30–40 dB	1–2	10	Level at which 2 consecutive words are missed	10 dB above level at which 2 words were missed	2 or 5	Same procedure and criteria as used in Wilson, Morgan, and Dirks	2 or 5	Same procedure and criteria as used in Wilson, Morgan, and Dirks

Abbreviation: PAL, Harvard Psychoacoustic Lab, Auditory Test # 9.
Source: Rintelmann, W.F. *Hearing Assessment*, 2nd ed. © 1991. Reprinted by permission of Pearson Education, Inc., Upper Saddle River, NJ.

Middle Ear Measures

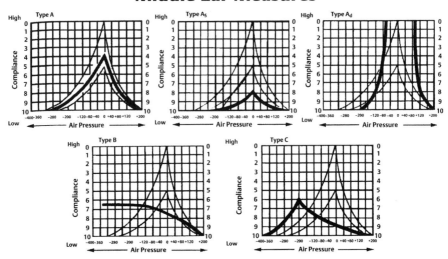

Fig. 4.15   The classic classification of tympanograms (after Jerger, 1970). (From Roeser, R.J., Valente, M., Hosford-Dunn, H. (2007), *Audiology Diagnosis,* 2nd ed. New York: Thieme. Reprinted by permission.)

Table 4.52 Tympanogram types and their description using the classic and absolute systems

Tympanogram Type	Compliance (mL)	Static Admittance	Peak Pressure (daPa)	Clinical Audiologic Findings
Type A	0.4 to 1.5	0.27 to 2.8	+50 to −150	Represents normal middle ear function; the peak (point of maximum compliance) occurs within normal static admittance limits and at pressures between +50 to −150 mm H_2O
Type A_s	0.4 to 1.5	<0.27	+50 to −150	Represents abnormal stiffness in the middle ear system, resulting in a fixation of the ossicular chain as in otosclerosis; static admittance measures are abnormally low
Type A_d	0.4 to 1.5	>2.8	+50 to −150	Represents a flaccid tympanic membrane resulting from scar tissue or a possible disarticulation of the middle ear ossicles; compliance measures are abnormally high
Type B (perf)	>1.5	<0.27	No peak	Represents some pathological condition exists in the middle ear; static compliance (admittance) measures are abnormally low, but initial compliance values are high
Type B (o.m.)	<0.4	<0.27	No peak	Represents restricted tympanic membrane mobility and would indicate that some pathological condition exists in the middle ear; static compliance measures are abnormally low
Type C	0.4 to 1.5	0.27 to 2.8	−200 or worse	Represents significant negative pressure in the middle ear cavity (considered significant for treatment when more negative than −200 mm H_2O); this may indicate a precursor or resolution of otitis media; compliance measures are usually within normal limits

Abbreviations: o.m., otitis media; perf, perforation.
Source: Roeser, R.J., Valente, M., Hosford-Dunn, H. (2007). *Audiology Diagnosis*, 2nd ed. New York: Thieme. Reprinted by permission.

Table 4.53   Normative values: Vector tympanometry

	Peak Y (mmho or cm³)		V_{ec} (cm³)		TW (daPa)	
	Mean	90% range	Mean	90% range	Mean	90% range
Children	0.5	0.2–0.9	0.7	0.4–1.0	100	60–150
Adults	0.8	0.3–1.4	1.1	0.6–1.5	80	50–110

Source: American Speech-Language-Hearing Association (ASHA). (1990), Guidelines for screening for hearing impairment and middle-ear disorders. Asha (Suppl. 2)32:17–24. Reprinted by permission.

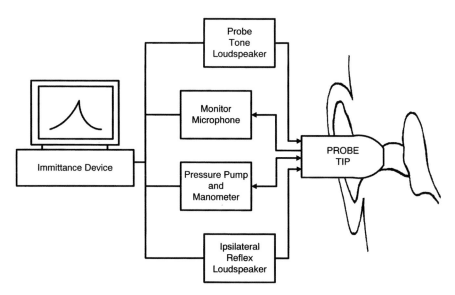

Fig. 4.16   Block diagram of the major components of a clinical acoustic immittance device. (From Gelfand, S.A. (2001), *Essentials of Audiology,* 2nd ed. New York: Thieme. Reprinted by permission.)

Acoustic Reflex Arc

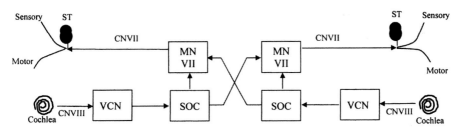

Fig. 4.17 Schematic of the acoustic reflex neural pathways. CN VII, seventh cranial nerve; CN VIII, eighth cranial nerve; MNVII, motor nucleus of the seventh cranial nerve; SOC, superior olivary complex; ST, stapedius muscle; VCN, ventral cochlear nucleus. (From Clark, JL, Roeser, RJ, Mendrygal, M (2007). Middle Ear Measures. In Roeser, RJ, Valente, MH, Hosford-Dunn, H (Eds). *Audiology Diagnosis*, 2nd ed. New York: Thieme. Reprinted by permission.)

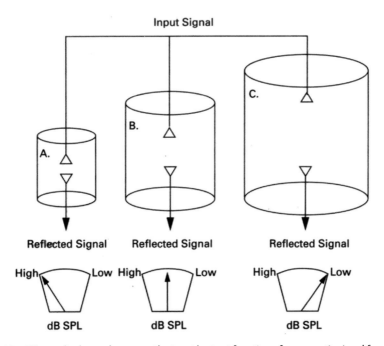

Fig. 4.18 Effects of volume change on the input/output function of an acoustic signal for a small cavity (A), a medium cavity (B), and a large cavity (C). (From Clark, JL, Roeser, RJ, Mendrygal, M (2007). Middle Ear Measures. In Roeser, RJ, Valente, MH, Hosford-Dunn, H (Eds). *Audiology Diagnosis*, 2nd ed. New York: Thieme. Reprinted by permission.)

Table 4.54 **The mean (or median) contralateral, 226-Hz acoustic-reflex thresholds (dB HL re: ANSI–1969 or ISO–1964 for the pure-tone activators and dB SPL re: 20 μPa for the broadband noise activators) from seven studies**

Study, Number of Subjects, Type of Statistic, and Standard Deviation (SD)	Reflex-Activator Signal (Hz)					
	250	500	1,000	2,000	4,000	Noise
Anderson and Wedenberg, 1968						
N = 200, median	84.2	87.4	85.6	85.5	90.7	
Chiveralls, 1977						
N = 100, median	89.9					
N = 200, median		83.6	82.8	81.5	82.8	
Gelfand and Piper, 1981						
N = 12, mean		81.5	82.4	83.1		76.2
SD		(4.2)	(5.2)	(4.9)		(6.5)
Handler and Margolis, 1977						
N = 17, mean		82.5	83.0	83.0	86.5	75.0
SD		(6.1)	(5.1)	(5.2)	(9.0)	(8.4)
Osterhammel and Osterhammel, 1979						
N = 65, mean		90.1	90.2	89.8	93.8	
Peterson and Liden, 1972[a]						
N = 88, mean	84.6	85.2	85.4	84.0	84.4	
SD	(7.1)	(7.0)	(6.7)	(5.5)	(7.2)	
Wilson, 1981						
N = 18, mean	78.8	79.4	82.8	82.1	83.3	71.7
SD	(6.3)	(4.7)	(4.5)	(4.6)	(5.9)	(8.6)

[a]800 Hz probe, ascending, amplitude measurement.

Table 4.55 **Comparison of crossed and uncrossed acoustic reflex patterns as a function of probe and stimulus reference ear**

Reflex Pattern	Reference Ear Probe		Stimulus		Consistent with
	R	L	R	L	
Crossed	□	□	□	□	Normal middle ear function bilaterally
Uncrossed	□	□	□	□	
Crossed	□	■	■	□	Left cranial nerve (CN) VII disorder or mild left
Uncrossed	□	■	□	■	middle ear disorder
Crossed	■	□	□	■	Left CN VIII disorder or severe left cochlear loss
Uncrossed	□	■	□	■	
Crossed	■	■	■	■	Left middle ear disorder, intra-axial brainstem lesion
Uncrossed	□	■	□	■	eccentric to the left, or a combined CN VII and CN VIII disorder
Crossed	■	■	■	■	Extra-axial or intra-axial brainstem disorder having
Uncrossed	□	□	□	□	bilateral effects
Crossed	■	□	□	■	Extra-axial or intra-axial brainstem disorder
Uncrossed	□	□	□	□	eccentric to the left

Note: In the uncrossed condition, patterns are the same for both reference systems; however, crossed patterns change for the two systems
Source: Collier, C. and Roeser, R., unpublished, 2012.

Table 4.56 Tympanometric configuration of some common middle ear pathologies

| | | | Shape | |
Middle Ear Disorder	Pressure Peak	Amplitude	High-Frequency Probe Tone	Low-Frequency robe Tone
Acute serous otitis media	None to severe negative	None to shallow	Flat to slight rising Converging	Flat to falling
Serous otitis resolving	Moderate to negative	Shallow to normal	Normal	Normal
"Glue" ear	Moderate to severe negative	Flat to shallow	Flat	Flat to falling
Cholesteatoma	Normal-negative to absent	Nonshallow	Converging Flattened Converging	Lower at negative pressure
Acute otitis media	Positive	Normal	Normal	Normal
Blocked eustachian tube	Mild to moderate negative	Normal	Normal	Normal
Glomus tumor	Nonnormal	Extremely shallow	Vascular perturbations	Vascular perturbations
Otosclerosis	Normal	Shallow	Normal	Normal
Malleolar fixation	Normal	Shallow	Normal	Normal
Incudostapedial interruption	Normal	Large	Peaked to normal	Deep notches, peaked and undulating
Crural interruption	Normal	Large	Peaked to normal	Deep notches, peaked and undulating
Healed TM perforation	Normal	Large	Normal to peaked	Notch to peaked
Perforated TM	None	Elevated baseline	Flat	Flat
Stapedectomy	Normal	Large	Normal	Notched and undulating

Abbreviation: TM, tympanic membrane.
Source: Feldman, A.S. and Wilber, L.A. *Acoustic Impedance and Admittance—The Measurement of Middle Ear Function.* Baltimore: Lippincott Williams & Wilkins, 1976. Reprinted by permission.

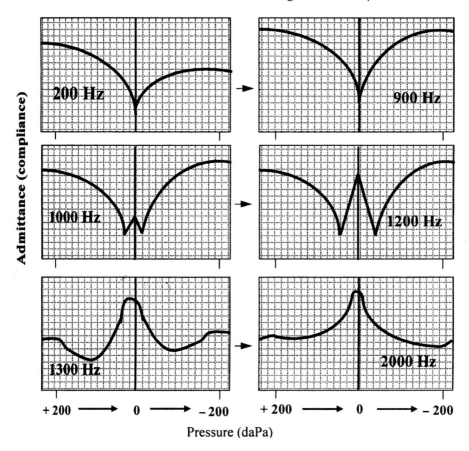

Fig. 4.19 Multifrequency tympanometry recordings. (From Clark, JL, Roeser, RJ, Mendrygal, M (2007). Middle Ear Measures. In Roeser, RJ, Valente, MH, Hosford-Dunn, H (Eds). *Audiology Diagnosis*, 2nd ed. New York: Thieme. Reprinted by permission.)

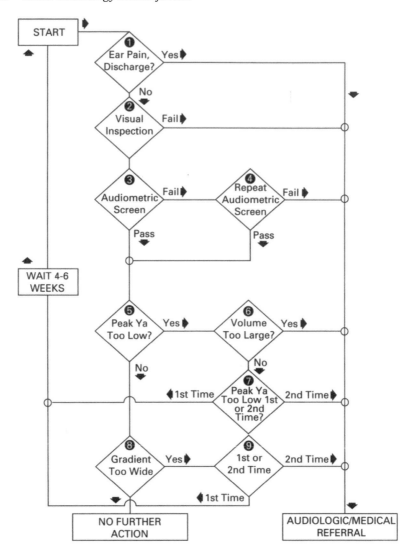

Fig. 4.20 Flowchart for determining audiological/medical referral for hearing and middle ear screening. (From American Speech-Language-Hearing Association (ASHA) (1990), Guidelines for screening for hearing impairments and middle-ear disorders. *Asha* 32(Suppl 2):17–24. Reprinted by permission.)

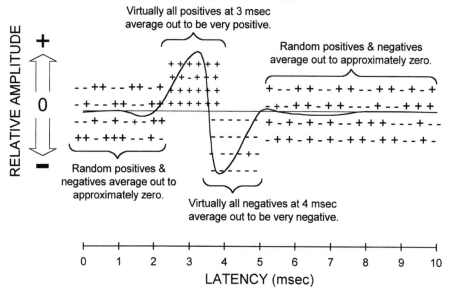

Fig. 4.21 Illustration of the averaging concept. (From Gelfand, S.A. (2009), *Essentials of Audiology*, 3rd ed. New York: Thieme. Reprinted by permission.)

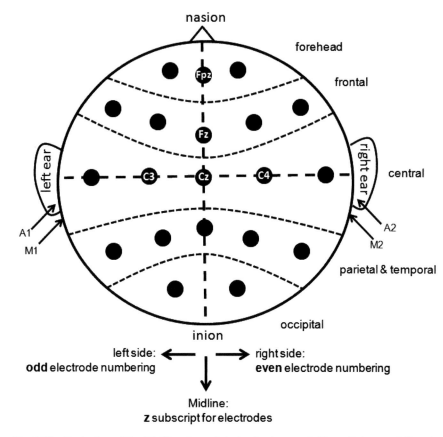

Fig. 4.22 Illustration of the 10–20 system of electrode placement. (From Atcherson, S.R. and Stoody, T.M. (2012), *Auditory Electrophysiology*. New York: Thieme. Reprinted by permission.)

Table 4.57 Typical findings for electroacoustic and electrophysiological measures across categories of hearing loss or auditory disorder

| Test | *Type of Hearing Loss or Auditory Disorder* | | | |
| | *Conductive* | *Neural* | *APD* | |

Test	Conductive	Neural	APD
Immittance				
Tymp	Abnormal	Normal	Normal	Normal
AR	Absent or abnormal	Abnormal or absent	Absent or abnormal	Normal (contra-lateral may be abnormal)
OAE	Absent or abnormal	Abnormal or absent	Normal or absent	Normal
ECochG				
SP	Abnormal	Abnormal or absent	Present	Normal
CM	Abnormal or absent	Abnormal or absent	Present	Normal
AP	Abnormal	Present or abnormal	Absent	Normal
ABR	Abnormal (i.e., elevated threshold, delayed latency)	Abnormal (i.e., elevated threshold)	Absent or abnormal	Normal (speech evoked ABR may be abnormal)
ASSR	Abnormal (i.e., elevated threshold)	Abnormal (i.e., elevated threshold)	Absent or abnormal (i.e., elevated threshold)	Normal

Abbreviations: ABR, auditory brainstem response; AP, action potential; APD, auditory processing disorder; AR, acoustic reflex; ASSR, auditory steady-state response; CM, cochlear microphonic; ECochG, electrocochleography; OAE, otoacoustic emission; SP, summating potential; Tymp, tympanic.

Source: Objective Assessment of Hearing (p. 142) by J.W. Hall and D.W. Swanepoel. Copyright © 2010 Plural Publishing, Inc. all rights reserved. Used by permission.

Table 4.58 Classification of human auditory evoked potentials

			Relationship to Stimulus		
Function	Anatomy	Latency	Transient	Steady State	Sustained
Sensory	Cochlear and eighth nerve	First (0–5 milliseconds)	Eighth nerve CAP, ABR waves I,II	Cochlear microphonic	Summating potential
	Brainstem	Fast (2–20 milliseconds)	ABR (waves III, IV, V)	FFR, > 60-Hz ASSR	Pedestal of FFR
	Early cortical	Middle (10–100 milliseconds)	Middle-latency AEP (MLAEP: Na, Pa, Nb)	–40-Hz ASSR	
	Cortical	Slow (50–300 milliseconds)	Slow "vertex" potential (P1, N1, P2, N2)	< 20-Hz ASSR	Cortical sustained potential
Processing Contingent potentials	Cortical	Late (150–1,000 milliseconds)	Mismatch negativity (MMN) Processing negativity (Nd) N2b P3a, P3b N400, P600		CNV

Abbreviations: ABR, auditory brainstem response; AEP, auditory evoked potential; ASSR, auditory steady-state response; CAP, compound action potential; CNV, contingent negative variation; FFR: frequency following response; MLAEP, middle latency auditory evoked potential.

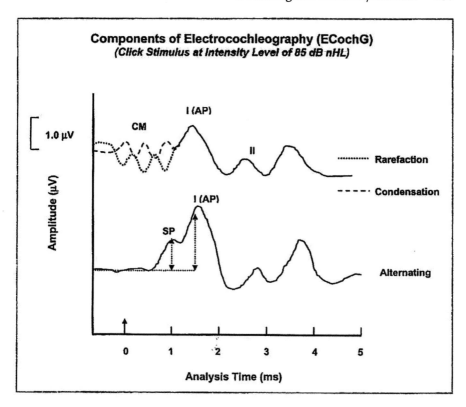

Fig. 4.23 Different electrocochleography (ECochG) components (cochlear microphonic [CM], summating potential [SP], action potential [AP]) can be enhanced with different stimulus polarity conditions (e.g., rarefaction, condensation, or alternating). (From *Objective Assessment of Hearing* (p. 63) by J.W. Hall and D.W. Swanepoel. Copyright © 2010 Plural Publishing, Inc. All rights reserved. Used by permission.)

Table 4.59 Advantages and disadvantages of electrocochleography (ECochG) in the diagnosis of auditory neuropathy (AN) in comparison to other electroacoustic and electrophysiological auditory measures

	Typical test finds in auditory neuropathy	Advantages	Disadvantages
ECochG	• Cochlear potentials are generally present • Different patterns of summating and compound action potentials suggest different sites of lesion • CM present, sometimes enlarged, and may persist for several milliseconds	• Information on multiple anatomic sites (outer hair cells, inner hair cells, eighth CN) • Can differentiate pre- versus postsynaptic auditory neuropathy • Minimally affected by middle ear disease	• No information on central auditory nervous system • Invasive transtympanic EcochG is best for differentiating pre- and postsynaptic lesion
OAEs	• Present OAEs but may disappear over time	• Information on outer hair cell status • Measurement is quick and simple • Common technique in clinical audiology	• No information on structures other than outer hair cells • Not present in middle ear disease • May disappear over time in AN • Not present in middle ear disease
Acoustic reflexes	• Mostly absent but may be elevated in some cases	• Information on multiple anatomic sites (cochlea, eighth CN, auditory brainstem) • Independent of synchronous neural activity • Widely available in audiology clinics	• Not present in middle ear disease
ABR	• Absent at maximum intensities or grossly abnormal neural peaks at elevated intensities (peaks uncorrelated with hearing thresholds) • CM present and inverting with condensation and rarefaction polarity and may persist for several milliseconds	• Information on multiple anatomic sites (cochlea, eighth CN, auditory brainstem) • Important for diagnosis of AN (CM presence and absent or abnormal neural peaks) • Can be recorded in middle ear disease	• May be absent in other disorders
ASSR	• Absent or elevated responses uncorrelated with hearing thresholds	• Sensitive measure of neural activity	• May be absent in other disorders • No clinical role in diagnosing AN at this stage

Abbreviations: ABR, auditory brainstem response; ASSR, auditory steady-state response; CM, cochlear microphonic; CN, cranial nerve; ECochG, electrocochleography; OAE, otoacoustic emissions.

Note. Clinical advantages shared by all electroacoustic and electrophysiological auditory measures are not cited.

Source: Objective Assessment of Hearing (p. 65) by I.W. Hall and D.W. Swanepoel. Copyright © 2010 Plural Publishing, Inc. All rights reserved. Used by permission.

Table 4.60 Classification of auditory evoked potentials

Common Name	Latency Range (msec)	Analysis Method	Physiological Description	Anatomic Generator	Stimulus Response	Exogenous or Endogenous
ECochG (CM, SP, CAP)	0–2	Time	Cochlear, neurogenic	Hair cells, auditory nerve	Steady state, transient	Exogenous
ABR (I, III, V)	1–10	Time	Neurogenic	Auditory nerve, brainstem	Transient	Exogenous
FFR	NA	Time, frequency	Neurogenic	Brainstem	Steady state	Exogenous
MLR (Na, Pa)	15–80	Time	Neurogenic	Subcortical, cortical	Transient	Exogenous
LAEP (or LLR) (P1, N1, P2)	50–250	Time	Neurogenic	Cortical	Transient	Exogenous,* endogenous
MMN	150–300	Time, subtraction	Neurogenic	Cortical	Transient	Exogenous, endogenous*
P300	250–400	Time	Neurogenic	Cortical	Transient	Exogenous, endogenous*
N400	350–500	Time	Neurogenic	Cortical	Transient	Exogenous, endogenous
ASSR (< 20, ~40, > 60 Hz)	10–30	Frequency, phase	Neurogenic	Brainstem, subcortical, cortical	Steady state	Exogenous,* endogenous
VEMP (P1, N1)	12–27	Time	Myogenic	Vestibulocolic reflex	Transient	Exogenous

Abbreviations: ABR, auditory brainstem response; ASSR, auditory steady-state response; CAP, compound action potential; CM, cochlear microphonic; FFR, frequency-following response; LAEP, late auditory evoked potential; LLR, late latency response; MLR, middle latency response; MMN, mismatch negativity; NA, not available; SP, summating potential; VEMP, vestibular evoked myogenic potential
*Predominant classification of the two descriptions.
Source: Atcherson, S.R. and Stoody, T.M. (2012). *Auditory Electrophysiology*. New York: Thieme. Reprinted by permission.

Table 4.61 Parameters to obtain single-channel recording of auditory evoked potential (AEP)

AEP	Stimulus Type	Stimulus Repetition Rate (No./Second)	Preamplification Gain (X)	Low- and High-Pass Filter Settings (Hz)	Averaging Window (Msec)	No. of Samples
SLR						
ECochG[a]	BBC/TB	9–11	20,000–100,000	1 to 10 and 3,000	5–10	1,000 to 2,000
ABR	BBC/TB	11–33	100,000–250,000	30 to 100 and 3,000	10–20	2,000 to 3,000
MLR						
MLR	BBC tone bursts	8–10	50,000–100,000	1 to 20 and 1,000	50–100	1,000 to 2,000
40-Hz SSP	Tone bursts	40	50,000–100,000	1 to 20 and 1,000	50–100	1,000 to 2,000
LLR						
N1-P2	Tone bursts	0.5–1.0	20,000–50,000	1 and 100	500	50 to 100
P300	Two different tone bursts	0.5–1.0	20,000–50,000	1 and 100	500 to 750	100 to 200

Abbreviations: ABR, auditory brainstem response; BBC, broadband click; ECochG, electrocochleography; LLR, late latency response; MLR, middle latency response; SLR, short latency response; SSP, steady-state potential.
[a]Extratympanic.

Source: Ferraro, J.A., and Durrant, J.D. Auditory evoked potentials: Overview and basic principles. In: Kate, J. (ed.), *Handbook of Clinical Audiology*, 4th ed., 1994, page 332. Baltimore: Lippincott Williams & Wilkins. Reprinted by permission.

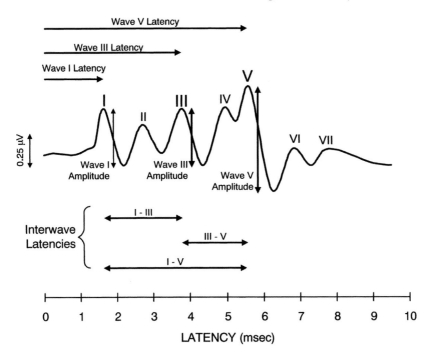

Fig. 4.24 An idealized auditory brainstem response (ABR). Arrows indicate the wave I, II, and III absolute latencies and amplitudes, and the interwave latencies between waves I and V, I and III, and III and V. (From Gelfand, S.A. (2001), *Essentials of Audiology,* 2nd ed. New York: Thieme. Reprinted by permission.)

Table 4.62   Protocol for bone conduction auditory brainstem response (ABR) measurement

Parameter	Selection	Comment
Stimulus parameters		
Bone oscillator	B-70 or B-71	Dedicated for ABR measurement
Type	Click	Tone bursts can also be used
Duration	0.1 millisecond (100 µs)	
Polarity	Alternating	To minimize stimulus artifact
Rate	11.1/sec	Slower if wave I is not clear
Intensity	Variable	Maximum is ~50 dB nHL
Repetitions	Variable	Dependent on signal-to-noise ratio
Masking	Sometimes	Not needed if wave I is present
Mode	Monaural	Always delivered to mastoid
Acquisition parameters		
Electrodes		
Noninverting	Fz	High forehead preferred vs vertex
Inverting	Ai	Ipsilateral earlobe or TIPtrode; two channel electrode array (Fz-Ai and Fz-A2) with contralateral inverting electrode helps to identify wave I
Ground	Fpz	Low forehead is convenient
Filters		
HP (high pass)	30 Hz	Bone conduction ABR contains substantial low frequency energy
LP (low pass)	1,500 or 2,000 Hz	
Notch	None	Notch filter reduces response energy
Amplification	× 100,000	
Analysis Time	15 milliseconds	
Pre-stimulus baseline	–1 millisecond	Inspection of pre-stimulus time to estimate background noise
Sweeps (No. of stimuli)	Variable	Dependent on signal-to-noise ratio

Table 4.63 **A protocol used for measurement of frequency-specific auditory brainstem responses (ABRs)**

Stimulus Parameter	Suggestion	Comment
Transducer	Insert	Insert earphones offer many advantages in clinical ABR measurement, especially with infants and young children.
Polarity	Alternating	Instead of the usual rarefaction polarity, alternating polarity stimuli can be used to minimize the possibility of a frequency following type response.
Ramping	Blackman	Ramping refers to how the rise/fall portions of the tone burst are shaped. Some nonlinear ramping or windowing technique reduce spectral splatter and increase frequency specificity of tone burst stimulation. Blackman windowing is the best, and most current auditory evoked response (AER) systems include it in their stimulus package.
Duration	Variable	The rise/fall and plateau times for the tone burst stimuli vary depending on the frequency. As a rule, it is desirable to use longer times for lower frequencies so as to include more cycles to increase the chance that the stimulus sounds like the desired frequency, and not a click. However, the use of a very brief (0.5 cycles or 2 milliseconds) 250-Hz tone burst will generate a more well-formed and distinct ABR, albeit not quite as frequency specific (an energy band within the frequency range of 100 to 600 Hz). The most common approach for signal duration is to use cycle rise time, 0 cycle plateau, and 2 cycles fall time. or, in milliseconds (ms): • 500 Hz: 4 milliseconds rise/fall and 0 milliseconds plateau • 1,000 Hz: 2 milliseconds rise/fall and 0 milliseconds plateau • 2,000 Hz: 1 millisecond rise/fall and 0 milliseconds plateau • 4,000 Hz: 0.5 millisecond rise/fall and 0 milliseconds plateau

(*continued on next page*)

Table 4.63 *(Continued)*

Stimulus Parameter	Suggestion	Comment
Intensity	Variable	Keep in mind that the intensity levels on the screen for your ABR system will usually not be defined in dB nHL, as they are for a click. More often, the values are in dB SPL. That is, 95 dB may be selected, but the intensity range for the tone burst frequency may go as high as 115 dB. Always obtain behavioral threshold data for each tone burst stimulus to be used for ABR recording (with the earphones specific to the evoked response system and in the room where ABRs will be recorded), and then develop biological normative data for tone-burst intensity. For example, if the maximum dial setting for a 500-Hz tone burst is 115 dB, but normal subjects have an average threshold of 30 dB for this stimulus, then at 115 dB on the dial the intensity level is really 85 dB nHL (referenced to the normal behavioral threshold for the stimulus). With most evoked response systems, these "correction factors" can be incorporated into the intensities displayed on the screen so that all intensity values are in dB nHL according to clinic normative data. It is then advisable to actually record ABRs for this 500-Hz stimulus from a few of these normal-hearing subjects to estimate the lowest intensity level that produces an observable and reliable ABR wave V.

Source: Objective Assessment of Hearing (p. 84) by J.W. Hall and D.W. Swanepoel. Copyright © 2010 Plural Publishing, Inc. All rights reserved. Used by permission.

Table 4.64 **Clinical decisions made from the initial analysis of an auditory brainstem response (ABR) elicited with high- and low-intensity click stimuli**

ABR Pattern	Clinical Decision
Normal latencies and amplitudes	• Record tone burst ABR and or otoacoustic emissions (OAEs) to confirm normal auditory sensitivity • Begin a frequency-specific ABR recording with a 500-Hz tone burst
Delayed wave I latency at high intensity	• Suspect conductive auditory dysfunction • Prepare to record a bone conduction ABR • Consider tympanometry if it has not already been reformed • Consider a referral to otolaryngology
Normal for high intensity but abnormal or absent ABR for low intensity	• Suspect a mild or moderate sensory hearing loss • Estimate auditory thresholds with tone burst signals • Verify sensory auditory dysfunction with OAEs
Abnormal or no ABR for high intensity level	• Suspect severe sensory hearing loss • Record an ABR for the maximum click stimulus intensity level • Consider recording an auditory steady-state response (ASSR)
No clear ABR	• Suspect auditory neuropathy (auditory neuropathy spectrum disorder) • Record an ABR with rarefaction and condensation stimulus polarity • Inspect waveforms for evidence of cochlear microphonic (CM) activity • Record OAEs to verify integrity of outer hair cells

Table 4.65 **Commonly used neurodiagnostic criteria for auditory brainstem response (ABR)**

	Clinical Utility	Comments
Monaural		
Absolute latencies for waves I, III, and V	• Measurement of latency at peak relative to stimulus onset • Wave V latency may be the most useful • 1.5, 3.5, and 5.5 msec, respectively, for waves I, III, and V are commonly used, but gender-specific local norms are ideal • Any absolute latency that exceeds 2 standard deviations is considered diagnostically significant	• Take into account time delay of insert earphones compared with TDH headphones • Wave I usually unaffected by vestibular schwannomas, but can be diminished or absent in the presence of hearing loss • Though debatable, may need to consider prolongations of wave V caused by cochlear hearing loss
Interwave (interpeak) latency interval (IWI) for waves I–III, III–V, and I–V	• Calculate difference between subsequent waves • 2 msec for I–III and III–V and 4 msec for I–V are commonly used, but gender-specific local norms are ideal • Any IWI that exceeds 2 standard deviations is considered diagnostically significant	• Generally better diagnostically than absolute latencies • Depends on wave I presence (which may be absent in cochlear hearing loss)
V/I amplitude ratio	• Divide wave V amplitude by wave I amplitude • < 0.75 is considered diagnostically significant	• Amplitudes can be variable and unreliable • Wave IV/V complexes can be problematic
Binaural		
Interaural latency difference (ILD or IT5) for wave V	• Calculating difference in wave V latency between ears • > 0.3 or 0.4 msec is considered diagnostically significant	• Differences in intensity between right and left earphone placements could complicate measurement • Presence of hearing loss (cochlear or conductive) could complicate measurement • Selters and Brackmann (1977) correction for hearing loss could be used

Source: Atcherson, S.R. and Stoody, T.M. (2012), *Auditory Electrophysiology.* New York: Thieme. Reprinted by permission.

Table 4.66   Summary of nonpathological and auditory ("pathological") factors that may influence the outcome of auditory brainstem response (ABR) measurement in children

Factor	Influence
Nonpathological	
Age	Latency, particularly for wave V and interwave latencies, decreases and morphology changes from premature infancy through 18 months postterm birth. Analysis of ABR findings for children under the chronological age of 18 months (corrected for premature birth) must be done with age-corrected normative data.
Gender	Differences in ABR findings for males versus females are insignificant in children before puberty.
Body temperature	Hyper- and hypothermia exert important and indirect influences on ABR latencies. Wave V latency and the wave I-V latency interval increase by ~0.2 milliseconds for every degree of temperature decrease from normal body temperature (37.0ºC or 98.6ºF). A corresponding decrease in ABR latency is associated with increased body temperature (hyperthermia).
State of arousal	State of arousal, including attention, sleep, and sedation, has no significant effect on the ABR.
Movement	Bodily movement, including myogenic artifact, has a significant negative influence on the quality of ABR recordings.
Drugs	Most drugs have no effect on the ABR, including sedatives commonly used in children (e.g., chloral hydrate and Versed). Selected anesthetic agents (e.g., propofol and sevoflurane) produce a modest increase in ABR interwave latency values. Nitrous oxide, a gas that is sometimes used to induce anesthesia, can inflate the middle ear space and produce a transient (intraoperative) conductive hearing loss producing a prolongation of absolute ABR latencies.
Auditory	
Middle ear dysfunction	Even a modest degree of conductive hearing loss may produce a delay in absolute ABR latencies, beginning with wave I. Conductive hearing loss has no important effect on ABR interwave latencies. Middle ear dysfunction has no influence on ABRs evoked with bone conduction stimulation.
Sensory (cochlear) dysfunction	High-frequency cochlear auditory dysfunction and resulting hearing loss typically is associated with poorer waveform morphology and reduction of wave I amplitude. With moderate to severe sensory nearing loss, wave I may be absent. An ABR is rarely recorded with sensory hearing loss exceeding 80 dB HL within the 1,000- to 4,000-Hz frequency region. Isolated low-frequency sensory hearing loss with preservation of hearing above 2,000 Hz has little or no effect on the ABR. A click-evoked ABR can be recorded if hearing sensitivity is within normal limits at some frequencies (including interactive frequencies) within the region of 1,000 to 4,000 Hz.

(*continued on next page*)

Table 4.66 (*Continued*)

Factor	Influence
Neural	An abnormal ABR will typically be recorded in retrocochlear and neural auditory dysfunction. The pattern of ABR abnormality will depend on the location and extent of the lesion or dysfunction. A tumor in the cerebellopontine angle (CPA) characteristically results in an ABR characterized by normal wave I latency and amplitude, and either a delay of interwave latencies or absence of ABR wave III and/or wave V.
Auditory neuropathy	The neurophysiological signature of auditory neuropathy (also now known as auditory neuropathy spectrum disorder [ANSD]) is the absence of all ABR components with evidence of cochlear microphonic (CM) activity for single polarity (rarefaction and condensation) click stimuli.

Note: The influence of stimulus and acquisition parameters on the ABR is not included in the table.
Source: Objective Assessment of Hearing (p. 97) by J.W. Hall and D.W. Swanepoel. Copyright © 2010 Plural Publishing, Inc. All rights reserved. Used by permission.

Table 4.67 Means (M) and standard deviations (SD) of interpeak latency differences for each of 11 age groups*

Interpeak Latency Difference	Age Group (months)	Number	M (msec)	SD	r
I–III	3–6	78	2.523	0.215	0.99
	6–9	65	2.416	0.225	0.99
	9–12	89	2.313	0.235	0.95
	12–15	14	2.313	0.149	0.99
	15–18	70	2.258	0.157	0.99
	18–21	27	2.29	0.238	0.96
	21–24	27	2.168	0.206	0.97
	24–27	17	2.278	0.172	0.87
	27–30	17	2.099	0.137	0.94
	30–33	58	2.210	0.157	0.99
	33–36	24	2.171	0.197	0.95
III–V	3–6	79	2.128	0.215	0.99
	6–9	67	2.082	0.215	0.99
	9–12	89	1.992	0.199	0.99
	12–15	47	2.006	0.219	0.98
	15–18	71	1.999	0.163	0.99
	18–21	28	1.992	0.189	0.98
	21–24	27	1.959	0.195	0.98
	24–27	18	1.912	0.182	0.91
	27–30	17	1.915	0.155	0.88
	30–33	58	1.904	0.180	0.99
	33–36	24	1.937	0.174	0.98
I–V	3–6	78	4.653	0.287	0.98
	6–9	65	4.502	0.270	0.99
	9–12	89	4.306	0.285	0.99
	12–15	48	4.320	0.240	0.99
	15–18	71	4.252	0.224	0.99
	18–21	27	4.182	0.227	0.98
	21–24	28	4.140	0.248	0.95
	24–27	17	4.197	0.171	0.94
	27–30	17	4.015	0.215	0.96
	30–33	58	4.117	0.226	0.97
	33–36	25	4.121	0.251	0.93

*Note: The number of subjects in each group is given, along with the proportion of variance accounted for by a normal ogive approximation to the observed cumulative distributions.
Source: Bess. F.H. and Gravel, J.S. (2006), *Foundations of Pediatric Audiology*. Plural Publishing, Inc. Copyright Fred H. Bess. Reprinted by permission.

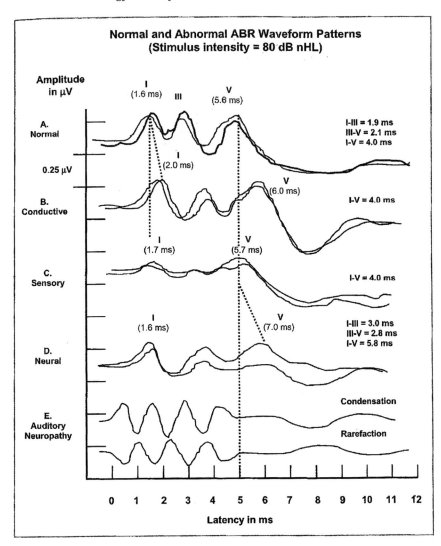

Fig. 4.25 Illustration of representative ABR waveforms recorded with click stimulation for different types of auditory dysfunction. Basic ABR analyses calculations are shown for the normal (top) waveform. (From *Objective Assessment of Hearing* (p. 91) by J.W. Hall and D.W. Swanepoel. Copyright © 2010 Plural Publishing, Inc. All rights reserved. Used by permission.)

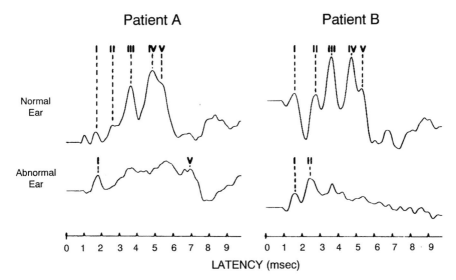

Fig. 4.26 Two examples of abnormal ABR results in cases of retrocochlear pathology. (Adapted from American Speech-Language-Hearing Association (ASHA). (1987), *The Short Latency Auditory Evoked Potentials*. Rockville Pike, MD: ASHA. Reprinted by permission of ASHA.)

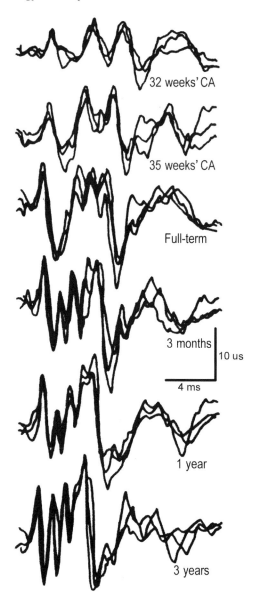

Fig. 4.27 Normal maturation of the auditory brainstem response from 32 weeks' conceptional age (CA) to 3 years of age. (From Salamy, A. (1984), Maturation of the auditory brainstem response from birth through early childhood. Journal of Clinical Neurophysiology 1(3):293. American Electroencephalographic Society. Baltimore: Lippincott Williams & Wilkins. Reprinted by permission.)

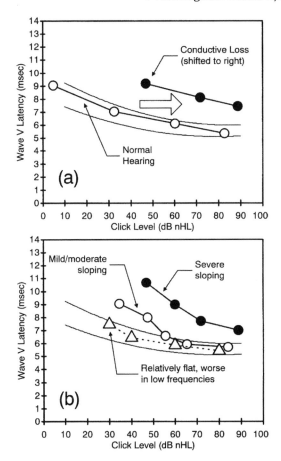

Fig. 4.28a,b Representative clinical wave V latency-intensity functions. The paired curved lines in each panel are normal confidence limits. (**a**) Results for a normal ear and a case of conductive loss. Notice the conductive function is shifted to the right, represented by the arrow. (**b**) Functions for cochlear sensorineural loss generally converge toward the normal latency range as click intensity is raised, but this is affected by shape and degree of loss. (From Gelfand, S.A. (2009), *Essentials of Audiology*, 3rd ed. New York: Thieme. Reprinted by permission.)

Table 4.68 Recommended clinical protocols for obtaining and evaluating middle latency responses

Parameter	Recommendation	Comment
Stimulus type	Clicks, tone bursts	Depends on purpose of MLR
Stimulus duration	< 10 msec	
Stimulus rate	7.1–17.1/s	Depends on maximum length sequence
Stimulus intensity	70 dB nHL	
Stimulus mode	Monaural	
Time window	0–70 msec	
Signal averages	500–1,000	May need more replications with lower numbers of responses averaged
High-pass cutoff	10 Hz	
Low-pass cutoff	300 Hz	
50- or 60-Hz notch filter	Off	
Number of electrode channels	2–4	Minimum of one electrode over each hemisphere for neural exam
Noninverting electrodes	Cz, C3, C4	
Inverting electrode	Ai/nose/nape	Earlobe better than mastoid
Artifact rejection	± 100 µV	Set to reject 10% of averages
Eye-blink rejection	Electrodes above/below eye	
Subject state	Awake, relaxed, and still	Light sleep OK
Latency measures	Na and Pa absolute latencies	
Amplitude measures	Na-Pa peak to peak (µV)	
Hemispheric differences	Na-Pa from C3 inverting vs C4 inverting	≥ 50% considered abnormal
Ear differences	Na-Pa from right ear vs left ear stimuli	≥ 50% considered abnormal

Abbreviations: MLR, middle latency response; nHL, normal hearing level.
Source: Atcherson, S.R. and Stoody, T.M. (2012), *Auditory Electrophysiology.* New York: Thieme. Reprinted by permission.

Table 4.69 Description of the middle and long latency auditory evoked potentials

Component	Classification	Latency (msec)	Amplitude (μV)	Response Features
Na	MLAEP exogenous	18–25	5–7	May be present even when the Pa is absent
Pa	MLAEP exogenous	24–36	8–12	
Nb	MLAEP exogenous	34–47	8–12	Not always fully developed until 8–10 years of age
Pb	MLAEP exogenous	55–80	5–7	Sensitive to changes in stimulus parameters (i.e, frequency, intensity, "on" and "off" effects); amplitude changes with sleep state
ASSR	Exogenous	9–38*	0.3–1.8*	This is a "frequency following" type of response using a combination of both AM and FM
P50 gating response	MLAEP exogenous/ gating response	40–70	3–8 (S1) 0–6 (S2)	S2 amplitude is 60% or less of the S1 amplitude in normal individuals; absent in AD/HD and schizophrenia
P1	LLAEP† exogenous	55–80	5–7	Sensitive to changes in stimulus parameters (i.e., frequency, intensity, "on" and "off" effects); amplitude changes with sleep state
N1	LLAEP exogenous	80–150	5–10	Sensitive to changes in the acoustic features of the stimulus (i.e., spectrum); amplitude changes with sleep state and attention
P2	LLAEP exogenous	145–180	3–6	Sensitive to changes in the acoustic features of the stimulus (i.e., spectrum); amplitude changes with sleep state and attention
N2	LLAEP endogenous	180–250	3–6	Sensitive to change in the acoustic features of the stimulus; amplitude significantly affected by attention as well as sleep state
MMN	Exogenous	200–300	30–50	Not affected by attention; subject sleep state will vary in both amplitude and latency
P300, P300a, P300b	Endogenous cognitive	220–380	12	P300a is related to stimulus novelty; P300b is related to task response; the amplitude is affected by attention as well as sleep state
N400	Endogenous linguistic	390–510	–10	Sensitive to linguistic content; amplitude changes with low versus high predictability sentences

Abbreviations: AD/HD, attention deficit/hyperactivity disorder; AM, amplitude modulation; ASSR, auditory steady-state response; FM, frequency modulation; LLAEP, long latency auditory evoked potential; MLAEP, middle latency auditory evoked potential; MMN, mismatch negativity.

*Designated as an MLAEP when labeled Pb. If labeled P1, then it is associated with the LLAEP.
†Designated as an LLAEP when labeled P1. If labeled Pb, then it is associated with the MLAEP.

Note: Amplitude and latency values vary with carrier frequency and type of modulation.
Source: Roeser, R.J., Valente, M., Hosford-Dunn, H. (2007). *Audiology Diagnosis*, 2nd ed. New York: Thieme. Reprinted by permission.

Table 4.70   Middle latency auditory evoked potential (AEP) recording parameters

Electrodes	
Type	Ag-AgCl, silver, gold
Montage	Single channel
	Cz (noninverting)
	Ai (inverting)
	Fpz (ground).
	Multichannel
	Cz, T3, and T4 (noninverting)
	C7–noncephalic (inverting)
	Fpz (ground)
Recording parameters	
Channels	One channel is standard
	Two or more channels for hemispheric specificity
Time base	80–100 msec, with a 10-msec preanalysis
No. of averages	500–1,000
Filter (bandpass)	3–1500 Hz
Artifact rejection	Three quarters maximum sampling amplitude
Stimuli	
Type	100 msec acoustic clicks may be used but are not preferred
	Brief tone with a 2–1–2 cycle
	Blackman 5-cycle brief tone
Transducer	Tubal insert phones
	Calibrated earphones (e.g., TDH-39)
	Sound field speakers
Polarity*	Rarefaction
Level	75–80 dB nHL for a robust response showing all of the subcomponents
	Brief tones may be used to estimate hearing sensitivity, and the actual level would vary
Rate	Up to 11 per second, but lower rates are preferable (5 per second)
	In young children, rates as low as 2 to 3 per second yield best results
ISI	90–200 msec, with the longer ISI preferred
	300–500 msec in young children

Abbreviations: ISI, interstimulus interval; nHL, normal hearing level; TDH, TDH-39.

*In children, it is sometimes necessary to reverse the polarity for better morphology.

Source: Roeser, R.J., Valente, M., Hosford-Dunn, H. (2007), *Audiology Diagnosis,* 2nd ed. New York: Thieme. Reprinted by permission.

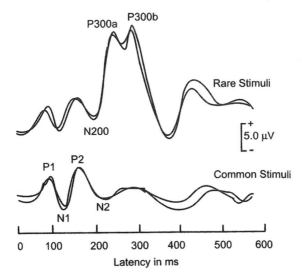

Fig. 4.29 P300 event-related auditory potential in response to the phoneme /ba/ (rare or oddball stimulus) and /da/ (common or frequent stimulus). The rare stimulus was presented with a probability of 0.20, and presentation of the stimulus did not occur in two consecutive trials. (From Roeser, R.J., Valente, M., Hosford-Dunn, H. (2007), *Audiology Diagnosis,* 2nd ed. New York: Thieme. Reprinted by permission.)

Table 4.71   P300 recording parameters

Electrodes	
Type	Ag-AgCl, gold (not preferred)
Montage	Single channel (not preferred)
	Cz (noninverting)
	C7 (inverting)
	Fpz (ground)
	Multichannel
	Fz (noninverting)
	Cz (noninverting)
	Pz (noninverting)
	C7 (inverting)
	Fpz (ground)
Eye movement	Superior orbit of one eye to the inferior orbit of the opposite eye (polarity not specified)
Recording parameters	
Channels	One channel (not recommended)
	Three channels for best localization of the response
	The target, or oddball (rare), stimuli are averaged in one buffer, and the common or frequent stimuli are averaged in a second buffer
Time base	500 msec, with a 100-msec preanalysis
No. of averages	200–250
Filter (bandpass)	0.05–50.0 Hz
Artifact rejection	Three-quarters maximum sampling amplitude
Stimuli	
Type	Tone bursts with 10 msec rise/fall time and a 25–50 msec plateau time
	Brief duration speech material (i.e., CVC) may be used
	The target, or oddball (rare) stimuli, should occur not more than 20% of the time, randomly presented, and not occurring in succession
Transducer	Tubal insert phones
	Calibrated earphones (e.g., TDH-39)
	Sound field speakers
Polarity	Not specified
Level	75–80 dB nHL for a robust response showing all of the subcomponents
Rate	0.9 per second or less, depending on the stimulus length
ISI	1.1 seconds or longer, depending on the stimulus length

Abbreviations: CVC, consonant-vowel-consonant; ISI, interstimulus interval; nHL, normal hearing level.

Source: Roeser, R.J., Valente, M., Hosford-Dunn, H. (2007), *Audiology Diagnosis,* 2nd ed. New York: Thieme. Reprinted by permission.

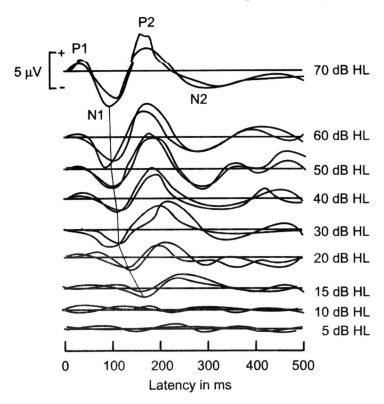

Fig. 4.30 The long latency auditory evoked potential (AEP) to different intensities. Notice that the latency of the response shows little variation at high to moderate levels, then quickly increases near threshold. In contrast, the amplitude shows a graded response with intensity. (From Roeser, R.J., Valente, M., Hosford-Dunn, H. (2007), *Audiology Diagnosis*, 2nd ed. New York: Thieme. Reprinted by permission.)

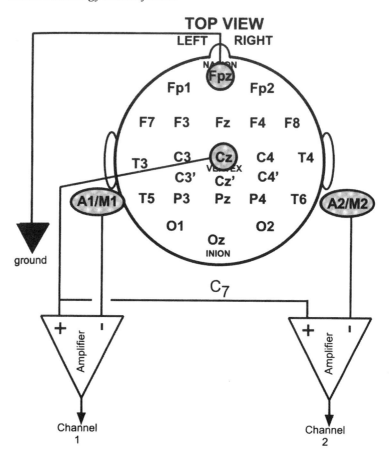

Fig. 4.31 Electrode montage for the long latency auditory evoked potential (AEP) (Cz-A1 and Cz-A2). (From Roeser, R.J., Valente, M., Hosford-Dunn, H. (2007), *Audiology Diagnosis*, 2nd ed. New York: Thieme. Reprinted by permission.)

Table 4.72   Suggested stimulus parameters and recording considerations for late auditory evoked potentials (AEP)

Stimulus parameters	
Type	Tone bursts (audiogram frequencies) and other nonlinguistic stimuli (10–20 msec rise/fall time, 20–60 msec plateau, linear, or Blackman ramp)
	Speech or speechlike (words, consonant-vowel, or vowel stimuli)
	Clicks (though generally not recommended)
Intensity	60–80 dB nHL (normal hearing level, suprathreshold)
	Variable in 5- to 10-dB steps (threshold estimation)
Polarity	Rarefaction, but generally not relevant
Rate	1.7 to 0.7/sec (will depend on stimulus duration and time window)
Presentations	500 per trial (as few as 50 to as many as 1,000 may be needed, depending on the patient characteristics during the test and amount of noise)
Transducer	ER-3A (or loudspeaker with hearing aids and cochlear implants)
Recording considerations	
Electrodes	Cz (noninverting), ipsilateral, or contralateral earlobe (inverting and not linked), and Fpz (ground)
	Above or below one eye (with two-channel system, and if more channels are available an electrode lateral to one eye)
Amplification	50,000 to 75,000 times
Artifact rejection	± 100 µV
Data points	256 points (~426 samples/s) or 512 points (~853 samples/s)
Time window	–100 to 500 msec or longer (will depend on stimulation rate and desired component latencies)
Filters	0.1 to 100 Hz during acquisition and offline digital filtering of 1 to 15 Hz or 1 to 30 Hz
Replications	A minimum of two

Source: Atcherson, S.R. and Stoody, T.M. (2012), *Auditory Electrophysiology.* New York: Thieme. Reprinted by permission.

Table 4.73   Long latency auditory evoked potential (AEP) recording parameters

Electrodes

Type	Ag-AgC
Montage	Single channel
	Cz (noninverting)
	Ai (inverting)
	Fpz (ground)
	Multichannel
	Cz (noninverting)
	A1 (inverting)
	A2 (inverting)
	Fpz (ground)
Eye movement	Superior orbit of one eye to the inferior orbit of the opposite eye (polarity not specified)

Recording parameters

Channels	One channel is standard
	Two or more channels for hemispheric specificity
Time base	300 msec, with a 50-msec preanalysis
No. of averages	200–250
Filter (bandpass)	1–300 Hz
Artifact rejection	Three-quarters maximum sampling amplitude

Stimuli

Type	Tone bursts with a 5–10 msec rise–fall time and a 25–50 msec plateau time
	Brief duration speech material (i.e., CVC) may be used
Transducer	Tubal insert phones
	Calibrated earphones (e.g., TDH-39)
	Sound field speakers
Polarity*	Rarefaction
Level	75–80 dB nHL for a robust response showing all of the subcomponents
	Tone bursts may be used to estimate hearing sensitivity, and the actual level would vary
Rate	0.9–2.9 per second (we prefer the lower rate of ~0.9–1.3 per second)
ISI	300 msec–1.1 seconds, with the longer ISI preferred

Abbreviations: CVC, consonant-vowel-consonant; ISI, interstimulus interval; nHL, normal hearing level.

*In children, it is sometimes necessary to reverse the polarity for better morphology.

Source: Roeser, R.J., Valente, M., Hosford-Dunn, H. (2007), *Audiology Diagnosis,* 2nd ed. New York: Thieme. Reprinted by permission.

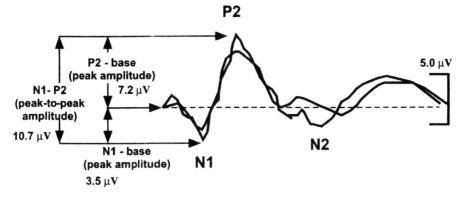

Fig. 4.32 Long latency auditory evoked potential showing the measurement of the N1 peak amplitude, the P2 peak amplitude, and the N1-P2 peak-to-peak amplitude. Note the asymmetry in the amplitudes between the peak amplitudes of the N1 and P2. (From Roeser, R.J., Valente, M., Hosford-Dunn, H. (2007), *Audiology Diagnosis*, 2nd ed. New York: Thieme. Reprinted by permission.)

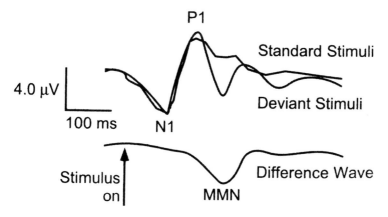

Fig. 4.33 The mismatch negativity (MMN) to the phonemes /ba/ (standard stimulus) and /do/ (deviant stimulus). The bottom tracing shows the MMN as a difference wave; however, the MMN is clearly seen when the two waveforms (standard and deviant) are so overlaid, as seen in the top tracing. (From Roeser, R.J., Valente, M., Hosford-Dunn, H. (2007), *Audiology Diagnosis*, 2nd ed. New York: Thieme. Reprinted by permission.)

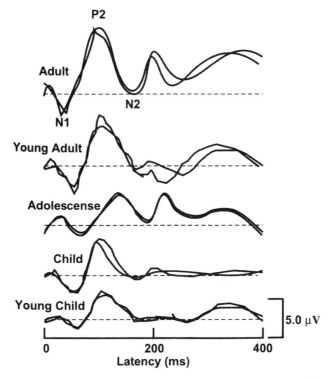

Fig. 4.34 Developmental changes in the P2 from young child (3 years old) to adult (42 years old). (From Roeser, R.J., Valente, M., Hosford-Dunn, H. (2007), *Audiology Diagnosis,* 2nd ed. New York: Thieme. Reprinted by permission.)

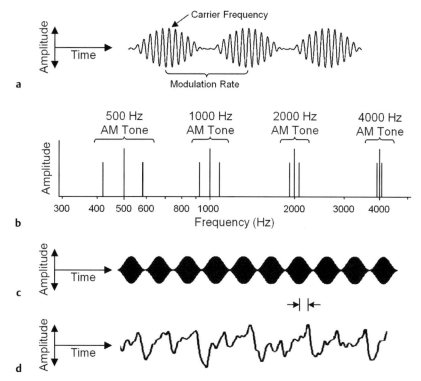

Fig. 4.35a–d   Idealized drawings. (**a**) Waveform of an amplitude modulation (AM) tone with a 1000-Hz carrier frequency and an 80-Hz modulation rate. (**b**) Spectra of 500-, 1000-, 2000-, and 4000-Hz AM tones with 90-Hz modulation rates (logarithmic scale). (**c**) Envelope of an amplitude-modulation tone (stimulus). (**d**) Auditory steady-state response (ASSR) waveform in which the electroencephalographic (EEG) activity is synchronized to the modulation rate of the stimulus, with a slight delay *(arrow)*. (Part d adapted from Grason-Stadler, Inc. (GSI). (2001), Auditory Steady-State Response: A New Tool for Frequency-Specific Hearing Assessment in Infants and Children. Eden Prairie, MN. Reprinted by permission. © 2001 Grason-Stadler, Inc.)

Table 4.74 Common terminology related to auditory steady-state response (ASSR) stimuli, response recording, and analysis

Term	Abbreviation	Definition
Related to stimuli		
Carrier frequency	Cf	Test stimulus that determines the site of stimulation on the basilar membrane
Modulation frequency	Mf	The rate at which the carrier or test frequency is being amplitude modulated into distinct pockets of energy
Amplitude modulation	AM	The test stimulus (or carrier frequency) is modulated in amplitude at a specific rate (modulation frequency)
40 Hz ASSR	40 Hz	ASSR technique with test stimuli modulated at a rate between 35 and 45 Hz
80 Hz ASSR	80 Hz	ASSR technique with test stimuli modulated at a rate between 70 and 110 Hz
Frequency modulation	FM	Modulation of the test signal in frequency (e.g., 10% FM of a 1,000-Hz tone results in frequency energy between 950 and 1050 Hz)
Mixed modulation	MM	Combined amplitude and frequency modulation of a test (carrier) stimulus
Exponential modulation	AM2	Amplitude modulation with a steep slope (exponential) for stimulus cycle
Modulation depth		The depth of the amplitude or frequency modulation (e.g., 20%)
Multiple stimuli technique		A presentation paradigm where multiple stimuli can be presented simultaneously to both ears (four frequencies per ear)
Single stimulus technique		A presentation paradigm where only one stimulus is presented at a time
Related to response recording and analysis		
Fast Fourier transform	FFT	Transforms EEG activity in the time-domain (amplitude and latency) to the frequency-domain (frequency, amplitude, and phase information)
Phase analysis		Analysis of the response phase at the frequency of modulation to determine if a response is present (if present, phrases cluster together)
Phase coherence		Statistical test to determine if there is a significant difference between the distribution of phases in a recording compared with a random distribution
Spectral analysis		Considers response in frequency-domain to determine whether the response at the modulation frequency is significantly different from background EEG
F-test		Statistical test for spectral analysis, compares response amplitude at rate of stimulation to noise at adjacent frequencies for a significant difference
Physiological recruitment		Abnormally rapid growth in ASSR amplitude due to cochlear damage; physiological correlate to the perceptual phenomenon called recruitment

Table 4.75 Typical stimulus and response acquisition parameters for frequency-specific auditory steady-state response (ASSR)

Parameter	Selection	Comment
Stimulus parameters		
Carrier frequencies	500, 1,000, 2,000, 4,000 Hz	
Modulation frequencies	70–100 Hz for infants and sleeping adults	
40 Hz for awake adults		Multiple simultaneous stimuli carrier tones modulated at distinct rates more than ½ octave apart
Amplitude modulation (AM) depth	100%	
Frequency modulation (FM) depth	10–20%	
Advanced modulation options	Exponential modulation (AM2)—higher amplitudes Phase adjusted stimuli—higher amplitudes	
Stimulus intensity range	0–125 dB HL (depending on transducer and frequency)	
Transducers	Insert earphones, supra-aural earphones, sound-field speaker, bone oscillator	
Calibration reference	dB HL	
Recording parameters		
Electrode montage	Single-stimulus ASSR: Adults Noninverting = Cz or Fz Inverting = lower neck (inion in awake subject or ipsilateral mastoid Ground—contralateral mastoid Multiple-stimulus ASSR: Adults Midline electrodes essential Cz or Fz for noninverting and lower neck or inion for inverting	Infants Noninverting = Cz or Fz Inverting = ipsilateral mastoid Ground—contralateral mastoid Infants 2-channel ASSR: noninverting to ipsilateral side of each ear; 1 channel ASSR test multiple frequencies in one ear at a time
Electrode impedance	< 6 kOhms and interelectrode difference < 3 kOhms	
Filter settings	40 Hz ASSR: 10–100 Hz* 80 Hz ASSR: 30–300 Hz* 6 dB/octave slope	
Amplification	10,000–50,000	

(*continued on next page*)

Table 4.75 *(Continued)*

Parameter	Selection	Comment
Averaging periods	40 seconds to 15 minutes	
Analysis time (epoch)	Usually ± 1 second	
Epochs in sweep	16 (may vary)	
Sweeps	Variable	
Statistical tests	F-test for spectral analysis	
	Phase coherence for phase	
	and analysis	

*Generic settings (system-specific filters).

Source: Objective Assessment of Hearing (p. 112) by J.W. Hall and D.W. Swanepoel. Copyright © 2010 Plural Publishing, Inc. All rights reserved. Used by permission.

Table 4.76 Summary of subject factors affecting 40 Hz and 80 Hz auditory steady-state response (ASSR) recordings in adults and infants

Subject Factors	Effect		Clinical Implications	
	Adults	Infants	Adults	Infants
Age	Not significant	40 Hz unstable; 80 Hz consistent; significant amplitude; increase in neonatal period and in 1st year of life	40 Hz and 80 Hz reliable	80 Hz essential; test infants older than 4 weeks but be aware of variability through 1st year of life
Sleep	40 Hz and 80 Hz present in wakefulness; 40 Hz has largest amplitude but is reduced by 50% during sleep; in sleep, 40 Hz amplitude larger at ≤ 1 kHz and 80 Hz amplitude larger at > 1 kHz	40 Hz in asleep state is unstable; 80 Hz in asleep state stable	For awake adults use 40 Hz; for sleeping adults use 40 Hz for 0.5 and 1 kHz and 80 Hz for 2 and 4 kHz	80 Hz stable and reliable during sleep; in awake subject internal noise may mask response
Anesthesia	40 Hz reduced; 80 Hz no effect	40 Hz ASSR unstable; 80 Hz ASSR no effect	40 Hz to monitor effect on consciousness; 80 Hz to monitor peripheral hearing	80 Hz reliably recorded
Attention	40 Hz demonstrates some effect	No data	No effect on threshold estimation	No data
Internal noise	80 Hz response smaller in awake state and more easily masked by internal noise close to threshold; less noise during sleep but smaller amplitude responses	Internal noise during awake state easily masks response close to threshold; in quiet sleep 80 Hz easily recorded	Awake subjects must be relaxed for reliable recordings; strategies to encourage sleep	Natural sleep, conscious sedation, or anesthesia for reliable recordings

Table 4.77   Auditory steady-state response (ASSR) recording parameters

Electrodes
Type — Ag-AgCl
Montage — Monaural presentation
   Nasion (inverting)
   A1 (noninverting)
   A2 (noninverting
   Fpz (ground)
   Binaural presentation
   Cz (inverting)
   Nape of neck
   Cz (noninverting)
   Pz (noninverting)
   Fpz (ground)
Recording parameters
Channels — 2
Time base — 15–20 seconds
No. of averages — 48–50 sweeps
Filter (bandpass) — 10–300 Hz
Artifact rejection — Three quarters maximum sampling amplitude
*Stimuli**
Type — Modulated tones

	AUDERA		MASTER	
AM	100%		100%	
FM	20%		20%	
Presentation	Monaural		Binaural	
CF (Hz)	MF (Hz)		MF (Hz)	
	Awake	Asleep	Right Ear	Left Ear
500	46	74	86	82
1,000	46	81	94	90
2,000	46	88	102	98
4,000	46	95	110	106

Polarity — Not applicable
Level — 0–~110 dB HL (0–~100 dB SPL)
Rate — See above MFs
ISI — None (continuous tones)
Transducer — Tubal insert phones
   Calibrated earphones
Response detection — *F*-test (*p* < 0.05) (MASTER) and phase coherence (*p* < 0.01) (AUDERA)

Abbreviations: AM, amplitude modulation; AUDERA, VIASYS Healthcare (Warwick, UK); CF, carrier frequency; FM, frequency modulation; HL, hearing level; ISI, interstimulus interval; MASTER, Bio-logic Systems Corp., Mundelein, IL; MF, modulation frequency; SPL, sound pressure level.
*The following serves as an example of what is available on commercial units.
Source: Roeser, R.J., Valente, M., Hosferd-Dunn, H. (2007), *Audiology Diagnosis,* 2nd ed. New York: Thieme. Reprinted by permission.

Otoacoustic Emissions

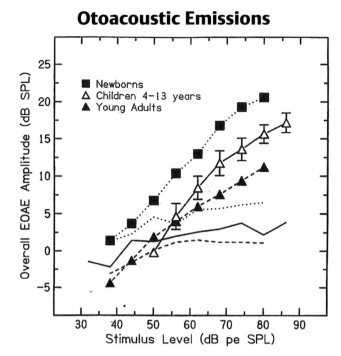

Fig. 4.36 Mean overall transient evoked otoacoustic emission (TEOAE) amplitude as a function of click stimulus level for three age groups. Open triangles, mean TEOAE amplitude (bar = 1 standard deviation) from 43 normally hearing children. Mean noise levels are depicted for infants *(dotted line)*, children *(solid line)*, and adults *(dashed line)*. (Adapted from data compiled by Susan Norton and Judith E. Widen, with permission).

Table 4.78 **Mean transient evoked otoacoustic emission (TEOAE) level (dB SPL), noise, and signal-to-noise ratio (SNR) along with the standard deviations for half-octave bands centered at 1,000, 1,500, 2,000, 3,000, and 4,000 Hz in newborns without risk factors for hearing loss**[*]

	Mean TEOAE Level (dB SPL)	Mean Noise (dB SPL)	Mean SNR (dB)
1,000 Hz	0.5 (7.5)	−2.0 (5.0)	2.5 (7.5)
1,500 Hz	6.0 (7.25)	−4.0 (4.5)	10.0 (7.0)
2,000 Hz	6.5 (9.0)	−6.0 (4.0)	12.5 (7.5)
3,000 Hz	8.0 (10.0)	−6.25 (4.25)	15.0 (7.75)
4,000 Hz	6.25 (10.0)	−8.25 (4.0)	14.5 (8.5)

[*]Databased from Norton et al, 2000. TEOAEs were collected using a customized click at 80 dB pSPL.
Source: Glattke, T.J. and Robinette, M.S. (2007), *Otoacoustic Emissions: Clinical Applications,* 3rd ed. New York: Thieme. Reprinted by permission.

Table 4.79 **Mean transient evoked otoacoustic emission (TEOAE) levels (Response) for newborns cared for in the well-baby nursery**[*]

Type of Recording	Number of Ears	Right Ear	Left Ear	Both Ears
		Mean (SD)		
Standard recording				
Aidan et al (1997)	1164	22.4 (5.4)	21.1 (5.4)	21.8 (5.4)
Kok et al (1993)	1036	—	—	20.2 (−)
Paludetti et al (1999)	640	21.5 (5.1)	21.8 (5.6)	—
Welch et al (1996)	87	—	—	22.5 (5.2)
QuickScreen recording				
Hancur (1999)	154	18.1 (5.3)	18.3 (5.4)	18.2 (5.3)
Welch et al (1996)	87	—	—	20.1 (4.8)

[*]For all studies TEOAEs were evoked by click stimuli of ~80 dB pe SPL, and the nonlinear mode of stimulus presentation and averaging on the Otodynamics ILO 88 was used in all studies.
Source: Glattke, T.J. and Robinette, M.S. (2007), *Otoacoustic Emissions: Clinical Applications,* 3rd ed. New York: Thieme. Reprinted by permission.

Table 4.80 **Transient evoked otoacoustic emission (TEOAE) in normal-hearing children**

Study	Age in Years Range	Mean	Number of Ears/Subjects	Overall Amplitude in dB SPL Mean	(SD)	Reproduced (%) Mean	(SD)
Norton and Widen, 1990	0–9.9	(5.4)	32	20.0	(5.4)	90.4	(12.3)
	10–19.9	(12.6)	37	17.0	(4.2)	90.6	(10.4)
	20–29.9	(23.7)	37	10.9	(4.3)	83.4	(14.8)
Spektor et al, 1991	4–10	(7.5)	13	13.5			
	22–29	(26)	11	9.1			
Glattke et al, 1995	0–10		277	12.5		75	
	10–20		93	10.1		80	
	20–30		6	11.8		85	
Nozza et al, 1997	5–10		112/56	13.2	(~4.3)	72.4	(~21.4)
Qiu et al, 1998	7 days–12 months		/20	17.3	(5.4)	85.3	(14.3)
	6–16		/40	15.1	(4.2)	84.2	(14.5)
	18–65		/30	12.1	(3.4)	86.1	(13.5)

Source: Glattke, T.J. and Robinette, M.S. (2007), *Otoacoustic Emissions: Clinical Applications,* 3rd ed. New York: Thieme. Reprinted by permission.

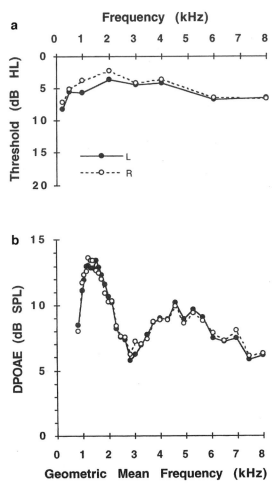

Fig. 4.37a,b   Distortion product otoacoustic emissions (DPOAE) amplitudes as a function of ear: Left *(solid circles)* versus right *(open circles)* ears. (**a**) Mean behavioral thresholds were slightly better for the right than for the left ear, particularly for the middle frequencies. (**b**) Mean DPOAE amplitudes in 0.1-octave steps showing insignificant differences between right and left ears. To determine the statistical significance ($p < 0.05$) of the observed differences, analyses of variance (ANOVA) and t-tests were used. (From Glattke, T.J. and Robinette, M.S. (1997), *Otoacoustic Emissions: Clinical Applications.* New York: Thieme. Reprinted with permission.)

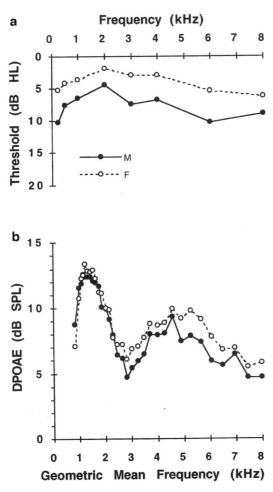

Fig. 4.38a,b DPOAE amplitudes as a function of gender: Male *(solid circles)* versus female *(open circles)* ears. (**a**) Mean behavioral thresholds were better in women than in men at all frequencies. (**b**) Mean DPOAE amplitudes in 0.1-octave steps were greater for women, particularly for frequencies above approximately 2.5 kHz. To determine the statistical significance ($p < 0.05$) of the observed differences, analyses of variance (ANOVA) and *t*-tests were used. (From Glattke, T.J. and Robinette, M.S. (1997), *Otoacoustic Emissions: Clinical Applications.* New York: Thieme. Reprinted by permission.)

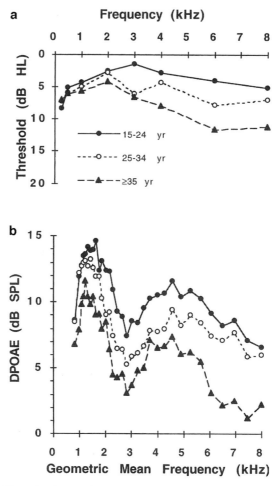

Fig. 4.39a,b DPOAE amplitudes as a function of age: 15–24 *(solid circles)*, 25–34 *(open circles)*, and 35 *(solid triangles)* years. (**a**) Mean behavioral thresholds increased with age above 2 kHz. (**b**) Mean DPOAE amplitudes in 0.1-octave steps were smaller with increasing age, particularly for frequencies above 2 kHz. To determine the statistical significance ($p < 0.05$) of the observed differences, analyses of variance (ANOVA) and t-tests were used. (From Glattke, T.J. and Robinette, M.S. (1997), *Otoacoustic Emissions: Clinical Applications.* New York: Thieme. Reprinted by permission.)

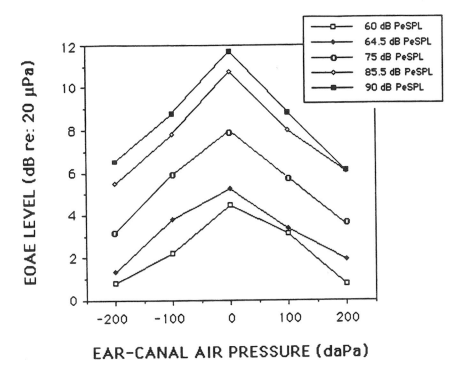

EAR-CANAL AIR PRESSURE (daPa)

Fig. 4.40 Effect of ear-canal pressure on TEOAE response amplitudes for click stimuli presented at the indicated levels *(inset)*. (From Naeve, S.L., Margolis, R.H., Levine, S.C., Fourneir, E.M. (1992), Effect of ear-canal air pressure on evoked otoacoustic emissions. J. Acoust. Soc. Am. 91, 2091.)

Auditory Processing Disorders

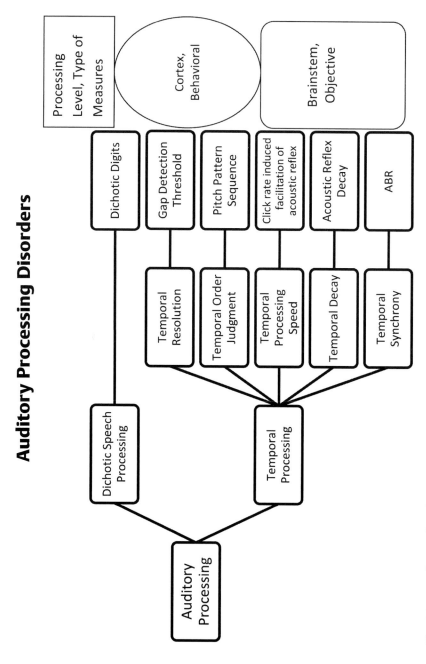

Fig. 4.41 Test battery flow chart for evaluation of auditory processing deficits. (From Rawool, V. (2011), *Hearing Conservation*. New York: Thieme. Reprinted by permission.)

Table 4.81 Central auditory tests: Summary of site of lesion[a,b]

Type of Test	Low Brainstem	High Brainstem	Cortex/hemispheric	Interhemispheric
Monotic and/or low redundancy monaural speech tests (i.e., speech in noise, compressed speech, filtered speech, etc.)	Ipsilateral ear deficit (3)	Contralateral (2), bilateral (2), ipsilateral (1)	Contralateral ear deficit (3)	No deficit
Phase tests (i.e., tonal and speech MLDs)	Moderate to severe bilateral deficits (3)[c]	Little or no deficit	No deficit	No deficit
Binaural interaction tests (i.e., RASP, binaural fusion)	Mild to moderate bilateral deficits (2)[c]	?	Little or no deficit	Little or no deficit
Localization-lateralization tasks	Moderate deficit (2)	Moderate deficit (2)	Moderate contralateral lateral ear deficit (3)	No deficit
Dichotic tasks (i.e., digits, SSW, competing CVs, etc.)	Moderate ipsilateral ear deficit (3)	Contralateral (2), bilateral (2), ipsilateral (2) ear deficits	Moderate contralateral ear deficit (3)	Severe left ear deficit (3)
Pattern tasks (i.e., frequency, intensity patterns)	?	?	Moderate to severe bilateral deficits (3)	Severe bilateral deficits (3)

Abbreviations: CV, consonant-vowel; MLD, masking level difference; RASP, rapidly alternating speech perception; SSW, staggered spondee word.

[a]The author's interpretation of expected findings for some common types of central auditory tests for lesions occurring at various anatomic sites in the central auditory nervous system.

[b]Key: 3, high probability of occurrence; 2, moderate probability of occurrence; 1, low probability of occurrence.

[c]Scored and interpreted as a binaural test.

Source: Musiek, F.E. Application of central auditory tests: An overview. In: Kate, J. (ed.). *Handbook of Clinical Audiology*, 4th ed., 1994, page 325. Baltimore: Lippincott Williams & Wilkins. Reprinted by permission.

Table 4.82 A proposal for a differential diagnosis of (central) auditory processing disorders

Auditory processing disorder must be differentiated from . . .	In contrast to the disorder, the other condition . . .
Normal variations in auditory processing abilities	Is not substantially below what is expected for a child's age level
Peripheral hearing impairment	Is characterized by a unilateral or bilateral conductive or sensorineural hearing loss of any degree, from mild to severe
Language impairment	Is characterized by a phonological impairment, limited vocabulary, difficulty in acquiring new words, shortened sentences, simplified grammatical structure, and slow rate of language development
Learning disorder	Is characterized by an impairment confined to a specific area of academic achievement (i.e., reading, arithmetic, writing skills)
Borderline intellectual functioning	Is characterized by a degree of intellectual impairment
Attention deficit/hyperactivity disorder	Is a persistent pattern of inattention and/or hyperactivity that is more frequent and severe than is typically observed in individuals at a normal level of development

Source: Roeser, R.J., Valente, M., Hosford-Dunn, H. (2007), *Audiology Diagnosis,* 2nd ed. New York: Thieme. Reprinted by permission.

Table 4.83 Identification of auditory processing disorders according to comprehensive approach

Deficit Profile	Buffalo Model	Bellis/Ferre	Chermak/Musiek
Decoding	Decoding deficit	Decoding deficit	Auditory discrimination Auditory closure
Temporal processing		Prosodic deficit	Temporal analysis Temporal synthesis
Binaural listening	Integration deficit	Integration deficit	Binaural separation Binaural summation Binaural integration Interhemispheric transfer
Tolerance fading memory	Tolerance fading memory		
Auditory language		Auditory association	Metalinguistics
Executive control	Organization deficit	Organization/output deficit	Metacognition

Source: Roeser, R.J. and Downs, M.P. *Auditory Disorders in School Children,* 4th ed. New York: Thieme. Reprinted by permission.

Table 4.84   Management components for auditory decoding/closure deficits

Direct therapy/auditory training
   Auditory vigilance training
   Auditory discrimination of frequency, intensity, and duration
   Phonemic analysis and synthesis training/phoneme discrimination activities
   Speech-in-noise training
   Fast ForWord™/Earobics™
Compensatory strategies
   Metalinguistic strategies: vocabulary building, auditory closure activates, discourse cohesion,
   schema and scripts
   Speech/language therapy
Metacognitive strategies
   Modifications to environment
   Preferential seating
   Supplement with visual cues (notes, outlines)
   Repeat/rephrase
   Preteach new words, concepts
   Naturally clear speech
   Assistive listening devices to improve signal-to-noise ratio
   Bilateral earplugs to minimize noise
   Tape lectures
   Changes to physical environment to reduce noise and reverberation
At home
   Listening games: Telephone, Simon Says, and alphabet games
   Games to enhance vocabulary/relationship among words: Catch Phrase™, Scattergories™,
   Taboo™, Wheel of Fortune™, word puzzles/searches
   Phonemic analysis: MadGab™
   Read "popular" magazines to help provide social context
   Read age-appropriate joke and riddle books together
   Review/discuss upcoming movies to aid in comprehension of plots
   Select several "words of the week" from school material and use them daily
   Prepare/rehearse for new situations
   Avoid important communication from a different room or in background noise

Source: Roeser, R.J. and Downs, M.P. *Auditory Disorders in School Children,* 4th ed. New York: Thieme. Reprinted by permission.

Table 4.85   Management components for temporal processing deficits

Direct therapy/auditory training
  Gap detection
  Pattern recognition training: pitch, duration, intensity
  Prosody/segmentation training
  Fast ForWord™/Earobics™
  Auditory memory enhancement
Compensatory strategies
  Vocabulary building: key word extraction; language and humor, discourse cohesion
  Schema/scripts
  Counseling if social/emotional concerns
  Speech-language therapy
  Reading program
  Music activities
  Metacognitive strategies
Environmental modifications
  Animated teacher
  Naturally clear speech
  Repetitions with key word emphasis
  Preteach material
  Visual aids as supplements
  Untimed tests
  Examination with closed-set questions
At home
  Games that require sequencing, synthesis pattern recognition: Simon™, SuperSimon™,
    Bop-It™, Bop-It Extreme™, Taboo™, Guesstures™ (charades), Pictionary™
  Games/activities that require following auditory directions: Simon Says, Say After Me
    (child as leader and participant)
  Read aloud together
  Recite poems, limericks, and rhymes
  Review jokes and riddles together
  Avoid plays on words and sarcasm
  Keep instructions short and simple
  Check for understanding
  Prepare/rehearse for new social situations

Source: Roeser, R.J. and Downs, M.P. *Auditory Disorders in School Children,* 4th ed. New York:
Thieme. Reprinted by permission.

Table 4.86 Management components for binaural listening: Integration deficit

Direct therapy/auditory training
  Auditory vigilance training
  Interhemispheric transfer exercises
  Phoneme training
  Prosody training
  Speech-in-noise training
  Auditory memory enhancement
Compensatory strategies
  Linguistic: vocabulary building
  Speech/language intervention
  Reading program
  Content mastery/tutoring for academic weaknesses
  Memory aids: mnemonics, rote memory, drills, chinking, rehearsal
  Metacognitive strategies
Environmental modifications
  Preferential seating
  Evaluate use of assistive listening devices
  Unilateral earplug to minimize weak-ear effect
  Untimed tests
  Examinations with closed-set questions
  Quiet environment for test taking
  Content mastery/tutoring for specific academic weaknesses
  Reduce need to listen and write: note-taking assistance, provide outlines
  Repetition might be preferable to rephrasing
  Avoid visual cues as concurrent supplement
At home
  Activities to strengthen verbal and motor coordination: Name That Tune, Bag of Surprises
    (child must identify unseen/unnamed objects or search for target item); have child talk
    about a picture while drawing it
  Activities to strengthen multimodality processing: Bop-It™, Bop-It Extreme™, Simon™,
    Super Simon™, Charades, Pictionary™
  Listen to imbalanced stereo to detect loudness differences
  Reduce to single modality in face of comprehension difficulty: listen, then look

Source: Roeser, R.J. and Downs, M.P. *Auditory Disorders in School Children,* 4th ed. New York:
Thieme. Reprinted by permission.

Table 4.87   Management components for tolerance fading memory

Direct therapy/auditory training
   Noise desensitization training
   Auditory memory training
   Compensatory strategies
   Memory strategies
   Chema/scripts
Environmental modifications
   Outlines/note-takers/tape recorders
   Assistive listening devices
   Preferential seating
   Earplugs
   Test taking in quiet
At home
   Memory games: Simon™, SuperSimon™, alphabet sequencing games ("I went to the store, and I bought . . .")
   Organizational/memory strategies: use of calendar; daily planner; dry-erase board for messages; review class work and create mnemonics where appropriate
   Listening games in noise: maintain high success
   Prepare/rehearse for new situations

Source: Roeser, R.J. and Downs, M.P. *Auditory Disorders in School Children,* 4th ed. New York: Thieme. Reprinted by permission.

5

Tinnitus

Table 5.1 Tinnitus classification taxonomy, associated functional domains, and representative assessment tools based on the World Health Organization's International Classification of Functional, Disability, and Health (WHO-ICF, 2004)

Category	Definition	Functional Domains	Assessment Tools
Impairment	Dysfunction of the auditory system resulting in the perception of tinnitus	Perception of pitch/loudness/location/quality	Psychoacoustic measures, direct estimation ratings, visual analogue scales
Activity limitation	Effect of impairment on reducing an individual's ability to function in a normal manner	Emotional effects (e.g., depression, annoyance), hearing interference, intrusiveness or persistence of tinnitus, sleep disturbance, rest or relaxation interference, cognitive effects (e.g., reduced concentration), loss of control	Self-report tinnitus questionnaires, psychological tests, diaries
Participation restriction	Psychosocial manifestation of impairment and activity limitation resulting in the need for extra effort and reduced independence	Difficulty participating in social events; difficulty performing work or home obligations; interference with leisure activities; interference with relationships with family, friends, coworkers; reduced overall quality of life	Self-report tinnitus questionnaires, diaries

Source: Newman, C.W. and Sandridge, S.A. Tinnitus management. In: Montano, J.J. and Spitzer, J.B. (eds.), *Adult Audiologic Rehabilitation* (p. 402). Copyright © 2009 Plural Publishing, Inc. All rights reserved. Used with permission.

Table 5.2   Psychoacoustic measurements conducted as part of the tinnitus assessment

Measurement	Definition
Pitch match	Ability of the patient to equate the pitch of an externally generated pure tone (or narrow-band noise) to the most prominent pitch of patient's perceived tinnitus
Loudness match	Ability of the patient to equate the loudness of an externally generated pure tone (or narrow-band noise) to the overall loudness of patient's perceived tinnitus.
Minimum masking level	Minimum level of a broadband noise (BBN) required to completely mask the patient's tinnitus; if the tinnitus cannot be masked, the minimum level of a BBN that changes the perception of the tinnitus (e.g., louder or softer)
Residual inhibition	Period of time when the patient's tinnitus has been partially or completely suppressed after the externally produced masking stimuli has been turned off
Loudness discomfort level	The threshold level of discomfort for pure tones, BBN, or cold running speech

Source: Newman, C.W. and Sandridge, S.A. Tinnitus management. In: Montano, J.J. and Spitzer, J.B. (eds.), *Adult Audiologic Rehabilitation* (p. 414). Copyright © 2009 Plural Publishing, Inc. All rights reserved. Used with permission.

Table 5.3 Comparison of salient features underlying masking therapy and habituation/retraining therapy

Feature	Masking Therapy	Habituation/Retraining Therapy
Rationale	To mask or partially mask perception of tinnitus	To promote habituation of tinnitus
Counseling	Not to attend to tinnitus; provide control	Do not fear tinnitus
Types of ear-level devices used	Maskers or tinnitus instruments (masker + hearing aid housed in same device); used monaurally or binaurally; trial-and-error procedure in clinic to determine most effective device	Sound generator or combination unit (sound generator + hearing aid housed in same device); used binaurally; device selection based on prescribed category (0, 1, 2, 3, or 4)
Spectral characteristics of sound	Noise varies depending on patient's perception of most effective	Stable broadband noise
Sound therapy regimen	Use of ear-level device with masking noise adjusted to patient's preference, typically at the lowest level to mask (or partially mask) tinnitus; wear as desired	Use of ear-level device with noise adjusted to just below "mixing point" at the beginning of the day; use during waking hours
Follow-up visits	Typically at 6 months and 1 year to ensure proper use of maskers	Typically at 3 and 6 weeks, and 3, 6, 12, and 18 months
Long-term use	Use as long as necessary to provide masking relief	Use until habituation is achieved, typically 1 to 2 years

Source: Newman, C.W. and Sandridge, S.A. Tinnitus management. In: Montano, J.J. and Spitzer, J.B. (eds.), *Adult Audiologic Rehabilitation* (p. 425). Copyright © 2009 Plural Publishing, Inc. All rights reserved. Used with permission.

Table 5.4 The ten-question screening version of the tinnitus handicap inventory

Because of your tinnitus is it difficult for you to concentrate?
Do you complain a great deal regarding your tinnitus?
Do you feel as though you cannot escape your tinnitus?
Does your tinnitus make you feel confused?
Because of your tinnitus do you feel frustrated?
Do you feel that you can no longer cope with your tinnitus?
Does your tinnitus make it difficult for you to enjoy life?
Does your tinnitus make you upset?
Because of your tinnitus do you have trouble falling asleep at night?
Because of your tinnitus do you feel depressed?

Source: Newman, C.W. and Sandridge, S.A. Tinnitus management. In: Montano, J.J. and Spitzer, J.B. (eds.), *Adult Audiologic Rehabilitation* (p. 406). Copyright © 2009 Plural Publishing, Inc. All rights reserved. Used with permission.

Table 5.5   Representative models and mechanisms underlying the generation of tinnitus

Generator	Investigator	Mechanism
Peripheral contribution	Penner (1990)	Spontaneous otoacoustic emissions
	Jastreboff (1990)	Discordant inner and outer hair cells; damaged outer hair cells with relatively intact inner hair cells result in increased neural spontaneous activity from the cochlea
	Patuzzi (2002)	Damaged outer hair cells cause excessive release of neurotransmitter (glutamate) from inner hair cells producing sustained cochlear activity
	Sahley and Nodar (2001)	Increase of endogenous dynorphins (associated with stress) potentiates excitatory function of glutamate resulting in increased spontaneous neural activity
	Chery-Croze, Truy, and Morgon (1994)	Loss of lateral efferent connectivity between inner and outer hair cells result in an imbalance between inhibitory and excitatory cochlear events causing an increase of spontaneous neural activity
	Moller (1984)	Cross-talk between nerve fibers results from ephaptic coupling (interneural synchrony)
Brainstem contribution	Kaltenbach (2000)	Hyperactive spontaneous activity in the dorsal cochlear nucleus
	Salvi, Wang, and Powers (1996)	Hyperactive spontaneous activity in the inferior colliculus and dorsal cochlear nucleus result in tonotopic reorganization (auditory plasticity) of these structures
Cortical contribution	Salvi, Lockwood, and Burkard (2000)	Cortical reorganization following changes in the auditory periphery result in a disproportionately large number of neurons becoming sensitive (tuned) to frequencies at the upper and lower borders representing peripheral hearing loss
	Arnold, Bartenstein, Oestreicher, Romer, and Schwaiger (1996)	Hyperactivity in the left transverse temporal gyrus
	Lockwood et al (1998)	Abnormal activation of auditory cortex and amygdale

Table 5.5   *(Continued)*

Generator	Investigator	Mechanism
Somatic modulation	Levine (2004)	Modulation of tinnitus results from an interaction of auditory perception and somatosensory links between the dorsal cochlear nucleus and medullary somato-sensory nucleus
Psychological factors	Sweetow (1986, 2000)	Cognition—inappropriate ways of thinking about tinnitus result from maladaptive strategies and cognitive distortions
	Hallam, Rachman, and Hinchcliffe (1984)	Habituation—intolerance to tinnitus results from individual's failure to habituate (adapt) to the tinnitus sensation
	Hallam et al (1984); Hallam and McKenna (2006)	Attention—disturbing tinnitus is a failure to shift attention away from tinnitus
	Hallam et al (1984); Jastroboff and Hazell (1993); McKenna (2004)	Learning—enhanced tinnitus perception is a learned response resulting from negative emotional reinforcement involving the limbic system and autonomic activation

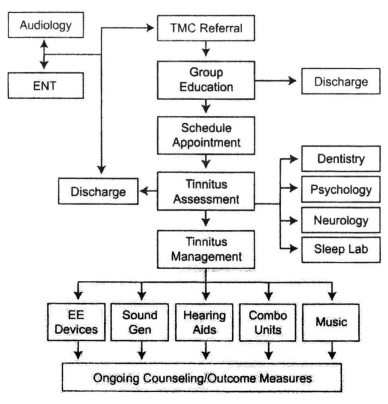

Fig. 5.1 Tinnitus Management Clinic (TMC) clinical pathway. Combo, combination; EE, environmental enhancement; ENT, ear, nose, and throat physician (otolaryngologist); Gen, generators. (From Newman, C.W., Sandridge, S.A., Bolek, L. (2008), Developmental and psychometric adequacy of the screening version of the Tinnitus Handicap Inventory. *Otol. Neurol.* 29:276–281. Reprinted with permission of Lippincott Williams and Wilkins.)

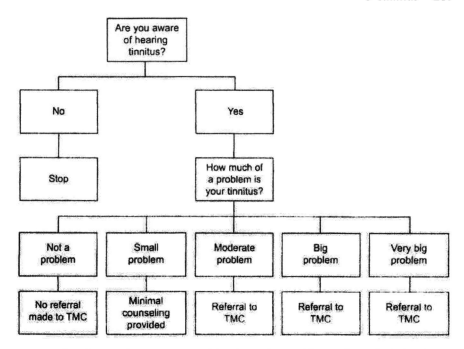

Fig. 5.2 Flow chart used as screening model to determine need for enrollment in the Tinnitus Management Clinic (TMC). (From Newman, C.W. and Sandridge, S.A. Tinnitus management. In: Montano, J.J. and Spitzer, J.B. (eds.), *Adult Audiologic Rehabilitation* (p. 405). Copyright © 2009 Plural Publishing, Inc. All rights reserved. Used with permission.)

Table 5.6 Examples of self-report tinnitus questionnaires

Questionnaire/Authors	Content	Scoring/Interpretation	Psychometrics	Strengths/Weaknesses
Tinnitus Questionnaire/ Tinnitus Effects Questionnaire (TQ/TEQ; Hallam, Jakes, and Hinchcliffe, 1998)	52 items: sleep disturbance, emotional distress, auditory perceptual difficulties, inappropriate or lack of coping skills ("absolutist" beliefs)	Level of agreement with each statement: true (2 points), partly true (1 point), not true (0 points); score range: 0–104 points, with higher scores reflecting greater tinnitus complaints	High internal consistency and reliability (Cronbach's α = 0.91–0.95); high test retest reliability (r = 0.91–0.94); convergent validity with the THQ and TRQ	Stable measure over time making it a useful outcome measure; no data available regarding what is considered a clinically or statistically significant change in score following intervention for a given patient
Tinnitus Handicap Questionnaire (THQ; Kuk, Tyler, Russell, and Jordan, 1990)	27 items: Factor 1: physical, emotional, social consequences of tinnitus; Factor 2: effects on hearing; Factor 3: patient's view of tinnitus	Level of agreement with each statement between 0 (strongly disagrees) and 100 (strongly agrees); mean scores calculated, with high scores reflecting greater handicap; individual scores can be compared against normative percentile data	High internal consistency and reliability for total scale (Cronbach's α = 0.95 with factors ranging from 0.47 to 0.95); high test-retest reliability for total (r = 0.89), factor 1 (r = 0.89), and factor 2 (r = 0.90); low for factor 3 (r = 0.50); adequate construct validity (r > 0.50) with tinnitus loudness judgments, life satisfaction, hearing, depression, and general health	Percentile ranking for given patient is useful in determining individual severity; application of factor 3 as an independent measure is questionable; scoring on a 100-point scale may be difficult for some individuals
Tinnitus Severity Scale (TSS; Sweetow and Levy, 1990)	15 items: intrusiveness, distress, hearing loss, sleep disturbance, and medication	Multiple-choice format for each item; range in score 1 (no impact) to 4 (most impact); each item weighted 1 to 3 points (total = 39 points); total score calculated by multiplying item score by weight and summing the	Adequate test-retest reliability (r = 0.86)	Item analysis may be useful in determining treatment goals; limited psychometric data available

Instrument	Content	Scoring	Psychometric properties	Comments
Subjective Tinnitus Severity Scale (STSS; Halford and Anderson, 1991)	16 items: severity defined as intrusiveness, prominence, and distress	Yes/no response format; 10 items earn 1 point for Yes response; 6 items earn 1 point for No response; scoring range: 0–16, with high scores reflecting greater overall severity	High internal consistency and reliability (Cronbach's α = 0.94); criterion validity determined by significant correlations with clinician rating of severity	Brief and simple to administer and score; no severity classification schemes developed; no test-rest reliability available required for measuring outcome
Tinnitus Reaction Questionnaire (TRQ Wilson, Henry, Bowen, and Haralambous, 1991)	26 items: distress consequences including anger, confusion, annoyance, helplessness, activity avoidance, and panic	5-point scale (0 = not at all; 4 = almost all of the time); score range: 0–104, with higher scores reflecting greater distress	High internal consistency and reliability (Cronbach's α = 0.96); high test-retest reliability (r = 0.88); construct validity supported by moderate to high correlations with clinician ratings and self-report measures of anxiety and depression; four factors emerged using principal components analysis: general distress, interference, severity, and avoidance	Global measure of distress; brief and simple to administer and score; test-rest data helpful in determining treatment outcome; however, only short-term (3 day to 3 weeks) data available; no data available regarding what is considered a clinically or statistically change in score following intervention for a given patient
Tinnitus Handicap/Support Scale (TH/SS; Erlandsson, Hallberg, and Axelsson, 1992)	28 items: Factor 1: perceived attitudes or reactions of others; Factor 2: social support; Factor 3: personal and social handicaps	5-point scale (1 = strongly disagree, 5 = strongly disagree)	Construct validity assessed with the Rinnitus Severity Questionnaire (TSQ) showing significant relationships between tinnitus severity and perceived attitudes (factor 1) and between severity and personal and social handicaps (factor 3)	Only questionnaire assessing influence of significant other in management process; lacks test-retest reliability data; factor 2 is not sufficiently sensitive to quantify complexity of social support

(continued on next page)

Table 5.6 *(Continued)*

Questionnaire/Authors	Content	Scoring/Interpretation	Psychometrics	Strengths/Weaknesses
Tinnitus Handicap Inventory (THI; Newman, Jacobson, and Spitzer, 1996; Newman, Sandridge, and Jacobson, 1998)	25 items: Functional subscale: role limitations in mental, social/occupational, physical functioning; Emotional subscale: anger, frustration, irritability, depression; Catastrophic subscale: desperation, loss of control, inability to cope and escape, fear of grave disease	Response format: Yes (4 points); Sometimes (2 points); No (0 points); total score range: 0–100 points, with higher scores reflecting greater handicap; handicap severity categories: no handicap (0–16 points); mild (18–36 points); moderate (38–56 points); severe (58–100 points)	Excellent internal consistency and reliability (Cronbach's α = 0.096); high test-retest reliability: total (r = 0.92) and subscales (r = 0.84–0.94); 95% confidence interval = 20 points; convergent validity with Tinnitus Grading Questionnaire (TGQ) and TQ; construct validity with Beck Depression Inventory, Modified Somatic Perception Questionnaire, symptom rating scales (e.g., sleep, annoyance), tinnitus pitch and loudness	Helpful in identifying behaviors and thought patterns affected by tinnitus and the coping strategies used; test-retest data are not available; limited application for evaluating treatment outcome
Tinnitus Cognitions Questionnaire (TCQ; Wilson and Henry, 1998)	26 items: positive and negative thoughts	5-point scale: 0 = never, 4 = very frequently; negative items are scored 0–4; positive items are reverse scored 4 to 0; total score range: 0–104, with higher scores reflecting greater tendency to engage in negative thoughts and low engagement in positive thoughts	Excellent internal consistency and reliability (Cronbach's α = 0.91); excellent test-retest reliability (r = 0.88); factor analysis supported positive and negative subscales; construct and convergent validity assessed: TCQ showed moderate correlations with TRQ, THQ, and TQ	Useful index of cognitive responses; psychometrically robust; useful as an outcome measure; measures the extent to which patients actually engage in the reported cognition/thoughts

				TCQ; negative subscale showed high correlations with tinnitus (tinnitus-related distress, handicap, complaint behavior) and nontinnitus (general depression, automatic thoughts, locus of control) measures
Tinnitus Functional Index (TFI; Meikle, Henry, et al, 2008; Meikle, Steward, et al, 2008)	25 items 8 domains/subscales: intrusive, feeling, thinking, hearing, relaxing, sleeping, managing, quality of life	11-point scale (0 to 10); all responses summed, divided by number of questions answered, and multiplied by 10; total score range: 0–100	High test-retest reliability (short-term, $r = 0.82$; long-term, $r = 0.76$); excellent internal consistency reliability (Cronbach's $\alpha = 0.98$); good construct validity with THI ($r = 0.87$), visual analogue scale for severity ($r = 0.75$), THQ ($r = 0.83$); high responsiveness to treatment-related changes in the severity of tinnitus (0.79 effect size for overall TFI score)	Developed in a large sample of patients (327 for prototype 1; 347 for prototype 2); excellent measurement and psychometric properties; valid for measuring treatment-related changes

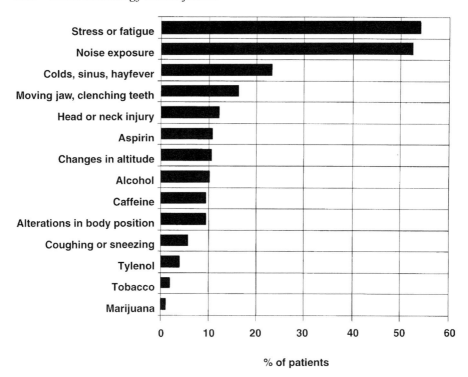

% of patients

Fig. 5.3 Factors that can increase the loudness of tinnitus. (From Valente, M., Hosford-Dunn, H., Roeser, R.J. (2008), *Audiology Treatment,* 2nd ed. New York: Thieme. Reprinted with permission.)

Table 5.7 Tinnitus severity index questions

Directions: For the questions below, please CIRCLE the number that best describes you.

	Never	Rarely	Sometimes	Usually	Always
Does your tinnitus:					
1. Make you feel irritable or nervous?	1	2	3	4	5
2. Make you feel tired or stressed?	1	2	3	4	5
3. Make it difficult for you to relax?	1	2	3	4	5
4. Make it uncomfortable to be in a quiet room?	1	2	3	4	5
5. Make it difficult to concentrate?	1	2	3	4	5
6. Make it harder to interact pleasantly with others?	1	2	3	4	5
7. Interfere with your required activities (work, home, care, or other responsibilities)?	1	2	3	4	5
8. Interfere with your social activities or other things you do in your leisure time?	1	2	3	4	5
9. Interfere with your overall enjoyment of life?	1	2	3	4	5
10. Interfere with your ability to sleep?	1	2	3	4	5
11. How often do you have difficulty ignoring your tinnitus?	1	2	3	4	5
12. How often do you experience discomfort from tinnitus?	1	2	3	4	5

Source: Valente, M., Hosford-Dunn, H., Roeser, R.J. (2008), *Audiology Treatment,* 2nd ed. New York; Thieme. Reprinted with permission.

6

Hearing Loss Prevention

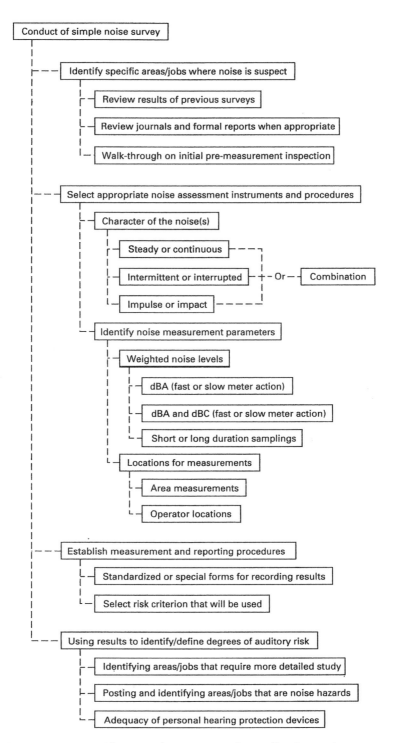

Fig. 6.1 Noise survey: Considerations when using a simple sound level meter. (From Gasaway, DG. *Hearing Conservation: A Practical Manual and Guide,* 1st ed. © 1985. Reprinted by permission of Pearson Education, Inc., Upper Saddle River, NJ.)

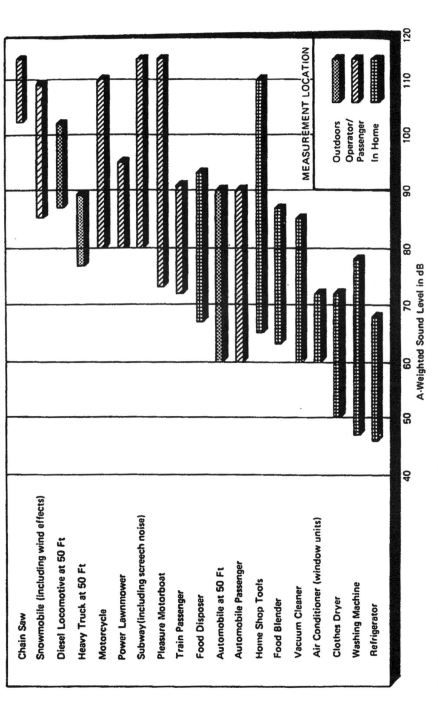

Fig. 6.2 Typical ranges of sound levels emitted by various products. (From Environmental Protection Agency, 1978, Protective Noise Levels. EPA 550/9–79–100. Washington, DC: U.S. Environmental Protection Agency.)

Table 6.1   Steps for checking Occupational Safety and Health Administration (OSHA) compliance assuming noise exposures in dBA

Step Number	Procedure	Result
1	Measure 8-hour TWA dBA	96 dBA
2	Labeled NRR of HPD	20 dB
3	Subtract 7 dB from the NRR (correction for dBA measures)	20 – 7 = 13 dB
4	Derate the corrected NRR in step 3 by 50% (divide by 2)	13/2 = 6.5
5	Subtract the expected HPD attenuation from the unprotected noise exposure to estimate protected noise exposure	96 – 6.5 = 89.5
6	Compare the estimated protected exposure to the permissible exposure limit (PEL)	
	If the worker has no standard threshold shift (STS), then the protected levels should be at most 90 dBA and preferably even lower	88.5 is below 90; the protected exposure in step 5 suggests effective noise control
	If the worker has had a STS, then the protected level should be at most 85 dBA or lower	88.5 is above 85; in the presence of STS additional noise controls appear to be necessary

Abbreviations: HPD, hearing protection device; NRR, noise reduction rating; TWA, time-weighted average.
Source: Rawool, V. (2012), *Hearing Conservation: in Occupational, Recreational, Educational, and Home Settings.* New York: Thieme. Reprinted by permission.

Table 6.2   Steps for following NIOSH (1998) recommendations assuming noise exposures in dBA

Step Number	Procedure	Result
1	Measure 8-hour TWA dBA	96 dBA
2	Labeled NRR of preformed earplug (not foam)	20 dB
3	Subtract 7 dB from the NRR (correction for dBA measures)	20 – 7 = 13 dB
4	Subtract 70% from the corrected NRR in step 3	13 – (13 × 0.7) = 3.9 dB
5	Subtract the expected HPD attenuation from the unprotected noise exposure to estimate protected noise exposure	96 – 3.9 = 92.1 dBA
6	Compare the estimated protected exposure to the NIOSH recommended exposure limit (REL) The protected exposure level should be below 85 dBA	92.1 dBA is above 85 dBA TWA; thus the current HPD is inadequate.

Abbreviations: HPD: hearing protection device; NRR: noise reduction rating; TWA: time-weighted average; NIOSH hearing protector derating formulas: Foam Earplug Derating: Protected exposure (dBA) = Unprotected exposure (dBA) – [0.5 (NRR-7)]; Preformed Earplug Derating: Protected exposure (dBA) = Unprotected exposure (dBA) – [0.3(NRR-7)] Earmuff Derating: Protected exposure (dBA) = Unprotected exposure (dBA) – [0.75 (NRR-7)]
Source: Rawool, V. (2012), *Hearing Conservation: in Occupational, Recreational, Educational, and Home Settings.* New York: Thieme. Reprinted by permission.

Table 6.3 Percentage of hearing handicap: Comparison of three procedures

	Procedure		
	Three Frequencies[a]	*Four Frequencies*[b]	*High Frequencies*[c]
Frequency (Hz)	500, 1,000, 2,000	500, 1,000, 2,000, 3,000	1,000, 2,000, 3,000, 4,000
Method of calculation	Average	Average	Average
Low fence (ANSI–1969)	25 dB	25 dB	25 dB
High fence (ANSI–1969)	92 dB	92 dB	75 dB
Percent per decibel loss	1.5	1.5	2
Relationship of better ear to poorer ear	5:1	5:1	5:1

Example using four-frequency average:

	500	1,000	2,000	4,000
Right ear	15	25	45	55
Left ear	30	45	60	85

1. Calculate average hearing threshold level:

$$\text{Right Ear} = \frac{15 + 25 + 45 + 55}{4} = \frac{140}{4} = 35 \text{ dB}$$

$$\text{Left Ear} = \frac{30 + 45 + 60 + 85}{4} = \frac{220}{4} = 55 \text{ dB}$$

2. Calculate monaural impairment:
   Right ear: 35 dB – 25 dB = 10 dB × 1.5% = 15%
   Left ear: 55 dB – 25 dB = 30 dB × 1.5% = 45%

3. Calculate percentage of binaural hearing handicap:

$$\text{Formula} = \frac{\text{Better ear (Smaller number)} \times 5 + \text{Worse ear (Larger number)} \times 1}{6}$$

$$= \frac{(15 \times 5) + (45 \times 1)}{6} = \frac{75 + 45}{6} = \frac{120}{6} = 20\%$$

[a]*Trans. Am. Acad. Ophthalmol. Otolaryngol.* 63, 236–238, 1959.
[b]*JAMA* 241(19), 2055–2059, 1979.
[c]*Asha* 23, 293–297, 1981.

Table 6.4 Noise exposure level and exchange rate comparisons

Exchange Rate Comparisons (Duration and Dose)

Noise Exposure Level dBA	3 dB (NIOSH)				5 dB (OSHA, MSHA, FRA)			
	Hours	Minutes	Seconds	% Noise Dose	Hours	Minutes	Seconds	% Noise Dose
>140	–	–	0	>32,500,000	–	–	0	>102,400
130	–	–	<1	3,276,800	–	1	52	25,600
129	–	–	1	2,600,798	–	2	10	22,286
128	–	–	1	2,000,000	–	2	27	19,401
127	–	–	1	1,600,000	–	2	49	16,890
126	–	–	2	1,300,400	–	3	14	14,703
125	–	–	3	1,000,000	–	3	47	12,800
124	–	–	3	800,000	–	4	19	11,143
123	–	–	4	650,000	–	4	55	9,701
122	–	–	6	500,000	–	5	30	8,445
121	–	–	7	400,000	–	6	36	7,352
120	–	–	9	325,100	–	7	30	6,400
119	–	–	11	250,000	–	8	24	5,571
118	–	–	14	200,000	–	9	36	4,850
117	–	–	18	162,550	–	11	24	4,222
116	–	–	22	129,016	–	13	12	3,676
115	–	–	28	100,000	–	15	–	3,200
114	–	–	35	80,000	–	17	24	2,786
113	–	–	45	64,508	–	19	48	2,425
112	–	–	56	50,000	–	22	48	2,111
111	–	1	11	40,000	–	26	24	1,838
110	–	1	29	32,254	–	30	–	1,600
109	–	1	53	25,000	–	34	12	1,393
108	–	2	22	20,000	–	39	36	1,213

dB(A)								
107	–	2	59	16,000	–	45	36	1,056
106	–	3	45	12,800	–	52	12	920
105	–	4	43	10,000	1	–	–	800
104	–	5	57	8,000	1	6	–	700
103	–	7	30	64,000	1	18	–	610
102	–	9	27	5,000	1	30	–	530
101	–	11	54	4,000	1	42	–	460
100	–	15	–	3,200	2	–	–	400
99	–	18	59	2,500	2	18	–	350
98	–	23	49	2,000	2	36	–	303
97	–	30	–	1,600	3	–	–	264
96	–	37	48	1,270	3	30	–	260
95	–	47	37	1,000	4	–	–	200
94	1	–	–	800	4	36	–	175
93	1	16	–	635	5	18	–	152
92	1	35	–	500	6	6	–	132
91	2	–	–	400	7	–	–	115
90	2	31	–	317	8	12	–	100
89	3	10	–	250	9	36	–	87
88	4	–	–	200	10	6	–	76
87	5	2	–	159	12	6	–	66
86	6	21	–	126	13	54	–	57
85	8	–	–	100	16	–	–	50
84	10	5	–	80	18	24	–	44
83	12	42	–	63	21	6	–	38
82	16	–	–	50	24	3	–	33
81	20	10	–	40	27	9	–	29
80	25	24	–	32	32	–	–	25

Abbreviations: FRA, Federal Railroad Administration; MSHA, Mine Safety and Health Administration; NIOSH, National Institute for Occupational Safety and Health; OSHA, Occupational Safety and Health Administration.

ITALICS. Numbers above 115 dB(A) are italicized to indicate that they are noise levels that are NOT permitted by regulatory agencies. The italicized numbers are included only because they are sometimes necessary for the computation of total noise dose or purely for comparison purposes.

Source: Meinke, DK (2012). Unpublished.

Table 6.5 Computation of the noise reduction rating (NRR)

Frequency (Hz)	125	250	500	1,000	2,000	3,000	4,000	6,000	8,000	
dB										
1. Assumed pink noise	100	100	100	100	100		100		100	
2. Correction for conversion to C-weighted levels	-.2	0	0		-.2		-.8		-3	dBC = 107.9
3. Unprotected dBC levels	99.8	100	100	100	99.8		99.2		97	
4. Corrections for conversion to A-weighted levels	-16.1	-8.6	-3.2	0	1.2		1.0		-1.1	
5. Unprotected dBA levels	83.9	91.4	96.8	100	101.2		101		98.9	
6. Average attenuation	32.1	30.6	34.5	31.4	30.8	37.3	36.3	34.1	36.3	
						Ave = 36.8		Ave = 35.2		
7. Standard deviation	5.9	6.1	6.5	5.5	4.1	5.3	6.1	6.7	6.9	
	×2	×2	×2	×2	×2	5.3 + 6.1 = 11.4		6.7 + 6.9 = 13.6		
	11.8	12.2	13	11	8.2					
8. APV$_{98}$ (line 6 – line 7)	20.3	18.4	21.5	20.4	22.6		25.4		21.6	
9. Protected ear dBA (line 5 – line 8)	63.9	73	75.3	79.6	78.6		75.6		77.3	dBA = 84.91
10. NRR = unprotected dBC – protected dBA – 3										107.9 – 84.9 – 3 = 20

Abbreviations: dBC, decibel C-weighted; Hz: Hertz.

Note: dBA and dBC levels in the last column were calculated using the following formula:

$$L = 10 \log \sum_{i=1}^{n} 10^{Li/10}$$

where

L = combined level in dB SPL

n = number of bands being combined

i = the ith band

Li = the octave band level of the ith band

Source: Rawool, V. (2012), *Hearing Conservation: in Occupational, Recreational, Educational, and Home Settings.* New York: Thieme. Reprinted by permission.

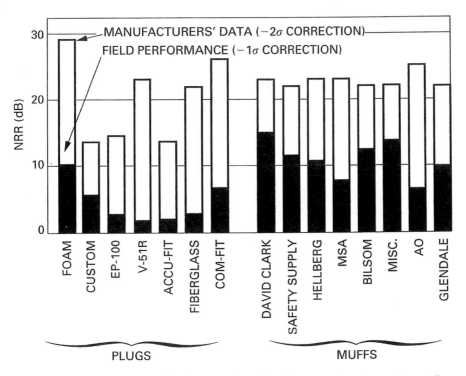

Fig. 6.3 Noise reduction rating (NRR) versus real-world performance of earplugs and earmuffs. (From Melnick, W., Industrial hearing conservation. In: Katz, J. (ed.), *Handbook of Clinical Audiology,* 4th ed. Baltimore: Williams & Wilkins, 1994:550. Reprinted by permission.)

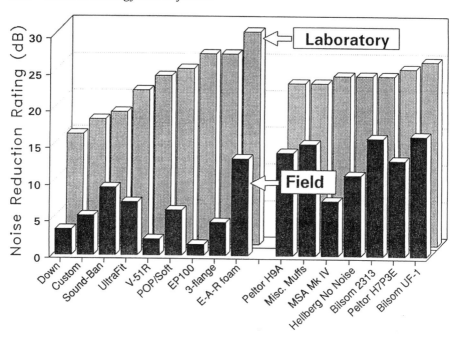

Fig. 6.4 Attenuation received in actual use (field) with that found in laboratory evaluations (as labeled). (From Berger, E.H., Royster, L.H., Royster, J.D., Driscoll, D.P., Layne, M. *The Noise Manual*, 5th ed., Chapter 10. Falls Church, VA: American Industrial Hygiene Association, 2003. Courtesy of E.H. Berger, 3M. Reprinted by permission.)

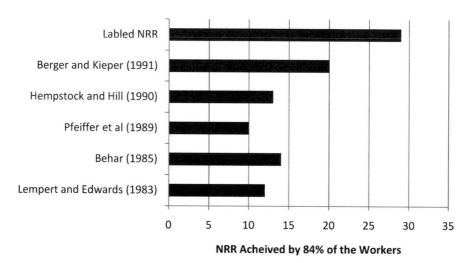

NRR Acheived by 84% of the Workers

Fig. 6.5 The NRRs achieved by 84% of the workers in different investigations for an earplug with an NRR of 29 (Behar, 1985; Berger and Kieper, 1991; Hempstock and Hill, 1990; Lempert and Edwards, 1983; Pfeiffer, Kuhnm, Specht, and Knipfer, 1989). (From Rawool, V. (2012), *Hearing Conservation: in Occupational, Recreational, Educational, and Home Settings.* New York: Thieme. Reprinted by permission.)

Table 6.6   Percent noise exposure (dose) for 8-hour time-weighted average (TWA)*

% or Dose	TWA	% or Dose	TWA	% or Dose	TWA	% or Dose	TWA
10	73.4	104	90.3	260	96.9	640	103.4
15	76.3	105	90.4	270	97.2	650	103.5
20	78.4	106	90.4	280	97.4	660	103.6
25	80.0	107	90.5	290	97.7	670	103.7
30	81.3	108	90.6	300	97.9	680	103.8
35	82.4	109	90.6	310	98.2	690	103.9
40	83.4	110	90.7	320	98.4	700	104.0
45	84.2	111	90.8	330	98.6	710	104.1
50	85.0	112	90.8	340	98.8	720	104.2
55	85.7	113	90.9	350	99.0	730	104.3
60	86.3	114	90.9	360	99.2	740	104.4
65	86.9	115	91.1	370	99.4	750	104.5
70	87.4	116	91.1	380	99.6	760	104.6
75	87.9	117	91.1	390	99.8	770	104.7
80	88.4	118	91.2	400	100.0	780	104.8
81	88.5	119	91.3	410	100.2	790	104.9
82	88.6	120	91.3	420	100.4	800	105.0
83	88.7	125	91.6	430	100.5	810	105.1
84	88.7	130	91.9	440	100.7	820	105.2
85	88.8	135	92.2	450	100.8	830	1053
86	88.9	140	92.4	460	101.0	840	105.4
87	89.0	145	92.7	470	101.2	850	105.4
88	89.1	150	92.9	480	101.3	860	105.5
89	89.2	155	93.2	490	101.5	870	105.6
90	89.2	160	93.4	500	101.6	880	105.7
91	89.3	165	93.6	510	101.8	890	105.8
92	89.4	170	93.8	520	101.9	900	105.8
93	89.5	175	94.0	530	102.0	910	105.9
94	89.6	180	94.2	540	102.2	920	106.0
95	89.6	185	94.4	550	102.3	930	106.1
96	89.7	190	94.6	560	102.4	940	106.2
97	89.8	195	94.8	570	102.6	950	106.2
98	89.9	200	95.0	580	102.7	960	106.3
99	89.9	210	95.4	590	102.8	970	106.4
100	90.0	220	95.7	600	102.9	980	106.5
101	90.1	230	96.0	610	103.0	990	106.5
102	90.1	240	96.3	620	103.2	999	106.6
103	90.2	250	96.6	630	103.3		

*From Occupational Noise Exposure; Hearing Conservation Amendment; Final Rule, *Federal Register*, 48(46):9737–9785 (March 8, 1983).

Source: Gasaway, DG. *Hearing Conservation: A Practical Manual and Guide*, 1st ed. © 1985. Reprinted by permission of Pearson Education, Inc., Upper Saddle River, NJ.

Table 6.7 Permissible noise exposures: Allowable minutes or hours of exposure for a single episode of noise for an 8-hour normal work period specified by OSHA–1983*

dBA	Minutes	Hours	dBA	Minutes	Hours
80	1,920	32	106	52	.87
81	1,674	27.9	107	46	.76
82	1,458	24.3	108	40	.66
83	1,266	21.1	109	34	.57
84	1,104	18.4	110	30	.50
85	960	16.0	111	26	.44
86	834	13.9	112	23	.38
87	726	12.1	113	20	.33
88	636	10.6	114	17	.29
89	552	9.2	115[a]	15	.25
90	480	8.0	116	13	.22
91	420	7.0	117	11	.19
92	372	6.2	118	10	.16
93	318	5.3	119	8	.14
94	275	4.6	120	8	.125
95	240	4.0	121	7	.11
96	210	3.5	122	6	.095
97	180	3.0	123	5	.082
98	156	2.6	124	4	.072
99	138	2.3	125	4	.063
100	120	2.0	126	3	.054
101	102	1.7	127	3	.047
102	90	1.5	128	3	.041
103	84	1.4	129	2	.036
104	78	1.3	130	2	.031
105	60	1.0			

*From Occupational Noise Exposure; Hearing Conservation Amendment; Final Rule, *Federal Register*, 48(46):9737–9785 (March 8, 1983).
[a]Upper limit for unprotected exposure to intermittent or steady-state noise.
Source: Gasaway, DG. *Hearing Conservation: A Practical Manual and Guide,* 1st ed. © 1985. Reprinted by permission of Pearson Education, Inc., Upper Saddle River, NJ.

Table 6.8 Age-correction values for males and females (according to tables F-1 and F-2, OSHA, 1983)

	Males					Females				
Frequency (Hz):	1,000	2,000	3,000	4,000	6,000	1,000	2,000	3,000	4,000	6,000
Age (Years)										
20 or younger	5	3	4	5	8	7	4	3	3	6
21	5	3	4	5	8	7	4	4	3	6
22	5	3	4	5	8	7	4	4	4	6
23	5	3	4	6	9	7	5	4	4	7
24	5	3	5	6	9	7	5	4	4	7
25	5	3	5	7	10	8	5	4	4	7
26	5	4	5	7	10	8	5	5	4	8
27	5	4	6	7	11	8	5	5	5	8
28	6	4	6	8	11	8	5	5	5	8
29	6	4	6	8	12	8	5	5	5	9
30	6	4	6	9	12	8	6	6	5	9
31	6	4	7	9	13	8	6	6	5	9
32	6	5	7	10	14	9	6	6	6	10
33	6	5	7	10	14	9	6	6	6	10
34	6	5	8	11	15	9	6	6	6	10
35	7	5	8	11	15	9	6	7	7	11
36	7	5	9	12	16	9	7	7	7	11
37	7	6	9	12	17	9	7	7	7	12
38	7	6	9	13	17	10	7	7	7	12
39	7	6	9	14	18	10	7	8	8	12
40	7	6	10	14	19	10	7	8	8	13
41	7	6	10	14	20	10	8	8	8	13
42	8	7	11	16	20	10	8	8	8	13
43	8	7	12	16	21	11	8	9	9	14
44	8	7	12	17	22	11	8	9	9	14
45	8	7	13	18	23	11	8	10	10	15

(*continued on next page*)

Table 6.8 (*Continued*)

Frequency (Hz):	Males					Females				
	1,000	2,000	3,000	4,000	6,000	1,000	2,000	3,000	4,000	6,000
Age (Years)										
46	8	8	13	19	24	11	9	10	10	15
47	8	8	14	19	24	11	9	10	11	16
48	9	8	14	20	25	12	9	11	11	16
49	9	9	15	21	26	12	9	11	11	16
50	9	9	16	22	27	12	10	11	12	17
51	9	9	16	23	28	12	10	12	12	17
52	9	10	17	24	29	12	10	12	13	18
53	9	10	18	25	30	13	10	13	13	18
54	10	10	18	26	31	13	11	13	14	19
55	10	11	19	27	32	13	11	14	14	19
56	10	11	20	28	34	13	11	14	15	20
57	10	11	21	29	35	13	11	15	15	20
58	10	12	22	31	36	14	12	15	16	21
59	11	12	22	32	37	14	12	16	16	21
60 or older	11	13	23	33	38	14	12	16	17	22

Note: Example of how to use age-correction values: Using 4,000 Hz as an example, suppose the threshold on the annual audiogram is 20 dB at age 32, and the threshold on the baseline audiogram was 5 dB at age 20. The uncorrected threshold shift would be as follows:

20 dB (annual) – 5 dB (baseline) = 15 dB (threshold shift).

Now find the age-correction values that apply to the baseline and annual audiogram. Find the difference between these age-correction values. For males at 4,000 Hz, these values are 10 dB at age 32 and 5 dB at age 20, and the difference between them is as follows:

10 dB (at age 32) – 5 dB (at age 20) = 5 dB (age correction).

This difference becomes the age correction. It is subtracted from the uncorrected threshold shift to find the age-corrected threshold shift. In our example, this is

15 dB (uncorrected) – 5 dB (correction) = 10 dB (age-corrected).

The age-corrected threshold shift is then used to find the (now age-corrected) standard threshold shift.

Source: Gelfand, S. (2001), *Essentials of Audiology*, 2nd ed. New York: Thieme. Reprinted by permission.

Table 6.9 **Example of calculation of a standard threshold shift (STS) using left ear air conduction thresholds (dB HL) of a hypothetical male worker**

	Age (Years)	*Frequency (kHz)*						
		500	*1,000*	*2,000*	*3,000*	*4,000*	*6,000*	*8,000*
Current confirmed thresholds	49	10	10	10	15	20	30	15
Baseline	21	0	0	5	5	5	10	10
Step 1	Calculate the average threshold shift at 2,000, 3,000, and 4,000 Hz for the current audiogram		10 + 15 + 20 = 45/3 = 15					
Step 2	Calculate the average threshold at 2,000, 3,000, and 4,000 Hz for the baseline audiogram		5 + 5 + 5 = 15/3 = 5					
Step 3	Determine if the current average thresholds at 2,000, 3,000, and 4,000 Hz are 10 dB or worse than the baseline thresholds		15 – 5 = 10. The current average thresholds are worse by 10 dB; thus there appears to be an STS.					

Source: Rawool, V. (2012), Hearing Conservation: in Occupational, Recreational, Educational, and Home Settings. New York: Thieme. Reprinted by permission.

Table 6.10 **Example of application on age-correction for determination of standard threshold shift (STS)**

	Age (Years)	Frequency (kHz)						
		500	1,000	2,000	3,000	4,000	6,000	8,000
Current	49	10	10	10	15	20	30	15
Baseline	21	0	0	5	5	5	10	10
Step 1	Locate expected values at the age of 49 years for men for 2,000, 3,000, and 4,000 Hz (Table F-1 of OSHA [1983] appendix F).			9	15	21		
Step 2	Locate expected values at the age of 21 years for men for 2,000, 3,000, and 4,000 Hz (Table F-1 of OSHA [1983] appendix F).			3	4	5		
Step 3	Calculate the difference between the values in step 1 and 2. This difference reveals the expected deterioration in thresholds due to the effect of aging from the age of 21 to 49 years.			6	11	16		
Step 4	Correct the current audiogram by subtracting the assumed age-related threshold shift obtained in step 3.			10 6 4	15 11 4	20 16 4	Current Age correction from step 3 Age corrected current threshold	
Step 5	Calculate the average threshold shift at 2,000, 3,000, and 4,000 Hz for the age corrected current audiogram.			4 + 4 + 4 = 12/3 = 4				
Step 6	Calculate the average threshold shift at 2,000, 3,000, and 4,000 Hz for the baseline audiogram.			5 + 5 + 5 = 15/3 = 5				
Step 7	Determine if the current average thresholds at 2,000, 3,000, and 4,000 Hz are 10 dB or worse than the baseline thresholds.			The current age-corrected thresholds are better than the baseline thresholds. Thus, there is no age-corrected STS.				

Abbreviation: OSHA, Occupational Safety and Health Administration

Source: Rawool, V. (2012), Hearing Conservation: in Occupational, Recreational, Educational, and Home Settings. New York: Thieme. Reprinted by permission.

Table 6.11   Reported methods for calculating hearing impairment

Impairment Formula	Impairment Formula Definition (Single Ear)	States or Jurisdictions Reporting Use/Comments
Medical evidence	Impairment rating determined by examining professional	AL, AZ, CT, DE, ID, IN, KY, LA, MA, MS, NE, NH, NM, OH, TN, VT, WY, Guam, New Brunswick, Prince Edward Island, Quebec
AAO-79/AMA	Average hearing levels > 25 dB at 500, 100, 2,000 and 3,000 Hz; 1.5% per dB	AK, AR, CA, CO, FL, IA, KS, MN, NV, NY, NC, ND, OK, PA, RI, SC, SD, TX, UT, VA, WA, WV, Washington, DC, U.S. Department of Labor's Federal Employees' Compensation Act (DOL-FECA), U.S. Department of Labor, Division of Longshore and Harbor Workers' Compensation, Ontario, Yukon Territories
AAOO-59	Average hearing levels > 25 dB at 500, 100, 2,000 and 3,000 Hz; 1.5% per dB	GA, HI, ME, MD, MO, MT
Illinois	Average hearing levels > 25 dB at 500, 100, 2,000, and 3,000 Hz; 1.82% per dB	IL
Michigan	Not applicable	Individuals are compensated only if an injury to the ear causes a loss of wages
New Jersey	Average hearing levels > 25 dB at 500, 100, 2,000, and 3,000 Hz; 1.5% per dB	NJ
Oregon	Average hearing levels > 25 dB at 500, 100, 2,000, 3,000, 4,000, and 6,000 Hz; 1.5% per dB	OR
Wisconsin	Average hearing levels ≥ 30 dB at 500, 100, 2,000, and 3,000 Hz; 1.6% per dB	WI, Northwest Territories, Saskatchewan
British Columbia	Average hearing levels > 25 dB at 500, 1,000, and 2,000 Hz; 2.5% per dB	British Columbia
Manitoba/Nova Scotia	Average hearing levels ≥ 35 dB at 500, 100, 2,000, and 3,000 Hz	Manitoba, Nova Scotia

Source: Used with permission from Megerson, SC (2001, April). *Current trends in workers' compensation practices for hearing loss.* Workshop at the annual conference of the American Association of Occupational Health Nurses, San Francisco. Data adapted from Dobie RA, Megerson SC. (2003). Workers Compensation. In E.H. Berger et al., eds., *The Noise Manual,* 5th ed. Falls Church, VA: American Industrial Hygiene Association. *Note:* Readers are encouraged to check current state statutes before use.

Table 6.12   Hearing loss statutes in the United States and Canada

Jurisdiction	1. Is occupational hearing loss compensable?	2. Is minimum noise exposure required for filing?	3. Schedule in weeks (one ear)	4. Schedule in weeks (both ears)	5. Maximum compensations (one ear)	6. Maximum compensation (both ears)	7. Hearing impairment formula	8. Waiting period
Alabama	Yes	No	53	163	$11,660	$35,860	ME	No
Alaska	Yes	No	*	*	*	*	AAO-79	No
Arizona	Yes	No	86	260	$23,100	$69,300	ME	No
Arkansas	Yes	No	42	158	$11,296	$42,502	AAO-79	No
California	Yes	No	50*	311*	$8,040*	$58,863*	AAO-79	No
Colorado	Yes	No	35	139	$5,250	$20,850	AAO-79	No
Connecticut	Yes	No	35	104	*	*	ME*	3 days
Delaware	Yes	No	75	175	$30,833	$71,944	ME	No
District of Columbia	Yes	No	39	150	$34,880	$134,170	AAO-79	6 months
Florida	Yes	No	18	105	$8,892	$51,870	AAO-79	No
Georgia	Yes*	Yes*	NA	150	NA	NR	AAOO-59	6 months
Hawaii	Yes	Yes	52	200	$26,416	$101,600	AAOO-59	No

9. Is deduction made for presbycusis?	10. Is award made for tinnitus?	11. Provision for hearing aid?	12. Credit for improvement with hearing aid?	13. Is hearing loss prior to employment considered in compensation claim?	14. Statute of limitations for hearing loss claim	15. Penalty for not wearing hearing protection devices?	16. Self-assessment of hearing impairment considered in rating/award?	Comments
No	Yes-I	Yes	No	Yes	2 years	Yes- D	Poss	
No	Yes-I	Yes	No*	No*	2 years	No	No	3–6: awards based on temporary disability and permanent partial impairment according to AMA guidelines; 12: unless hearing aid enables worker to return to work; 13: as long as there has been substantial aggravation at work
No	Yes- I	Yes	No	Yes	1 year	No	No	
Poss	No	Poss	No	Yes	Yes*	No	No	14: statute of limitations and other hearing loss issues currently before Board of Appeals
No	Yes	Yes	Yes	Yes	1 year	Yes-P	Yes	3–6: awards modified by age and occupation at time of injury
Yes	Yes	Yes	No	Yes	Yes	Yes-P	No	
Poss	Poss	Poss	Poss	Poss	1 year	Yes-P	Poss	5–6: no maximum reported; award is number of weeks of scheduled benefit at claimant's compensation rate; 7: case law has supported AAO-79
No	No	Yes	Yes	No	2 years	No	No	
Poss	Poss	Poss	Poss	Poss	1 year	Poss	Poss	
No	Yes-I	Yes	No	Yes	2 years	Yes-P	No	
NR	No	NR	NR	Yes	NR	Yse-D	NR	1: no awards granted for monaural hearing loss unless preexisting deafness in other ear; 2: 90 dBA for 90 days
No	Yes	Yes	No	No	2 years	No	No	

(*continued on next page*)

Table 6.12 *(Continued)*

Jurisdiction	1. Is occupational hearing loss compensable?	2. Is minimum noise exposure required for filing?	3. Schedule in weeks (one ear)	4. Schedule in weeks (both ears)	5. Maximum compensations (one ear)	6. Maximum compensation (both ears)	7. Hearing impairment formula	8. Waiting period
Idaho	Yes*	No	NR	175	NR	$42,639	ME	No
Illinois	Yes	Yes*	50–100	200	$43,989	$87,978	Other*	No
Indiana	Yes*	No	*	*	$12,500	$39,500	ME	No
Iowa	Yes	Yes	50	175	$43,600	$152,600	AAO-79	1 month
Kansas	Yes	No	30	110	$10,980	$40,260	AAO-79	No
Kentucky	Yes	No	520	Lifetime	*	*	ME	No
Louisiana	Yes*	No	100	100	NR	$36,700	ME	No
Maine	Yes	Yes	50	200	$20,100	$80,400	AAOO-59	30 days
Maryland	Yes	Yes*	125	250	NR	NR	AAOO-59	Yes
Massachusetts	Yes	No	*	*	*	*	ME	No

9. Is deduction made for presbycusis?	10. Is award made for tinnitus?	11. Provision for hearing aid?	12. Credit for improvement with hearing aid?	13. Is hearing loss prior to employment considered in compensation claim?	14. Statute of limitations for hearing loss claim	15. Penalty for not wearing hearing protection devices?	16. Self-assessment of hearing impairment considered in rating/award?	Comments
lo	Yes-I	No	No	Yes	1 year	No	No	1: only hearing loss due to work-related trauma/injury is considered
lo	Yes-I	Yes	No	Yes	2–3 years	No	No	2: 90 dBA TWA; 7: avg > 30 dB at 1,000, 2,000, and 3,000 Hz, 1.82% per dB
es	NR	No	NR	Yes	2 years	Yes-D	Yes	1: only hearing loss due to work-related trauma/injury is compensable, but case law evolving—likely to consider NIHL in future; 3–4: awards paid for temp. disability (up to 500 wks) or permanent partial impairment based on % of max. awards
es	Yes	Yes	No	Yes	2 years	Yes-D	No	
es	Yes-I	Yes	Yes	Yes	200 days	Yes-D	No	
lo	No	No	No	No	3–5 years	No	No	5–6: award based on % impairment and average weekly wage
lo	Yes-I	No	No	Yes	1 year	Yes-D	No	1: only hearing loss due to work-related trauma/injury is considered
es*	Yes-I	Yes	Yes	Yes	Yes	Yes-D	No	9: ½ dB for each year over 40 years of age
oss	Poss	Yes	No	Yes	Yes	NR	Poss	2: exposure to harmful noise for 90 days or more
es	Yes	Yes	NR	Yes	Yes	Yes	No	3–6: based on statewide average wage, with maximum of $700/week

(*continued on next page*)

Table 6.12 (*Continued*)

Jurisdiction	1. Is occupational hearing loss compensable?	2. Is minimum noise exposure required for filing?	3. Schedule in weeks (one ear)	4. Schedule in weeks (both ears)	5. Maximum compensations (one ear)	6. Maximum compensation (both ears)	7. Hearing impairment formula	8. Waiting period
Michigan	No*							
Minnesota	Yes	No	*	*	*	*	AAO-79	3 month
Mississippi	Yes	No	40	150	$11,191	$41,967	ME	No
Missouri	Yes	No	49	180	$14,442	$53,051	AAOO-59	6 month
Montana	Yes	Yes*	40	200	NR	NR	AAOO-59	6 month
Nebraska	Yes	No	50	*	$22,200	*	ME	No
Nevada	Yes	No	*	*	*	*	AAO-79	No
New Hampshire	Yes	No	30	123	$25,200	$103,320	ME	No
New Jersey	Yes	Yes*	60	200	$8,280	$48,200	Other*	4 weeks
New Mexico	Yes	No	40	150	$15,039	$56,397	ME	7 days
New York	Yes	Yes*	60	150	$24,000	$60,000	AAO-79	3 month

9. Is deduction made for presbycusis?	10. Is award made for tinnitus?	11. Provision for hearing aid?	12. Credit for improvement with hearing aid?	13. Is hearing loss prior to employment considered in compensation claim?	14. Statute of limitations for hearing loss claim	15. Penalty for not wearing hearing protection devices?	16. Self-assessment of hearing impairment considered in rating/award?	Comments
								1: no compensation for occupational hearing loss; employees are compensated only if an injury to the ear (that may or may not result in hearing loss) causes a loss of wages
No	No	Yes	No	Yes	3 years	No	No	3–6: hearing loss compensation is based on a percentage of body impairment (max. for one ear, 6% whole body; for both ears, 35% whole body)
No	Yes	Yes	No	No	Yes	No	Yes	
Yes*	Yes	Yes	No	Yes	No	Yes-P*	No	9: ½ dB per year over age 40 years; 15: results in 15% penalty
Yes*	No	No	No	Yes	No	No	No	2: 90 dB daily for 90 days or more; 9: ½ dB per year over age 40 years
No	Poss	Yes	No	Yes	2 years	No	No	4 and 6: average weekly wage multiplied by life expectancy
Poss	Yes	Yes	No	Yes	No	Yes-P	No	3–6: awards determined according to AMA guideline and state statute
No	No	Yes	No	Yes	2 years	No	No	
No	Yes	Yes	Yes	Yes	2 years	Yes-D	Yes	2: 90 dB TWA; 7: avg > 30 dB at 1,000, 2,000, and 3,000 Hz, 1.5% per dB
No	Yes	No	No	Yes	1 year	Poss-P	No	
No	No	No	No	Yes	90 days	No	No	2: exposure to harmful noise for 90 days or more

(*continued on next page*)

Table 6.12 (*Continued*)

Jurisdiction	1. Is occupational hearing loss compensable?	2. Is minimum noise exposure required for filing?	3. Schedule in weeks (one ear)	4. Schedule in weeks (both ears)	5. Maximum compensations (one ear)	6. Maximum compensation (both ears)	7. Hearing impairment formula	8. Waiting period
North Carolina	Yes	Yes*	70	150	$37,240	$79,800	AAO-79*	6 months
North Dakota	Yes	No	5	100	$695	$13,900	AAO-79	No
Ohio	Yes*	No	25	125	$13,525	$67,625	ME	No
Oklahoma	Yes	No	104	312	$22,194	$66,583	AAO-79	No
Oregon	Yes	No	*	*	$27,240	$87,168	Other*	No
Pennsylvania	Yes	No*	60	260	*	*	AAO-79	No
Rhode Island	Yes	Yes	17*	100*	$1,530*	$9,000*	AAO-79	6 months
South Carolina	Yes	No	80	165	$38,678	$79,773	AAO-79	No

9. Is deduction made for presbycusis?	10. Is award made for tinnitus?	11. Provision for hearing aid?	12. Credit for improvement with hearing aid?	13. Is hearing loss prior to employment considered in compensation claim?	14. Statute of limitations for hearing loss claim	15. Penalty for not wearing hearing protection devices?	16. Self-assessment of hearing impairment considered in rating/award?	Comments
No	No	Yes	No	Yes	2 years	Yes-D	No	2: 90 dBA for at least 90 days; 7: if hearing loss due to injury, then "medical evidence" is utilized
Poss	Yes-I	Yes	No	Yes	No	No	No	
No	No	Yes	No	No	2 years	No	No	1: only permanent total hearing loss in one or both ears is compensable
No	Yes*	Yes	No	Yes	2 years	Yes-D	No	10: up to 5% for tinnitus in cases of unilateral hearing loss
Yes	Yes	Yes	No	Yes*	1 year	No	No	3–4: one time permanent partial disability award based on impairment; 7: avg > 25 dB at 500, 1,000, 2,000, 3,000, 4,000, and 6,000 Hz, 1.5% per dB; 13: if baseline completed within 180 days of hire
No	No	No	No	Yes*	3 years	No	No	2: case law has adopted OSHA standards as employer defends; 5 and 6: No. of weeks × ⅔ average wage; 13: only if preemployment testing was performed at employer's expense
Yes	Poss-I	Poss	No	No*	2 years	No	No	3: 60 weeks if loss due to trauma; 4: 200 weeks for trauma; 5: $5,400 for trauma; 6: $18,000 for trauma; 13: current employer is solely responsible for occupational loss
No	No	No	No	Yes	No	No	No	

(*continued on next page*)

Table 6.12 (*Continued*)

Jurisdiction	1. Is occupational hearing loss compensable?	2. Is minimum noise exposure required for filing?	3. Schedule in weeks (one ear)	4. Schedule in weeks (both ears)	5. Maximum compensations (one ear)	6. Maximum compensation (both ears)	7. Hearing impairment formula	8. Waiting period
South Dakota	Yes	Yes*	50	150	$20,400	$61,200	AAO-79	No
Tennessee	Yes	No	75	150	$38,625	$77,250	ME	No
Texas	Yes	No	*	*	*	*	AAO-79	No
Utah	Yes	Yes*	NR	109	NR	$35,425	AAO-79	6 weeks
Vermont	Yes	No	24	142	$17,448	$103,052	ME	No
Virginia	Yes*	No	50	100	*	*	AAO-79	No
Washington	Yes	No	NA	NA	$10,837	$65,023	AAO-79	No
West Virginia	Yes	No	*	*	*	*	AAO-79	2 months
Wisconsin	Yes	No	36	216	*	*	Other*	7 days
Wyoming	Yes	No	*	*	*	*	ME	No
U.S. DOL FECA*	Yes	Yes	52	200	NR	NR	AAO-79	No

9. Is deduction made for presbycusis?	10. Is award made for tinnitus?	11. Provision for hearing aid?	12. Credit for improvement with hearing aid?	13. Is hearing loss prior to employment considered in compensation claim?	14. Statute of limitations for hearing loss claim	15. Penalty for not wearing hearing protection devices?	16. Self-assessment of hearing impairment considered in rating/award?	Comments
Yes*	No	Yes	No	Yes	2 years	Yes-D	No	2: 90 dB TWA; 9: ½ dB for each year over 45 years
Yes	Yes-I	Yes	Poss	Yes	1 year	Poss-D	Yes	
No	No	Yes	No	Yes	30 days	No	No	3–6: no maximum scheduled awards
NR	NR	NR	NR	Yes	180 days	NR	NR	2: 90 dBA TWA or impact/impulsive noise 140 dB or greater
No	Yes-I	Yes	No	No	Yes	Yes-D	No	
No	No	Poss	No	Yes	2–5 years	No	No	1: only hearing loss due to work-related trauma or injury is considered; 5–6: No. of weeks multiplied by average weekly wage
No	Yes-I	Yes	No	Yes	2 years	No	No	
Yes	No	Yes	No	Yes	3 years	No	No	3–6: hearing loss compensation is based on a percentage of whole body impairment (max. for both ears, 22.5% whole body)
No	No*	Yes	No	Yes	No	No	No	5–6: depends on year of retirement; 7: avg. ≥ 30 dB at 500, 1,000, 2,000, and 3,000 Hz; 10: not compensable since 1/1/92
NR	NR	No	No	Yes	Yes	Yes-D	NR	3–6: based on rating of impairment
No	No	Yes	No	No	3 years	No	No	DOL FECA, Department of Labor's Federal Employees Compensation Act

(*continued on next page*)

Table 6.12 (*Continued*)

Jurisdiction	1. Is occupational hearing loss compensable?	2. Is minimum noise exposure required for filing?	3. Schedule in weeks (one ear)	4. Schedule in weeks (both ears)	5. Maximum compensations (one ear)	6. Maximum compensation (both ears)	7. Hearing impairment formula	8. Waiting period
U.S. Department of Longshore and Harbor Workers' Compensation	Yes	No	52	200	*	*	AAO-79	No
Guam	Yes	No	52	200	$13,000	$50,000	ME	No
Alberta	Yes	Yes*	NA	NA	$3,184	$19,105	NR	No
British Columbia	Yes	Yes*	NA	NA	*	*	Other*	No
Manitoba	Yes	Yes*	NA	NA	*	*	Other*	No
New Brunswick	Yes	No	NA	NA	*	*	ME	No
NW Territories	Yes	Yes*	*	*	$147/ month	$887/ month	Other*	Yes*
Nova Scotia	Yes	Yes*	*	*	*	*	Other*	No

9. Is deduction made for presbycusis?	10. Is award made for tinnitus?	11. Provision for hearing aid?	12. Credit for improvement with hearing aid?	13. Is hearing loss prior to employment considered in compensation claim?	14. Statute of limitations for hearing loss claim	15. Penalty for not wearing hearing protection devices?	16. Self-assessment of hearing impairment considered in rating/award?	Comments
No	No	Yes	No	No	1 year	No	No	5–6: based on compensation rate, increasing annually
Yes	Yes-I	Yes	No	Yes	1 year	No	No	
No	Yes-I	Yes	No	Yes	5 years	No	No	2: 85 dBA for 8 hours
No	No	Yes	No	Yes	No	No	No	2: 85 dB Lex, 8 hours for 2 years; 5–6: based on % of annual wage; 7: avg > 28 dB at 500, 1,000, and 2,000 Hz; 2.5% per dB
Yes*	No	Yes	No	Yes	No	Poss-D	No	2: 85 dB for 2 years.; 5–6: lump sum paid based on %; 7: avg ≥ 35 dB at 500, 1,000, 2,000, and 3,000 Hz; 9: ½ dB per year over 60 years of age
No	Yes-I	Yes	No	Yes	Yes*	No	No	5–6: depends on percent of disability; 14: prior to retirement
No	No	Yes	No	Yes	1 year	No	No	2: 90 dB for 8 hour/day for 2 years; 3–4: no maximum time period; 7: avg ≥ 30 dB at 500, 1,000, 2,000, and 3,000 Hz; 8: when removed from exposure
Yes*	Yes*	Yes	No	Yes	5 years	No	No	2: 85 dB for 8 hour/day for 5 years; 3–6: awards based on preinjury wages and % impairment with no maximums; 7: avg ≥ 35 at 500, 1,000, 2,000, and 3,000 Hz; 9: ½ dB per year over age 60 years.; 10: 2–5% awarded if specific criteria are met

(*continued on next page*)

Table 6.12   (*Continued*)

Jurisdiction	1. Is occupational hearing loss compensable?	2. Is minimum noise exposure required for filing?	3. Schedule in weeks (one ear)	4. Schedule in weeks (both ears)	5. Maximum compensations (one ear)	6. Maximum compensation (both ears)	7. Hearing impairment formula	8. Waiting period
Ontario	Yes	Yes*	NA	NA	*	*	AAO-79	No
Prince Edward Island	Yes	Yes*	*	*	*	*	ME	No
Quebec	Yes	Yes*	*	*	*	*	ME	No
Saskatchewan	Yes	No	*	*	$1,130	$13,560	Other*	No
Yukon	Yes	Yes*	*	*	*	*	AAO-79	2–5 year

Abbreviations: AAO: American Academy of Otolaryngology – 1979; average > 25 dB at 500, 1000, 2000, and 3000 Hz; AAOO: American Academy of Ophthalmology and Otolaryngology – 1959; average > 25 dB at 500, 1000, and 2000 Hz; Avg., average; D, claim denied; DOL, U.S. Department of Labor; I, only if impairment is also present; ME, medical evidence; (hearing loss formula at discretion of consulting physician); NA, nonapplicable; NIHL, noise-induced hearing loss; NR, no response; OSHA, Occupational Safety and Health Administration; P, penalty applied; Poss., possible; Temp, temporary; TWA, time-weighted average.

*See comments in last column.

Source: Noise and Hearing Conservation Manual by Elliott H Berger. Copyright 2003 in the format Textbook via Copyright Clearance Center.

9. Is deduction made for presbycusis?	10. Is award made for tinnitus?	11. Provision for hearing aid?	12. Credit for improvement with hearing aid?	13. Is hearing loss prior to employment considered in compensation claim?	14. Statute of limitations for hearing loss claim	15. Penalty for not wearing hearing protection devices?	16. Self-assessment of hearing impairment considered in rating/award?	Comments
es*	Yes	Yes	No	Yes	6 months	No	No	2: 90 dB for 5 years.; 5–6: lump sum awards based on % impairment, age at date of accident, and maximum medical recovery; 9: ½ dB per year over age 60 years
es*	Yes*	Yes	No	Yes	No	No	No	2: 2 years minimum; 3–6: lump sum awards based on % impairment; 9: ½ dB per year over age 60 years; 10: 2% maximum
es	No	Yes	No	Yes	No	No	NR	2: 90 dB for 8 hour/day for 2 years; 3–6: lump sum award based on % impairment and age at time of injury
o	Yes-I	Yes	No	Yes	No	No	No	3–4: lump sum pension and hearing aid costs; 7: avg ≥ 30 dB at 500, 1,000, 2,000, and 3,000 Hz
s*	Yes-I	Yes	No	Yes	No	No	No	2: 85 dB for 8 hour/day; 3–6: awards based on % impairment and ability to return to work; 9: maximum 2% for each year over age 45 years

Table 6.13 International permissible exposure limits (PELs), exchange rates, and other requirements for noise exposure

Country and Year	PEL Equivalent 8-Hour dBA	Exchange Rate (dBA)	L_{ASmax} rms L_{pk} SPL	Level* (dBA) Engineering Control	Level* (dBA) Audiometric Test	Comment
Argentina	90	3	115 dBA**	85	85	
Australia, 1993	85	3	141 dB peak	85	85	See note 1
Austria	85		110 dBA	90		
Brazil, 1992	85	5	115 dBA 130 dB peak	90	85	See note 2
Canada, 1990	87	3		87	84	See notes 3, 4
Council of the European Communities (CEC), 1986	85	3	140 dBC peak	90	85	
Chile	85	5	115 dBA 140 dB peak			See note 5
China, 1985	70–90	3	115 dBA	90		
Finland, 1990	85	3			85	
France	85, 70, 55	3	135 dBC peak	90	85	See notes 3, 6
Germany, 1990	85	3	140 dBC peak	90		See note 7
Hungary	90	3	125 dBA 140 dBC peak	90		
India, 1989	85		115 dBA 140 dBC peak		85	
Israel, 1984	85		115 dBA 140 dBC peak		85	
Italy, 1990	85	5	140 dBC peak	90	85	See note 8
Japan, 1992	90	3		85	80	
Netherlands	85	3	140 dBC peak	90	85	
New Zealand, 1995	85	3	140 dBC peak	85	80	See note 9
Norway, 1982	85, 70, 55	3	110 dBA			See note 10
Poland	85	3	115 dBA 135 dBC peak		80	
Spain, 1989	85	3	140 dBC peak	90	85	
Sweden, 1992	85	3	115 dBA fast 140 dBC peak	85		
Switzerland	85 or 87	3	125 dBA 140 dBC peak	85	85	
United Kingdom, 1989	85, 90	3	140 dBC peak	90	90	See note 11
United States, 1983	90	5	115 dBA 140 dB peak	90	85	See note 12
Uruguay	90	3	110 dBA			
International Institute of Noise Control Engineering (I-INCE), 1995	85	3	140 dBC peak	85	85	See note 13

Abbreviations: dBC, decibels C-weighted; L_{ASmax} rms, level A-weighted, slow response, root mean square; L_{pk}, level peak measurement; PEL, permissible exposure level; SPL, sound pressure level.

*Like the PEL, the levels initiating the requirements for engineering controls and audiometric testing also, presumably, are average sound levels normalized to 8 hours.

**Unless otherwise stated, the Lmax is specified in terms of the slow meter response.

Data sources:

Jorge P. Arenas, Institute of Acoustics, Universidad Austral de Chile, Valdivia, Chile (for South American data; paper presented at the 129th meeting of the Acoustical Society of America, 1995).

Pamela Gunn, Department of Occupational Health, Safety, and Welfare, Perth, Western Australia (personal communication).

Tony F.W. Embleton, Technical assessment of upper limits on noise in the workplace. *Noise/News International*, I-INCE, Poughkeepsie, NY, 1997.

International Labor Office, Noise Regulations and Standards, CIS database. ILO, Geneva, Switzerland (summaries), 1994.

Published standards of various countries and papers as referenced below.

Notes:

1. The data listed are for the Australian national standard (Worksafe Australia, 1993); the various states issue their own standards. The national standard is supplemented by a code of practice, which includes goals and specific procedures for engineering controls, hearing tests, and other elements of the hearing conservation program. There is a recent standard developed jointly by noise and hearing conservation professionals from Australia and New Zealand (Standards Act/Standards New Zealand, 1998). It refers to "occupational noise management" and provides guidance on applying noise control measures to existing equipment and purchasing quieter equipment in the future.

2. There is some variation among the individual Canadian provinces: Ontario, Quebec, and New Brunswick use 90 dBA with a 5-dB exchange rate; Alberta, Nova Scotia, and Newfoundland use 85 dBA with a 5-dB exchange rate; and British Columbia uses 85 dBA with a 3-dB exchange rate. All require engineering controls to the level of the PEL. Manitoba requires certain hearing conservation practices above 80 dBA, hearing protectors, and training on request above 85 dBA, and engineering controls above 90 dBA.

3. The Council of the European Communities (CEC, 1986) and Germany (UVV Laerm, 1990) state that it is not possible to give a precise limit for the *elimination* of hearing hazard and the risk of other health impairments from noise.

4. The countries in the European Community were required to have standards that conformed to the CEC directive, or were at least as stringent, by January 1, 1990. This means that they must require the employer to reduce the noise level as far as possible, taking technical progress and the availability of control measures into account. They must also require the declaration of sound power levels of machinery to be purchased, and the use of reduced noise reflection in buildings, regardless of sound pressure or exposure levels.

5. China requires different levels for different activities: e.g., 70 dBA for precision assembly lines, processing workshops, and computer rooms; 75 dBA for duty, observation, and rest areas; 85 dBA for new workshops; and 90 dBA for existing workshops.

6. Germany also has noise standards of 55 dBA for mentally stressful tasks and 70 dBA for mechanized office work.

7. This is a recommendation only.

8. The Japanese standard makes the wearing of hearing protection mandatory at 90 dBA. It also states that efforts shall be made to reduce the noise level to 85 dBA, and employers whose workplaces exceed 90 dBA shall "forthwith tackle the noise level" to bring it below 90 dBA (Zusho and Miyakita, 1996).

(continued on next page)

Notes to Table 6.13 (Continued)

9. New Zealand has joined with Australia in a coordinated occupational noise management standard (SA/SNZ, 1998).

10. Norway requires a PEL of 55 dBA for work requiring a large amount of mental concentration, 70 dBA for work requiring verbal communication or great accuracy and attention, and 85 dBA for other noisy work settings. Recommended limits are 10 dB lower. Workers exposed to noise levels greater than 85 dBA should wear hearing protectors.

11. The United Kingdom "Noise at Work" regulation requires employers to reduce the risk to the lowest level reasonably practical. Two "action levels" are specified: 85 dBA is required for noise exposure assessment, training, the provision of hearing protection devices (HPDs) to workers who request them, and the mainte- nance and use of equipment; and 90 dBA is required for noise reduction by "means other than ear protectors" and mandatory provision and wearing of HPDs. Audiometric testing is not required but recommended at an L_{A8hn} of 90 dBA under separate regulations, the "Management of Health and Safety at Work Regulations, 1992." L_{A8hn}, level A-weighted average exposures normalized to 8 hours.

12. These levels apply to the OSHA noise standard, covering workers in general industry and maritime. As explained above, the U.S. military services require standards that are somewhat more stringent.

13. Reflects a consensus of the members of the International Institute of Noise Control Engineering.

Source: Dobie RA, Megerson SC. (2003). Workers Compensation. In E.H. Berger et al., eds., *The Noise Manual*, 5th ed. Falls Church, VA: American Industrial Hygiene Association. *Note:* Readers are encouraged to check current state statutes before use.

Table 6.14 Comparison of methods used in the United States, Canada, and the European Union for determining occupational noise-induced hearing loss

Country	Regulatory Jurisdiction or Recommended Noise Exposure Guideline	Steady-State Noise				Impulse/Impact Noise
		Action or Prevention Effort Implementation Level	Maximum Permissible Exposure Level (PEL) for 8 Hours	Exchange Rate	Maximum Permissible Level	Maximum Peak Sound Pressure Level
United States	NIOSH (1998)	85 dBA TWA* REL	85 dBA TWA* REL	3 dBA	140 dBA	140 dB SPL$_{pk}$ (integrated with continuous noise measurement)
United States	OSHA (1983)	85 dBA TWA	90 dBA TWA	5 dBA	115 dBA	140 dB SPL$_{pk}$ (integrated with continuous noise measurement)
United States	MSHA (2000)	85 dBA TWA	90 dBA TWA	5 dBA	115 dBA	140 dB SPL$_{pk}$ (integrated with continuous noise measurement)
United States	FRA (2007)	85 dBA TWA	90 dBA TWA	5 dBA	115 dBA* (exception: continuous exposure > 115 dBA are permissible provided total daily exposure is ≤ 5 seconds	140 dB SPL$_{pk}$ (integrated with continuous noise measurement)

(continued on next page)

Table 6.14 (Continued)

Country	Regulatory Jurisdiction or Recommended Noise Exposure Guideline	Steady-State Noise				Impulse/Impact Noise
		Action or Prevention Effort Implementation Level	Maximum Permissible Exposure Level (PEL) for 8 Hours	Exchange Rate	Maximum Permissible Level	Maximum Peak Sound Pressure Level
Canada	Alberta (2009)	85 dBA L_{ex}	90 dBA L_{ex}	3 dBA	115 dBA	Not specified
Canada	British Columbia	85 dBA L_{ex}	85 dBA L_{ex}	3 dBA	Not specified	140 dBC_{pk}
Canada	Federal	84 dBA L_{ex}	87 dBA L_{ex}	3 dBA	120 dBA	Not specified
Canada	Manitoba	80 dBA	80 dBA (hearing monitoring); 85 dBA (sound control)	3 dBA	Not specified	Not specified
Canada	New Brunswick	85 dBA L_{ex}	80 dBA L_{ex}	3 dBA	140 dBC	140 dBC limit 100 impacts per day
Canada	Newfoundland/Labrador	85 dBA L_{ex}	85 dBA L_{ex}	3 dBA	140 dBC	Not specified
Canada	Northwest Territories	85 dBA TWA (consistent with ACGIH noise threshold limit values)	82 dBA L_{ex}	3 dBA	140 dBC	140 dBC (integrated with continuous noise measurement)
Canada	Nova Scotia	85 dBA	85 dBA L_{ex}	3 dBA	140 dBC	140 dBC limit 100 impacts per day
Canada	Nunavut	85 dBA TWA	85 dBA TWA	5 dBA (3 dBA for mining)	140 dBC	140 dB SPL_{pk} limit 100 impacts per day
Canada	Ontario	85 dBA L_{ex}	85 dBA L_{ex}	3 dBA	140 dBC	140 dBC (integrated with continuous noise measurement)
Canada	Prince Edward Island	85 dBA L_{ex}	85 dBA L_{ex}	3 dBA	115 dBA	Not specified

Country	Jurisdiction					
Canada	Quebec	85 dBA TWA	85 dBA TWA	5 dBA	115 dBA	140 dBC peak impacts per day = 120; dB peak = 10,000; 130 dB peak = 1,000; 140 dB peak = 100
Canada	Saskatchewan	80 dBA	85 dBA L$_{ex}$ or regular exposure over 90 dBA	3 dBA	Not specified	Not specified
Canada	Yukon	85 dBA L$_{ex}$ and/or impact noise limit	85 dBA L$_{ex}$ and/or impact noise limit	3 dBA	140 dB SPL$_{pk}$	No. of impacts per dB SPL$_{pk}$ level per 24-hour period: 118 dB =14,000; 121 dB = 7,200; 124 dB = 3,600; 127 dB = 1,800; 130 dB = 900; 133 dB = 450; 136 dB = 225; 139 dB = 112; 140 dB = 90; >140 dB = 0
European Union	European Union Member	80 dBA TWA (lower action level) 85 dBA (upper action level) and impulse/impact criteria	87 dBA TWA	3 dBA	135 dBC (lower action level); 137 dBA (upper action level); 140 dBC exposure limit with protection	135 dBC (lower action level); 137 dBA (upper action level); 140 dBC exposure limit with protection

Abbreviations: ACGIH, American Conference of Governmental Industrial Hygienists; dBA, decibel A-weighted; dBC, decibel C-weighted; FRA, Federal Railroad Administration; L$_{ex}$, equivalent sound exposure level; MSHA, Mine Safety and Health Administration; NIOSH, National Institute for Occupational Safety and Health; OSHA, Occupational Safety and Health Administration; dB SPLpk, decibel peak sound pressure level; REL, recommended exposure level; SPL, sound pressure level; TWA, time-weighted average.

*NIOSH does not distinguish between an action level and permissible exposure level (PEL). Rather, a recommended exposure level (REL) is referenced for all components of the hearing conservation program.

Source: Adapted from Berger, E.H. 3M Corporation. Comparison of Noise Regulations Across Canada (http://www.e-a-r.com/hearingconservation/noise_main.cfm)

Table 6.15 Comparison of U.S. hearing conservation regulations, interpretations, and recommendations

Issue	Description and Definition	OSHA 29 CFR 1910.95	MSHA 30 CFR Part 62	NIOSH Publ. No. 98–126
Action level (AL)	The TWA exposure that requires program inclusion, hearing tests, training, and optional hearing protection	AL = 85 dBA TWA; AL is exceeded when TWA ≥ 85 dBA, integrating all sounds from 80 to 130 dBA	Similar to OSHA, except integration is for all sounds from 80 to at least 130 dBA	Does not have AL; rather has a single REL (see next row) for hearing loss prevention, noise controls, and HPDs
Permissible exposure limit (PEL)	The TWA, which when exceeded, requires feasible engineering and (MSHA)/or (OSHA) administrative controls, and mandatory hearing protection	PEL = 90 dBA TWA; PEL is exceeded with TWA > 90 dBA, integrating all sounds from 90 to 140 dBA, as inferred from Table G-16 of 1910.95 (b)	Similar to OSHA, except integration range is explicit in the regulation (62.101, Definitions), and is for all sounds from 90 to at least 140 dBA	REL = 85 dBA TWA; REL is exceeded with TWA ≥ 85 dBA, integrating all sounds from 80 to 140 dBA
Exchange rate	The rate at which exposure accumulates; the change in dB TWA for halving/doubling for allowable exposure time	5 dB	Same as OSHA	3 dB
Ceiling level	The limiting sound level above which employees cannot be exposed	No exposures > 115 dBA; there is evidence that this ceiling level is not being enforced	"P" code violation issued for any protected or unprotected exposures > 115 dBA	No protected or unprotected exposure to continuous, varying, intermittent, or impulsive noise > 140 dBA
Impulse noise	Noise with sharp rise and rapid decay in level, ≤ 1 second in duration, and if repeated, occurring at intervals > 1 second	To be integrated with measurements of all other noise, but should not exceed 140-dB peak SPL	To be integrated with measurements of all other noise	To be integrated with measurements of all other noise, but not to exceed 140 dBA

Monitoring	Assessment of noise exposure	Once to determine risk and HCP inclusion; from there as conditions change, resulting in potential for more exposure	Mine operator must establish system to evaluate each miner's exposure sufficiently to determine continuing compliance with rule	Every 2 years if any exposure ≥ 85 dBA TWA
Noise control	Investigation and implementation of feasible engineering and administrative control measures	Feasible controls required where TWA > 90 dBA; subsequent compliance policy (which may be changed/revoked by OSHA at any time) permits proven effective HCP in lieu of engineering where TWA < 100 dBA	Feasible engineering and administrative controls required for TWA > 90 dBA; even if controls do not reduce exposure to the PEL, they are required if feasible (i.e., ≥ 3-dBA reduction); administrative controls must be provided to the miner in writing and posted	Feasible controls to 85 dBA TWA; administrative controls must not expose more workers to noise
Hearing protection	Exposure requirements and conditions for use of HPDs	Optional for ≥ 85 dBA TWA; mandatory for > 90 dBA TWA, and for ≥ 85 dBA TWA for workers with STS; protect to 90 or to 85 with STS; choices must include a "variety," which is interpreted as at least one type of earplug and one type of earmuff	Use requirements same as OSHA, but amount of protection not specified, and choices must include two earplugs and two earmuffs; double hearing protection (muff plus plug) required at exposures > 105 dBA TWA	Mandatory for ≥ 85 dBA TWA; must protect to 85 dBA; double hearing protection (muff plus plug) recommended at exposures > 100 dBA TWA

(continued on next page)

333

Table 6.15 (Continued)

Issue	Description and Definition	OSHA 29 CFR 1910.95	MSHA 30 CFR Part 62	NIOSH Publ. No. 98–126
Evaluation of hearing protector effectiveness	Method of assessing adequacy of HPDs	Use manufacturer's labeled NRRs to assess adequacy, but subsequent compliance policy stipulates 50% derating of NRRs to compare relative effectiveness of HPDs and engineering controls	No method included in standard; preamble to regulation indicates that compliance guide will follow with suggested procedures	Labeled NRRs must be derated by 25% for muffs, 50% for foam plugs, and 70% for other earplugs unless data available from ANSI S12.6–1997 Method B
Supervisor of audiometric testing	The person who conducts or who is responsible for the conduct of audiometric testing and review	Licensed or certified audiologist, otolaryngologist, or other physician	Licensed or certified audiologist or physician	Audiologist or physician
Audiometric technician	The person who conducts audiometric testing and routine review under guidance of a professional supervisor	Must be responsible to supervisor (see above); CAOHC certified, or has demonstrated competence to supervisor; when microprocessor audiometers used, certification not required	Must be under direction of supervisor (see above); must be certified by CAOHC or equivalent certification organization	Must be under direction of supervisor (see above); must be certified by CAOHC or equivalent certification organization
Audiometry	Initial and ongoing hearing tests used to assess the efficacy of hearing conservation measures	Required annually for all workers exposed ≥ 85 dBA TWA; baseline test within 6 months of exposure, 12 months if using mobile testing service, with HPDs in the interim	Same as OSHA, but choice of whether or not to take an audiogram is at miner's discretion	Required for all workers exposed ≥ 85 dBA TWA; baseline test preplacement or within 30 days of exposure; best practice is to test workers exposed > 100 dBA TWA twice per year
Quiet period prior to baseline audiogram	Period of nonexposure to workplace noise required prior to baseline audiogram	14 hours; use of HPDs acceptable as alternative	Same as OSHA	No exposure to noise ≥ 85 dBA for 12 hours; HPDs cannot be used as alternative

		OSHA	MSHA	NIOSH
Background noise	Permissible noise in audiometric test chamber during testing	Levels specified as 40 dB @ 500 and 1,000 Hz, 47 dB @ 2,000 Hz, 57 dB @ 4,000 Hz, and 62 dB @ 8,000 Hz	According to scientifically validated procedures	Per ANSI S3.1–1999 or latest revision; 19 dB more stringent than OSHA at 500 Hz, and 13 to 25 dB more stringent at other frequencies
Audiogram review and employee notification	Required actions following audiograms	Not specified unless STS is detected; see STS follow-up	Audiograms must be reviewed within 30 days and feedback provided in writing to each miner within 10 days thereafter	Not specified unless STS detected; see STS follow-up
STS (OSHA/NSHA standard threshold shift; NIOSH significant threshold shift)	A change in hearing compared with an earlier (baseline) hearing test that requires follow-up action	≥ 10-dB average shift from baseline hearing levels at 2,000, 3,000, and 4,000 Hz in either ear	Same as OSHA	≥ 15-dB shift for the worse from baseline at any test frequency, in either ear, confirmed with follow-up test for same ear/frequency
STS retests	Follow-up audiogram that is permitted or required when initial STS is detected	May obtain retest within 30 days and substitute for annual audiogram; same as OSHA	Same as OSHA	Must provide confirmation audiogram within 30 days
STS follow-up	Required actions when an STS is detected	Notify worker within 21 days; unless STS is not work-related, must fit or refit employee with HPDs and select higher attenuation if necessary, refer for audio/ontologi-cal exam if more testing needed or problem due to HPDs, and inform employee of need for exam if problem unrelated to HPD usage is suspected	Within 30 days of receiving evidence or confirmation of STS, unless STS is not work-related, must retrain the miner, provide miner an HPD or a different HPD, and review effectiveness of any engineering and administrative controls to correct deficiencies	Notify worker within 30 days; must take action such as explain effects of noise, reinstruct and refit with HPDs, provide additional training in hearing loss prevention, or reassign to quieter area

(continued on next page)

Table 6.15 (Continued)

Issue	Description and Definition	OSHA 29 CFR 1910.95	MSHA 30 CFR Part 62	NIOSH Publ. No. 98–126
Baseline revision	Procedures for revising the baseline audiogram to reflect changes in hearing	Annual audio substituted for baseline when STS is persistent or thresholds show significant improvement	Annual audio substituted for baseline when STS is permanent or thresholds show significant improvement	Annual audio substituted for baseline when confirming audiogram validates an STS
Presbycusis or age correction	Adjustments for hearing levels for anticipated effects of age	Allowed	Same as OSHA	Not allowed
Recordable or reportable hearing loss	Amount of hearing loss triggering reporting requirements on workplace injury/illness logs	By OSHA directive, ≥ 25-dB average shift from original baseline at 2,000, 3,000, and 4,000 Hz, in either ear, with age correction; rule change pending	≥ 25-dB average shift from baseline, or revised baseline, at 2,000, 3,000, 4,000 Hz in either ear	Not indicated
Training and education	Description of the annual training and educational component of the hearing conservation program	Annual for all employees exposed to ≥ 85 dB TWA; include effects of noise, HPDs, and purpose and explanation of audiometry	Same as OSHA, except must begin within 20 days of enrollment in HCP, and include description of mine operator and miner's responsibilities for maintaining noise controls	Same as OSHA, but must also include psychological effects of noise, and roles and responsibilities of both employers and workers in program
Warning signs and postings	Requirements to post signs for noisy areas or to post regulations	Hearing conservation amendment shall be posted in workplace	No requirements for posting, but when administrative controls are utilized the procedures must be posted	Signs must be posted at entrance to areas with TWAs routinely ≥ 85 dBA

Record retention	Specification on retention of data and transfer requirements if employer goes out of business	Noise surveys for at least 2 years, hearing tests for duration of employment, with requirement to transfer records to successor if employer goes out of business	Employee noise exposure notices and training records for duration of enrollment in HCP + 6 months, and hearing tests for duration of employment + 6 months, with requirement to transfer records to successor mine operation	Noise surveys for 30 years, hearing tests for duration of employment + 30 years, calibration records for 5 years, with record transfer per 29CFR1910.20(h)

Abbreviations: ACGIH, American Conference of Governmental Industrial Hygienists; CAOHC, Council for Accreditation in Occupational Hearing Conservation; dBA, decibel A-weighted; dBC, decibel C-weighted; FRA, Federal Railroad Administration; HCP, hearing conservation program; HPD, hearing protection device; MSHA, Mine Safety and Health Administration; NIOSH, National Institute for Occupational Safety and Health; NRR, noise reduction rating; OSHA, Occupational Safety and Health Administration; REL, recommended exposure level; SPL, sound pressure level; STS, standard threshold shift; TWA, time-weighted average.

Note: This table is provided to permit a quick comparison of the hearing conservation requirements of U.S. general industry (OSHA, 1983a), mining (MSHA, 1999), and recommendations of the NIOSH (1998) Criteria for a Recommended Standard: Occupational Noise Exposure. Please note the following conditions for use of this table:

1. The MSHA regulation was published September 13, 1999, with an effective date of September 13, 2000. This table is current as of spring 2000 but litigation could cause changes before implementation. Check with MSHA (see Web address below) for latest status.
2. The Criteria Document is a NIOSH recommendation, not a compliance document, but can be construed as a "best practices" guide.
3. Recordable or reportable hearing loss is addressed under OSHA in 29 CFR 1904, and directly in the MSHA rule.

This analysis is not intended to be all-inclusive; please check with the applicable agency for updates and current status. OSHA information is available at http://www .osha.gov ; MSHA at http://www.msha.gov; and NIOSH at http://www.cdc.gov/niosh,

Source: Noise and Hearing Conservation Manual by Elliott H. Berger. Copyright 2003 in the format Textbook via Copyright Clearance Center.

Table 6.16   Internet hearing loss prevention program (HLPP) resources

American Academy of Audiology Position Statement Preventing Noise-Induced Occupational Hearing Loss	www.audiology.org/resources/document library/documents/niohlprevention.pdf
American Speech-Language-Hearing Association (ASHA) Resource Guide Hearing Conservation/Occupational Audiologists	www.asha.org/aud/occupational/
Council for Accreditation in Occupational Hearing Conservation (CAOHC)	www.caohc.org
Dangerous Decibels	www.dangerousdecibels.org
Department of Defense (U.S.)	www.dtic.mil/whs/directives/corres/pdf/605512p.pdf
E-A-R Hearing Conservation and Earlogs	www.e-a-r.com/hearingconservation
Mine Safety and Health Administration (MSHA) 30 CFR Part 62	www.msha.gov/30CFR/62.0.htm
MSHA Compliance Guide Noise	www.msha.gov/REGS/COMPLIAN/GUIDES/NOISE/GUIDE303COVER.HTM
National Hearing Conservation Association (NHCA)	www.hearingconservation.org
National Institute for Occupational Safety and Health (NIOSH) Criteria for a Recommended Standard—Occupational Noise Exposure	www.cdc.gov/niosh/98-126.html
NIOSH Hearing Protector Compendium	www.cdc.gov/niosh/topics/noise/hpcomp.html
NIOSH Noise and Hearing Loss Prevention	www.cdc.gov/niosh/topics/noise/
NIOSH Preventing Occupational Hearing Loss—A Practical Guide	www.cdc.gov/niosh/96-110.html/
Noise Pollution Clearing House	www.nonoise.org

Source: An Essential Guide to Hearing and Balance Disorders by R. Steven Ackley. Copyright 2007. Reprinted by permission of Taylor & Francis Group LLC—Books in the format Trade Book via Copyright Clearance Center.

7

Vestibular Assessment and Rehabilitation

Table 7.1 Causes of equilibrium disturbances

Otologic Conditions	Neurologic Conditions	Trauma	Other
Benign paroxysmal positional vertigo	Migraine	Head or cervico-spinal injury	Tumors; cerebello-pontine angle and posterior fossa cysts
Vestibular neuronitis	Stroke	Labyrinthine concussion	Chiari malformations type I and II
Labyrinthitis	Seizure disorders	Barotrauma	Aging; sensory loss, cerebral hypoxia, and deconditioning
Meniere's disease	Multiple sclerosis		Medication: prescription, over-the-counter, supplements, and polypharmacy
Superior canal dehiscence	Spinocerebellar degeneration		Ocular disorders: glaucoma, refractive errors, and low vision
Perilymph fistula			Metabolic disorders: diabetes, hypoglycemia, and thyroid disease
Vestibular schwannoma			Cardiovascular: aortic stenosis, low cardiac output, peripheral arterial disease, and postural hypotension
Acoustic neuroma			Musculoskeletal and orthopedic problems; anxiety and psychiatric disorders

Source: Roeser, R.J., Valente, M., Hosford-Dunn, H. (2007), *Audiology Diagnosis,* 2nd ed. New York: Thieme. Reprinted by permission.

Table 7.2   Advantages and disadvantages of videonystagmography testing

Advantages
1. Enables visual observation and videorecording of actual eye movement; advantageous for differential diagnosis of BPPV variants and visualization of rotatory-torsional nystagmus
2. Two-camera VNG systems provide evaluation of the ocular motility of each eye independently
3. Does not require patient preparation and electrode placement
4. Does not require calibrations, as are necessary with traditional ENG corneoretinal-based technology
5. Patient is not required to close eyes, eliminating Bell's phenomenon and need for tasking
6. No need to maintain darkened test room environment
7. Preferable for pediatric testing
8. Enables correlation between actual eye movement and graphic algorithm analysis
9. Provides increased educational/clinical understanding of the neurophysiological and neuromuscular basis of eye movement

Disadvantages
1. Video goggles can be weighty or slightly uncomfortable for some patients
2. Positioning of patient may require adjustment of camera angle(s)
3. Patients with dark eyelashes and blepharochalasis (drooped eyelids) may require their eyes to be taped open
4. Ophthalmic hemorrhages may pose difficulty for the camera's tracking of the pupil

Abbreviations: BPPV, benign paroxysmal positional vertigo; ENG, electronystagmography; VNG, videonystagmography.

Source: Roeser, R.J., Valente, M., Hosford-Dunn, H. (2007), *Audiology Diagnosis,* 2nd ed. New York: Thieme. Reprinted by permission.

Table 7.3 Videonystagmography test battery and description of findings

Test	Abnormality	Interpretation
Spontaneous nystagmus test	Involuntary, unprovoked nystagmus that can appear in any direction	Indicates the presence of pathological condition within the peripheral or central vestibular system
Saccade test	Ocular dysmetria, characterized by overshoot, undershoot, glissades, pulsions occurring over 50% of the time in the recording	CNS pathological condition, involving the cerebral cortex, brainstem, or cerebellum
Smooth pursuit test	Breakup of smooth pursuit	Cerebellar dysfunction, eye, and neurological disorder, as well as systemic conditions affecting the CNS
Optokinetic test	Asymmetry in amplitude of response	CNS pathological condition or uncompensated vestibular
Gaze test	Persistent nystagmus recorded for ocular displacements of 20 degrees or less	Peripheral or CNS pathological condition, indicating brainstem or cerebellar disturbance
Head-shake test	Provocable nystagmus following 20 seconds of head shaking	Peripheral lesions tend to produce a fast phase away from involved ear; CNS lesions may cause nystagmus toward or away from the lesion
Modified Dix-Hallpike positioning test	Onset of rotary nystagmus ~10 seconds after positioning, then diminishes	Peripheral site of disorder consistent with posterior canal benign paroxysmal positional vertigo
Positional nystagmus test	Nystagmus provoked by static position; may be in any direction	Consistent with lesions in the peripheral or central vestibular pathway, or both
Bithermal caloric tests	UW: SPV differs by 20–30% or more between ears	UW: peripheral (nerve and/or end-organ) vestibular site of lesion
	DP: nystagmus in one direction is more intense than responses in the other direction; if no UW, a difference of 20% or more between right- and left-beating nystagmus is significant; if UW is present, a difference of 30% or more between right- and left-beating nystagmus is significant	DP: finding suggesting either a peripheral or central vestibular abnormality
	BW: SPV on each side is less than ~12 degrees/s	BW: either CNS disorder or peripheral vestibular abnormality
Fixation suppression	Inability of CNS to attenuate caloric nystagmus with vision enabled	Brainstem and/or cerebellar disease

Abbreviations: BW, bilateral weakness; CNS, central nervous system; DP, directional preponderance; SPV, slow phase velocity; UW, unilateral weakness.
Source: Roeser, R.J., Valente, M., Hosford-Dunn, H. (2007), *Audiology Diagnosis*, 2nd ed. New York: Thieme. Reprinted by permission.

Table 7.4   Caloric test results calculations

Calculation of percentage of left-right difference
  For a bithermal caloric test:

$$\frac{(\text{Left cold} + \text{Left hot}) - (\text{Right cold} + \text{Right hot})}{\text{Left cold} + \text{Right cold} + \text{Left hot} + \text{Right hot}} \times 100\%$$

  When right < left, the result will be a positive number; when left < right, the result will be a negative number.
  For a single temperature caloric test:

$$\frac{\text{Left} - \text{Right}}{\text{Right} + \text{Left}} \times 100\%$$

Calculation of directional preponderance

$$\frac{(\text{Left cold} + \text{Right hot}) - (\text{Left hot} + \text{Right cold})}{\text{Left cold} + \text{Right hot} + \text{Left hot} + \text{Right cold}} \times 100\%$$

Table 7.5   Drug-associated eye movement abnormalities

Drug	Eye Movement Abnormality
Alcohol (ethanol)	Vestibular dysfunction: positional nystagmus
	Brainstem-cerebellar dysfunction pattern
Aminoglycoside antibiotics:	Vestibular dysfunction: permanent labyrinthine
Streptomycin	hypofunction
Gentamicin	
Anticonvulsants:	Brainstem-cerebellar dysfunction pattern
Dilantin (phenytoin)	
Tegretol (carbamazepine)	
Antidepressants:	Central sedation pattern
Tricyclics (e.g., Elavil)	Internuclear ophthalmoplegia
Phenothiazines (e.g., Pamelor)	Opsoclonus
Others (e.g., Prozac)	Partial or total gaze paresis
Lithium	Brainstem-cerebellar pattern
	Opsoclonus
Chemotherapeutic anticancer	Vestibular dysfunction: permanent labyrinthine
agents (e.g., cisplatin)	hypofunction
Diuretics:	Vestibular dysfunction: transient labyrinthine
Lasix	hypofunction
Ethacrynic acid	
Haldol (Haloperidol)	Opsoclonus
Industrial solvents:	Brainstem-cerebellar dysfunction pattern
Xylene	Vestibular dysfunction: central positional nystagmus
Trichloroethylene	Exaggerated vestibulo-ocular reflex (VOR)
Marijuana	Brainstem-cerebellar dysfunction pattern
Methadone	Brainstem-cerebellar dysfunction pattern
Quinine	Vestibular dysfunction: positional nystagmus
Salicylates:	Vestibular dysfunction: transient labyrinthine
Aspirin (acetylsalicylic acid)	hypofunction
Stimulants:	Impaired accommodation/convergence; reduced
Amphetamine	saccadic latency
Sedatives:	Brainstem-cerebellar dysfunction pattern
Barbiturates (e.g., Phenobarbital,	Vestibular dysfunction: central positional nystagmus
Seconal)	
Chloral hydrate	Central sedation pattern
Tobacco:	Upbeat nystagmus
Smoking or chewing	Square wave jerks
Nicotine gum	
Tranquilizers:	Central sedation pattern
Benzodiazepines (e.g., Valium,	Brainstem-cerebellar pattern
Ativan, Xanax)	
Vestibular suppressants:	Central sedation pattern
Meclizine	Vestibular dysfunction: transient labyrinthine
Benadryl	hypofunction
Scopolamine	
Phenergan	
Flunarizine	

Source: Kamran Barin, Ph.D. Otometrics VNG/ENG Course, GN Otometrics A/S, 9 Hoerskaetten, DK-2630 Taastrup Denmark, T: +45 45 75 55 55, F: +45 45 75 55 59, www.otometrics.com. Reprinted by permission.

Table 7.6   Electronystagmography (ENG) results and site of lesion

Abnormal ENG Findings	Possible Site of Lesion	Comments
Ocular dysmetria test		
Overshoot or undershoot	Cerebellum or brainstem	
Gaze test (eyes open)		
Nystagmus recorded at any fixation point	CNS (brainstem or cerebellum)	Spontaneous nystagmus greater than 8 degrees/s in the same direction with eyes closed; findings could be related to peripheral or vestibular pathology
Vertical nystagmus (generally beating up)	Brainstem	
Vertical nystagmus without horizontal nystagmus	Midline or bilateral, involving upper pons or midbrain	
Horizontal nystagmus equal bilaterally	Brainstem	Watch for barbiturates or alcohol, which may contribute
Horizontal nystagmus unequal	CNS	If unequal, not likely associated with drug toxicity
Oblique or rotatory nystagmus (nonrecordable)	CNS	
Sinusoidal tracking test		
Breakup of smooth sinusoidal tracking	Brainstem	
Optokinetic test		
Poorly formed or asymmetric vertical and/or horizontal nystagmus	CNS	Existence of intense spontaneous nystagmus can contribute to OKN asymmetry related to a peripheral ocular pathology
Vertical OKN asymmetry	Brainstem	
Bilaterally absent or weak horizontal OKN	Midline brainstem	
Abnormal OKN plus gaze nystagmus or gaze paresis	Brainstem or cerebellum	
Abnormal OKN plus normal gaze	Cerebral hemisphere	In cerebral hemisphere lesions, the predominant OKN beats toward the side of the lesion
Paroxysmal test (positive Dix-Hallpike test)		
Latent period before and nystagmus Nystagmus of limited duration Nystagmus fatigues with repeated maneuvers	Vestibular system (peripheral)	

(*continued on next page*)

Table 7.6 *(Continued)*

Abnormal ENG Findings	*Possible Site of Lesion*	*Comments*
Positional test		
Excessive or spontaneous nystagmus with eyes closed	When viewed singly cannot provide site of lesion	
Caloric test		
Unilateral weakness equals 20% difference in the nystagmus response between the right- and left-ear irrigations	Vestibular	
Bilateral weakness results when nystagmus responses less than 7.5 degrees/s for each ear	Possibly peripheral	
Directional preponderance results when a 30% difference in intensity of right- and left-beating nystagmus exists	Nonlocalizing information	
Failure of fixation suppression	CNS	

Abbreviations: CNS, central nervous system; OKN, optokinetic nystagmus.

Source: Northern, J.L. (ed.), (1984), *Hearing Disorders.* Boston: Little, Brown. Reprinted by permission.

Table 7.7   Risk factors and intervention suggestions

Intervention

Name _____ Date _____

Referring Physician _____

The following have been identified as possible factors in increasing this patient's risk of future falls.

___ *Vestibular pathology:* An impairment of the vestibular system can cause the patient to become dizzy or off-balance; associated with certain movements and certain visual environments. Vestibular rehabilitation can minimize the effects of this impairment.

___ *Polypharmacy:* The use of four or more prescription medications or the initiation of a new medication or dosage has been associated with an increased risk of falling. A review of all medications by the primary care physician is indicated.

___ *Use of tricyclic antidepressants or benzodiazepines:* Associated with increased risk of falls. Selective serotonin reuptake inhibitor (SSRI) antidepressants may have fewer side effects, but it is not clear that they result in a reduced risk of falling compared with tricyclics and benzodiazepines. A review of the patient's medications is indicated.

___ *Orthostatic (postural) hypotension:* Postural presyncope associated with orthostatic hypotension may result in an increased risk of falling when assuming the upright position. Diabetes and many medications used to regulate the heart rate and blood pressure can suppress the carotid sinus reflex and result in temporary cerebral hypoperfusion. Increased fluids, support hose, and/or brief exercise (fist clenching, etc.) before standing can reduce the effect of orthostatic hypotension. A review of medications is indicated.

___ *Impaired proprioception (somatosensation):* The sense of touch is an important contributor to balance and orientation. The stretch receptors in the legs, the fingertips, and the soles of the feet provide feedback. Balance retraining therapy can help the patient use vestibular and visual feedback to compensate for loss of proprioceptive information. Vestibular rehabilitation is recommended.

___ *Cerebellar dysfunction:* The integration of vestibular, visual, and proprioceptive information takes place in the cerebellum. Cerebellar dysfunction can result in slow or inappropriate reaction to self-movement and external visual stimuli. Vestibular rehabilitation can maximize the patient's potential, but benefit is often limited. Environmental assessment and reduction of fall hazards are recommended.

___ *Hearing loss:* Hearing loss reduces one's orientation and awareness of one's surroundings. A person with hearing loss is more likely to be startled by movement in the visual field, as he or she has fewer auditory warning signals. Amplification may be helpful.

___ *Impaired vision:* Vision plays an important role in balance, and patients with visual deficits have greater risk of falls. Visual problems associated with decreased postural stability include visual acuity less than 20/50, asymmetric vision-impairing binocular vision and depth perception, slow pupillary reaction causing increased adaptation time when going from a lighted to a dark room, and vice versa, and impaired peripheral vision. Ophthalmologic or optometric evaluation is recommended.

___ *Depression:* Depressed patients may be more internally (therefore less externally) aware. The use of antidepressant and anxiolytics increases the risk of falling. Psychiatric or psychological evaluation is recommended.

___ *Impaired cognition:* Patients with impaired cognition may be less aware of their surroundings or more likely to engage in risky activities. Neurologic evaluation is recommended.

___ *Impaired reaction time:* Many fall avoidance strategies are dependent on reaction time when postural stability is challenged. Slower reaction time may increase the risk of falls when the patient's limits of stability are exceeded. Neurologic evaluation is recommended.

Source: Valente, M., Hosford-Dunn, H., Roeser, R.J. (2008), *Audiology Treatment,* 2nd ed. New York: Thieme. Reprinted by permission.

Table 7.8   Fall risk questionnaire

Name _____ Date _____

Please answer all questions.

Yes No
1. ☐ ☐ Have you had a fall or near-fall in the past year?
2. ☐ ☐ Do you have a fear of falling that restricts your activity?
3. ☐ ☐ Do you experience dizziness or a sensation of spinning when you lie down, tilt your head back, or roll over in bed?
4. ☐ ☐ Do you feel uneasy or unsteady when walking down the aisle of a supermarket, for instance, or in an area congested with other people?
5. ☐ ☐ Do you have difficulty walking in the dark or on uneven surfaces, such as gravel or a sloped sidewalk?
6. ☐ ☐ Do your feet or toes frequently feel unusually hot or cold, numb, or tingly?
7. ☐ ☐ Do you wear bifocal or trifocal glasses, or is your vision notably better in one eye?
8. ☐ ☐ Do you experience loss of balance or a lightheaded/faint feeling when you stand up?
9. ☐ ☐ Do you take medication for depression, anxiety, nerves, insomnia (lack of sleep), or pain?
10. ☐ ☐ Do you take four or more prescription medications daily?
11. ☐ ☐ Do you feel as if your feet just won't go where you want them to go?
12. ☐ ☐ Do you feel as if you can't walk a straight line or are pulled to the side while walking?
13. ☐ ☐ Has it been longer than 6 months since you participated in a regular exercise program?
14. ☐ ☐ Do you feel that no one really understands how much dizziness and balance problems affect your quality of life?
15. ☐ ☐ Are you interested in improving your balance and mobility?

Source: Roeser, R.J., Valente, M., Hosford-Dunn, H. (2007), *Audiology Diagnosis,* 2nd ed. New York: Thieme. Reprinted by permission.

Table 7.9   Physician's guide to the fall risk questionnaire

Questions 1 and 2: A previous fall may indicate increased risk for future falls. Inquire as to the circumstances of the fall. Fear of falling can lead to restricted activity.

Questions 3, 4, and 5: A positive response to any of these questions indicates the possibility of a vestibular disorder. Patients with benign paroxysmal positional vertigo (BPPV) are at risk of falling if they tilt their head back. Patients with vestibular disorders tend to be more reliant on vision for postural control. When the visual feedback is unreliable (moving visual scene) or unavailable (dark), patients are at risk of loss of balance and falling. Vestibular evaluation may be indicated (e.g., electronystagmography, posturography, and rotary chair test).

Questions 5 and 6: The sense of touch is an important contributor to balance and orientation. The stretch receptors in the legs, the fingertips, and the soles of the feet provide sensory feedback for balance. An assessment for peripheral neuropathy may be indicated.

Question 7: Vision plays an important role in balance, and patients with visual deficits have a greater risk of falls. Visual problems associated with decreased postural stability include visual acuity less than 20/50, asymmetric vision-impairing binocular vision and depth perception, slow pupillary reaction causing increased adaptation time when going from a lighted to a dark room and vice versa, and impaired peripheral vision. Multifocal glasses have been shown to increase the risk of falling. Ophthalmology evaluation may be indicated.

Question 8: Orthostatic hypotension may result in an increased risk of falling when assuming the upright position. Diabetes and many medications used to regulate heart rate and blood pressure can lead to orthostatic hypotension.

Questions 9 and 10: The use of four or more daily prescription medications and the use of tricyclic antidepressants or benzodiazepines are associated with increased risk of falls.

Questions 11 and 12: Poor motor control is a sign of possible cerebellar dysfunction. The integration of vestibular, visual, and somatosensory information takes place in the cerebellum. Cerebellar dysfunction can result in slow or inappropriate reaction to self-movement or external visual stimuli.

Question 13: Inactive patients may have accelerated decrease in muscle mass and decreased reaction time when faced with a possible fall.

Question 14: Physicians often underestimate (compared with the patient) the impact that a balance problem has on the patient's quality of life.

Question 15: Therapy for improved balance requires motivation and commitment. Patient compliance is important to a successful fall prevention program.

Source: Roeser, R.J., Valente, M., Hosford-Dunn, H. (2007), *Audiology Diagnosis,* 2nd ed. New York: Thieme. Reprinted by permission.

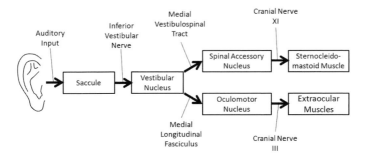

Fig. 7.1 A simple illustration of the two vestibular evoked myogenic pathways (VEMPs). Both pathways begin with the saccule, inferior vestibular verve, and vestibular nucleus. The cervical (cVEMP) pathway is on top, and the ocular (oVEMP) pathway is on the bottom. (From Atcherson, S. and Stoody, T. (2012), *Auditory Electrophysiology: A Clinical Guide.* New York: Thieme. Reprinted by permission.)

8

Hearing Instruments

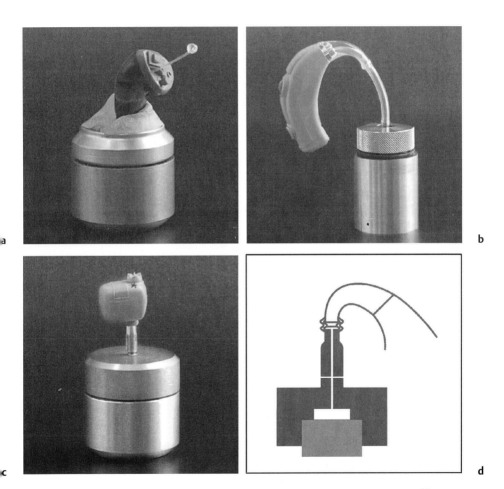

Fig. 8.1a–d Examples of 2-cc coupler commonly used for electroacoustic assessment of hearing aids. (**a**) HA-1. (**b**) HA-2. (**c**) HA-3. (**d**) HA-4. (From Valente, M., Hosford-Dunn, H., Roeser, R.J. (2008), *Audiology Treatment,* 2nd ed. New York: Thieme. Reprinted by permission.)

a

b

c

d

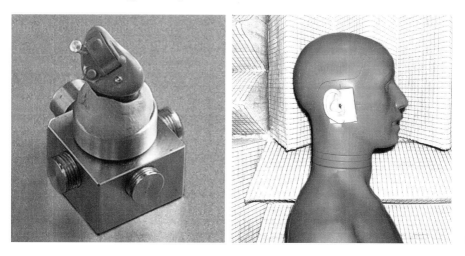

a   b

Fig. 8.2a,b (**a**) Zwislocki coupler. (**b**) Knowles Electronics Manikin for Acoustic Research (KEMAR). (From Valente, M., Hosford-Dunn, H., Roeser, R.J. (2008), *Audiology Treatment,* 2nd ed. New York: Thieme. Reprinted by permission.)

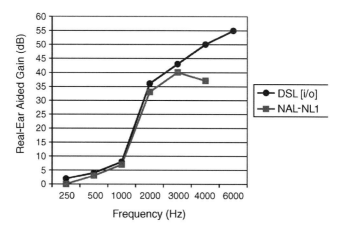

Fig. 8.3 Example of difference in real-ear aided gain between NAL-NL1 and desired sensation level (DSL) input/output (DSL [i/o]) indicating the desensitization factor applied to NAL-NL1 for a sloping hearing loss. (From Valente, M., Hosford-Dunn, H., Roeser, R.J. (2008), *Audiology Treatment,* 2nd ed. New York: Thieme. Reprinted by permission.)

Table 8.1 **A comparison of prescriptive methods**

Prescriptive Strategy	DSL [i/o] version 5	NAL-NL1
Audiometric data that can be used to derive targets	Thresholds obtained via headphones, insert earphones, sound field, and electrophysiological measures	Headphones and insert earphones
Adjustment for conductive/ mixed loss	Yes	Yes
Adjustments for binaural fitting	Yes	Yes
Individual-specific data can be entered and used in deriving targets	Yes: RECD, REDD, and REUR	Yes: RECD
Desensitization factor	No	Yes
Accounts for number of channels	Yes	Choose between 1 and 4 channels
Underlying rationale/goal	Loudness normalization, placement of acoustic cues available to normal-hearing listener into dynamic range of listener with hearing loss (given certain constraints)	Prescription designed to amplify speech such that at a given level, intelligibility is maximized with the constraints of normalizing overall loudness; resulting targets similar to those of an LE approach
Allows for choice of CT	Yes, but recommends CT based on degree of loss	Yes, but recommends midlevel CT
Adjustment for venting/ tubing	Yes	Yes
Age-related adjustments for ear canal characteristics	Yes	Yes
Age-related adjustments for audibility	Yes	No (for NAL-NL1)
Adjustment for hearing aid experience	No	No (for NAL-NL1)
Fitting information provided	Coupler targets, real-ear aided targets, real-ear gain targets, aided threshold targets, SPL-O-GRAM, and HA parameters (e.g., CT, CF, CR)	Coupler targets, real-ear gain targets, real-ear insertion gain, aided thresholds, Speech-O-Gram, and HA parameters

Abbreviations: CF, crossover frequency; CR, compression ratio; CT, compression threshold; DSL [i/o], desired sensation level input/output; HA, hearing aid; LDL, loudness discomfort level; LE, loudness equalization; LN, loudness normalization; NAL-NAL1, National Acoustic Laboratories' nonlinear fitting procedure, version 1; RECD, real ear-to-coupler difference; REDD, real ear-to-dial difference; REUG, real ear unaided gain; REUR, real ear unaided response.

Source: Data from National Center for Audiology (Canada), www.uwo.ca/nca; National Acoustic Laboratories (Australia), www.nal.gov.au.

**Table 8.2 Transformations that may be applied during selection of an appropriate 2-cc coupler response*

Measure	Definition	Application	Clinical Example
Audiometric information in real-ear dB SPL	Intensity value measured using a probe microphone near the eardrum at threshold, LDL, etc.	Eliminates need for average-based corrections in deriving real-ear targets	Data obtained in this format can be entered directly into fitting software
REDD	Difference between the intensity in dB HL on the audiometer dial and the intensity level in dB SPL measured near the eardrum	Can be applied to audiometric data obtained in dB HL (i.e., thresholds, LDLs) to transform to real-ear dB SPL	Can be entered directly into DSL[i/o], NAL-NL1, or real-ear equipment to transform data in dB HL to real-ear SPL
REUR	Outer ear canal resonance as measured using probe microphone	Can be used in deriving individual-specific insertion gain or coupler gain targets	Can be entered directly into NAL-NL1 fitting software; as a result, individual-specific coupler targets can be created; used in DSL [i/o] to customize sound-field threshold results that might be used with children
RECD	Difference between the output of a hearing aid, insert earphone, or earmold measured in the ear canal an identical input signal	Can be applied to insertion gain targets or real-ear output targets versus a 2-cc coupler with deriving appropriate 2-cc coupler targets; can be used to transform dB HL threshold to dB SPL threshold	Allows for verification of hearing aid settings in the coupler while accounting for individual ear canal characteristics
Coupler response for flat insertion gain (CORFIG)	REUR-RECD microphone location (i.e., BTE, CIC)	Correction factor that is added to REIG targets to obtain appropriate 2-cc coupler target	Adding CORFIG value to NAL-NL1 REIG target to derive 2-cc coupler target
Measure of dynamic range contour	Loudness discomfort levels; loudness	Determination of appropriate maximum output values and/or compression ratios for the hearing aid	These data can be entered into a real-ear system and used for verifying that maximum output of the hearing aid is set appropriately

Abbreviations: BTE, behind the ear; CIC, completely in canal; CORFIG, coupler response for flat insertion gain; DSL [i/o], desired sensation level input/output; HL, hearing level; LDL, loudness discomfort level; NAL-NL1, National Acoustic Laboratories' nonlinear fitting procedure, version 1; RECD, real ear to coupler difference; REDD, real ear to dial difference; REIG, real ear insertion gain; REUG, real-ear unaided gain; REUR, real-ear unaided response; SPL, sound pressure level.

* Transformations can be average-based or individual-specific data.

Source: Valente, M., Hosford-Dunn, H., Roeser, R.J. (2008). *Audiology Treatment*, 2nd ed. New York: Thieme. Reprinted by permission.

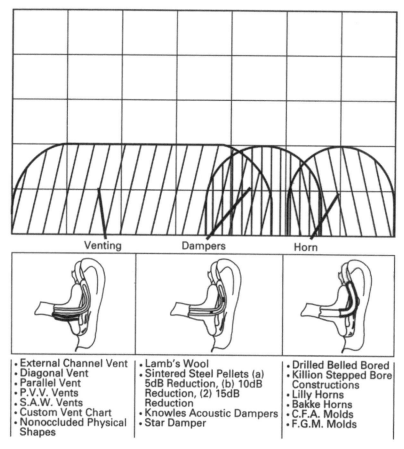

Venting	Dampers	Horn
• External Channel Vent • Diagonal Vent • Parallel Vent • P.V.V. Vents • S.A.W. Vents • Custom Vent Chart • Nonoccluded Physical Shapes	• Lamb's Wool • Sintered Steel Pellets (a) 5dB Reduction, (b) 10dB Reduction, (2) 15dB Reduction • Knowles Acoustic Dampers • Star Damper	• Drilled Belled Bored • Killion Stepped Bore Constructions • Lilly Horns • Bakke Horns • C.F.A. Molds • F.G.M. Molds

Fig. 8.4 Acoustical changes created by earmolds. (Courtesy of Microsonic Inc. Reprinted by permission.)

Table 8.3   Conversion from real-ear gain measurements to 2-cc coupler gain measurements

Hearing Aid Style (Coupler Type)	Frequency (Hz)						
	250	*500*	*1,000*	*2,000*	*3,000*	*4,000*	*6,000*
ITE (HA-1)[a]	−2.4	−2.0	+1.6	+1.2	+4.3	+2.8	−11.6
BTE (HA-2)[b]	−4.0	−4.0	−4.0	0.0	+7.0	−1.0	−3.0
Body (HA-2)[b]	−7.0	−7.0	+10.0	+11.0	+13.0	+13.0	+0.0

Abbreviations: BTE, behind the ear; ITE, in the ear.
[a]ITE corrections from Burnett, E.D. and Beck, L. (1987), A correction of converting 2 cm³ coupler responses to insertion gain responses for custom ITE non-directional hearing aids. *Ear and Hearing*, 7:257–265.
[b]BTE and body correction figures from Killion, M. and Monser, F.,"CORFIG. In: Studebaker, G. and Hochberg, I. (eds.), *Acoustical Factors Affecting the Hearing Aid Performance*. Baltimore: University Park Press, 1980; Lybarger, S., Physical and electroacoustical characteristics. In: Katz, J. (ed.), *Handbook of Clinical Audiology*, 3rd ed. Baltimore: Williams & Wilkins, 1985; and McCandless, G.A. and Lyregaard, P.E. (1983), Prescription of gain/output (POGO) for hearing aids. *Hear. Instr.* 34:16–21.

Table 8.4   Conversion values from dB HL to dB SPL in a 2-cc coupler for TDH-39, TDH-49, and TDH-50 earphones

Frequency (Hz)	TDH-39	TDH-49 and -50
250	20.7	21.7
500	9.9	11.9
750	7.3	7.8
1,000	5.5	6.0
1,500	2.5	3.5
2,000	5.2	7.2
3,000	5.7	5.2
4,000	−0.5	0.5
6,000	−0.2	−2.2

Source: Valente, M. (2002), *Strategies for Selecting and Verifying Hearing Aid Fittings*. New York: Thieme. Reprinted by permission.

Table 8.5 CORFIG corrections (average) for low-frequency venting effects

	Frequency (Hz)				
	250	*500*	*750*	*1,000*	*1,500*
Tight seal	—	—	—	—	—
Slit leak	2	2	1	—	—
1 mm	1	2	1	—	—
2 mm	7	1	—	—	—
Long open	17	10	4	1	—
Short open	26	21	14	10	5

Source: Valente, M. (2002), *Strategies for Selecting and Verifying Hearing Aid Fittings.* New York: Thieme. Reprinted by permission.

Table 8.6 Earmold response corrections (re: HA-2)

	Frequency (Hz)									
Earmold	*250*	*500*	*1,000*	*1,500*	*2,000*	*3,000*	*4,000*	*5,000*	*6,000*	*8,000*
Libby 4 mm	−1	−1	−2	0	0	2	3	0	0	1
Libby 3 mm	0	0	0	1	1	3	2	0	−4	−1
Macrae	−1	−1	−2	1	0	4	2	−3	−4	10
8CR	−1	−2	−3	−1	0	5	−3	−5	−2	8
6EF	0	0	0	0	0	2	2	−2	−3	−2
HA2	0	0	0	0	0	0	0	0	0	0
8B10	0	0	0	−1	−1	−2	−3	−4	−1	8
6R12	0	0	0	0	0	0	0	2	1	4
6B10	0	0	0	0	0	0	1	3	−5	−2
6B5	1	2	3	2	2	0	−1	−3	−2	2
6B0	0	1	1	0	0	−2	−5	−8	−7	−2
6C5	1	2	1	1	2	−5	−10	−13	−16	−10
6C10	1	3	0	−1	−3	−11	−17	−19	−22	−15
Cavity 1	−4	−2	1	−6	−15	−23	−30	−37	−35	−21
Cavity 2	−4	−3	−2	0	0	−12	−20	−28	−35	−21
Cavity 3	−2	−1	0	0	3	1	−11	−18	−24	−16

Source: Valente, M. (2002), *Strategies for Selecting and Verifying Hearing Aid Fittings.* New York: Thieme. Reprinted by permission. Adapted from Dillon H (2001). Hearing Aids. Sydney: Boomerang Press, pp xviii, 504.

Table 8.7 Common drill sizes and the resulting vent diameter

Drill Size	Vent Diameter (mm)
31	3.17
33	2.93
47	2.00
53	1.57
61	1.00
65	0.89
68	0.79
70	0.72
75	0.54
76	0.51
80	0.35

Source: Valente, M., Hosford-Dunn, H., Roeser, R.J. (2008), *Audiology Treatment*, 2nd ed. New York: Thieme. Reprinted by permission.

Table 8.8 Dimensions of Select-a-Vent (SAV), mini-SAV, and positive venting valve (PVV)

Type	(inch)	(mm)
SAV plug		
1	0.031	0.8
2	0.062	1.6
3	0.095	2.4
4	0.125	3.2
5	0.156	4.0
6	closed	closed
Mini-SAV plug		
1	0.020	0.5
2	0.030	0.8
3	0.040	1.0
4	0.060	1.6
5	0.075	1.9
6	closed	closed
PVV plug		
1	0.020	0.5
2	0.030	0.8
3	0.060	1.6
4	0.095	2.4
5	0.125	3.2
6	closed	closed

Source: Courtesy of Microsonic Inc. Reprinted by permission.

Table 8.9 Inside and outside diameters of tubing sizes as standardized by the National Association of Earmold Laboratories

	Inside Diameter		*Outside Diameter*	
Tubing Size	*(inch)*	*(mm)*	*(inch)*	*(mm)*
9	0.094	2.4	0.160	4.1
12	0.085	2.2	0.125	3.2
13 standard	0.076	1.9	0.116	2.9
13 medium	0.076	1.9	0.122	3.2
13 thick wall	0.076	1.9	0.130	3.3
13 double wall	0.076	1.9	0.142	3.6
14	0.066	1.7	0.116	2.9
15	0.059	1.5	0.166	2.9
16 standard	0.053	1.3	0.166	2.9
16 thin	0.053	1.3	0.085	2.2

Source: Valente, M., Hosford-Dunn, H., Roeser, R.J. (2008), *Audiology Treatment*, 2nd ed. New York: Thieme. Reprinted by permission.

Table 8.10 Mean and standard deviation (in parentheses) of the real-ear vent effects (dB) for three vent diameters (mm) relative to the occluded condition for ITE hearing aids when no sealing or sealing was placed around the shell of the ITE*

	Frequency				
Diameter	*200 Hz*	*500 Hz*	*1,000 Hz*	*1,500 Hz*	*2,000 Hz*
No sealing					
1.3 mm	−7.1(3.1)	0.3(2.9)	1.5(0.7)	0.5(0.6)	0.1(0.5)
2.0 mm	−11.1(3.9)	−0.9(3.6)	1.9(0.9)	0.7(0.7)	0.2(0.8)
3.0 mm	−21.9(4.0)	−10.5(3.2)	3.1(2.8)	2.6(1.7)	1.9(0.9)
Sealing with E-A-R rings					
1.3 mm	−6.8(2.2)	2.8(1.3)	0.8(0.6)	0.3(0.4)	−0.2(0.9)
2.0 mm	−12.1(2.5)	2.2(3.5)	1.7(0.7)	0.6(0.7)	0.3(0.9)
3.0 mm	−25.0(2.6)	−9.8(3.2)	5.1(2.0)	2.9(1.4)	2.0(0.7)
Diameter (mm) × length (mm)†					
0.45 × 22	−4.9(2.6)	0.5(2.0)	0.7(0.8)	0.1(0.9)	0.0(0.8)
0.95 × 22	−9.2(2.0)	2.8(2.5)	1.7(0.7)	0.6(1.1)	0.5(0.7)
1.45 × 22	−12.1(2.1)	1.5(3.9)	2.3(1.0)	1.0(1.1)	0.8(0.7)
2.0 × 22	−13.9(1.7)	0.6(4.0)	2.9(1.3)	1.4(1.1)	1.0(0.7)
2.0 × 16	−15.8(2.3)	−3.7(4.5)	2.5(1.4)	0.9(1.2)	0.3(1.0)
2.0 × 10	−18.9(2.5)	−7.9(3.7)	1.8(1.7)	1.0(1.2)	−0.1(1.5)
2.0 × 4	−22.6(2.9)	−11.4(4.7)	0.7(2.0)	1.5(2.0)	0.3(1.4)
3.0 × 4	−24.6(1.8)	−13.4(3.0)	0.1(2.6)	2.2(2.2)	0.9(1.2)

Abbreviation: ITE, in the ear.

*Data from Tecca, J. E. (1991). Real-ear vent effects in ITE hearing instrument fittings. *Hearing Instruments* 42(12), 12–12.

†Data from Tecca, J. E. (1992). Further investigation of ITE vent effects. *Hearing Instruments* 43(12), 8–10. Mean and standard deviations are given for real-ear vent effects (dB) for five bent diameters (mm) and four lengths (mm).

Source: Willard, F. Analysis of the development of the human auditory system. *Seminars in Hearing* 11(2):107–123. Reprinted by permission.

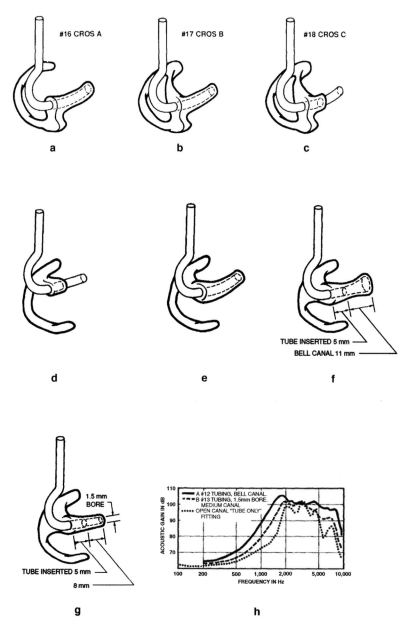

Fig. 8.5a–h Examples of eight nonoccluding earmolds. (**a**) Contralateral routing of signals (CROS) A. (**b**) CROS B. (**c**) CROS C. (**d**) Free field. (**e**) Janssen. (**f**) Extended range. (**g**) Another extended range. (**h**) Frequency response of three nonoccluding earmolds. (Courtesy of Microsonic Inc. Reprinted by permission.)

Fig. 8.6a–d   Earmold types.

(a) BASIC EARMOLD TYPES.

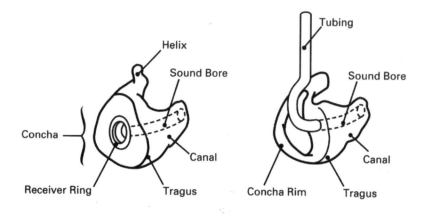

Typical Standard Mold   **Typical Skeleton Mold**

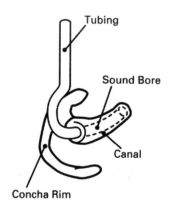

Fig. 8.6a–d *(Continued)*

(b) NATIONAL ASSOCIATION OF EARMOLD LABORATORIES (NAEL) TERMINOLOGY FOR PHYSICAL SHAPES.

Receiver (No. 1 Regular):
This mold style is characterized by a special receiver ring or clip that retains the external receiver of a body aid. The mold fills all the contours of the external ear for a tight seal. This type of mold can be made from hard or soft materials.

 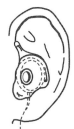

Receiver with Tube (No. 5X Full Concha):
Because a receiver mold gives a superior seal, this mold can be adapted to use with ear level and eyeglass aids.

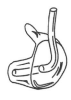 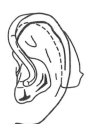

Receiver with a Hook:
This type was developed to retain a receiver and mold in the ear of a client whose external ear's cartilage will not hold the mold in place. The most common application is small children.

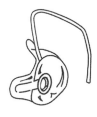 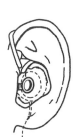

Skeleton (No. 2 Skeleton):
This is the most universal mold made. The design gives a good seal, and the cosmetic design is acceptable to most clients. Most acoustical options can be fitted into this physical shape.

 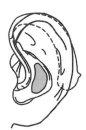

(continued on next page)

Fig. 8.6a–d *(Continued)*

(b) NATIONAL ASSOCIATION OF EARMOLD LABORATORIES (NAEL) TERMINOLOGY FOR PHYSICAL SHAPES.

Skeleton with D-90 Ring
(No. 7 D-90 Skeleton):
This mold is a duplicate of the skeleton with the exception of the ring. The tubing is now attached to the mold with a D-90 earmold adapter. This facilitates tubing changes.

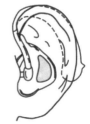

¾ Skeleton:
This mold is a reduction of the skeleton style. A portion of the concha rim has been removed. This would be used when the client's pinna had a shape in that area that made insertion or removal a problem.

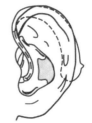

Semi-Skeleton (No. 6 Half Phantom):
This mold is a further reduction of the skeleton style. It again would relate to a problem in the external ear's shape.

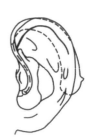

Canal:
This is the maximum reduction possible in the skeleton style. Only the canal portion remains. Cosmetically, this is the ultimate in conceal-ment. Because there is no retainer area on this mold in the helix or concha, there is a problem with retention.

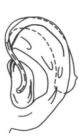

Fig. 8.6a–d *(Continued)*

(b) NATIONAL ASSOCIATION OF EARMOLD LABORATORIES (NAEL) TERMINOLOGY FOR PHYSICAL SHAPES.

Canal Lock (No. 3 Canal):
This mold is a modified canal shape. As you can see, a portion of the lower concha rim has been added to give more retention. The mold still is cosmetically very acceptable.

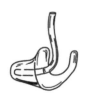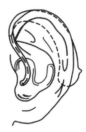

Shell (No. 5 Shell):
This mold was created from the design of the receiver mold, but with tubing. The receiver plate area of the mold has been belled in for cosmetic reasons. This mold will work in all cases because of its seal and design. Most acoustical options can be used with this physical shape.

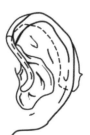

Half Shell (No. 4 Shell Canal):
This mold focuses on the very real client/ dispenser problem of earmold insertion. Some clients, due to advanced age or manual dexterity problems, do not easily learn the insertion technique. This mold simplifies insertion for the client and gives a good acoustic seal.

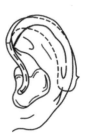

Modular All-in-the-Ear:
There are a series of different configurations available for the various "modular" all-in-the-ear hearing aids. Each manufacturer's aid has a different shape and each client's ear is different. One example of the many shapes is shown in the drawing.

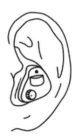

(continued on next page)

Fig. 8.6a–d *(Continued)*

(c) NON–NATIONAL ASSOCIATION OF EARMOLD LABORATORIES TERMINOLOGY FOR NONOCCLUDING PHYSICAL SHAPES.

Original CROS (No. 8 CROS):
Basically, a CROS mold is a reduction of a skeleton mold in the bridge area and the reduction of the canal portion of the mold so that the patient's canal is not occluded. Sound can pass around the retaining portions of a CROS mold. CROS molds are used in CROS and IROS fittings to significantly reduce an aid's response below 1000 Hz. It can be said that a CROS mold is the biggest vent.

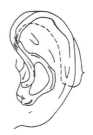

CROS with Changeable Tube Length:
This physical shape option's difference came about when measurement of the earmold's effect showed that the canal length changes for the frequency response.

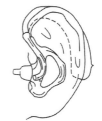

Wing CROS:
This type of CROS mold changes the location of the canal portion of the mold to the lower wall of the ear canal. Up to now, the canal portion of CROS molds was centered in the canal. It was felt by dispensers that more effective nonocclusion would occur if the bridge part of the mold was maximally reduced.

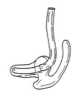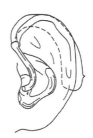

Janssen (No. 8-Q Janssen):
This nonoccluded earmold shape was developed to replace tube fittings. The Janssen mold has several design changes from earlier CROS-type configurations: (1) the canal length is as long as possible; (2) the tubing is heat molded around the tragus; (3) the canal of the mold can be soft material for greater client comfort; and (4) the canal portion of the mold runs along the top on the ear canal.

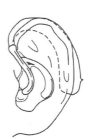

Fig. 8.6a–d *(Continued)*

Dual Diameter Nonoccluding (Proposed by Lybarger):

There are audiograms on which the hearing levels are normal out to 1,500 to 2,000 Hz and then fall off. Lybarger experimented with reverse horn theory and stepped bore constructions using tubing alone. This style of mold incorporated a piece of No. 13 tubing from the ear hook to a second piece of tubing with an inside diameter of 1/32", which then returns to a No. 13 tube that channels the sound down into the ear. These various-sized tubings are attached to a Janssen mold.

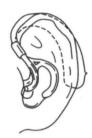

Nonoccluding Universal:

This is a new nonoccluding earmold shape that consolidates the features of other mold styles to maximize its effectiveness. This mold uses an S.A.V. Variable Vent System installed in the bridge of an almost Original CROS mold. The canal portion of this mold runs along the top of the ear canal like a Janssen mold. This mold offers the dispenser the benefits of a free-field mold, a Janssen mold, and variable venting.

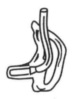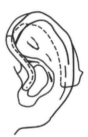

Tube Fittings:

This is the largest venting space it is possible to create with a hearing aid, to completely eliminate the body of the earmold and use a tube only. By not occluding the ear canal at all, natural ear canal resonance is not disturbed. There are audiological, otologic, psychological, and practical reasons to consider tube fittings.

When considering a tube fitting, the interior diameter of the tubing can be varied to create different acoustical effects. The tubing must be heat molded in the office to follow the contours of the pinna and canal. In practice, it has been found desirable to use a so-called no-mold tip at the end of the tubing to prevent irritation of the ear canal skin.

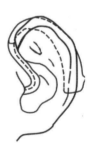

(continued on next page)

Fig. 8.6a–d *(Continued)*

(c) NON–NATIONAL ASSOCIATION OF EARMOLD LABORATORIES TERMINOLOGY FOR NONOCCLUDING PHYSICAL SHAPES.

Free-Field Variations (Free-Field Mold):
Nonoccluded earmold physical shapes have been subjected to a great deal of acoustical measurement. It was found by fitters that the more nonoccluded a earmold could be, the more acoustical reduction would occur in the low frequencies.

The free-field variations are a series of different physical shapes that have as their goal nonobstruction of the ear canal. A problem that arises from increasing nonobstruction is feedback. Some free-field molds attempt to solve this problem by occluding the concha but not the canal.

The free-field mold enables the audiologist to make tube fittings with the added security of retention on the ear.

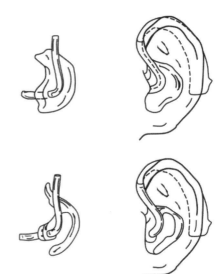

Fig. 8.6a–d *(Continued)*

(d) NON–NATIONAL ASSOCIATION OF EARMOLD LABORATORIES TERMINOLOGY FOR ANTI-FEEDBACK PHYSICAL SHAPES.

Shell Mold with Lucite® Body and Soft Canal:
This is one of the traditional methods in earmold selection for reducing the possibility of feedback. The soft canal portion may expand with body heat and thereby gives a tighter seal.

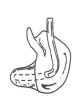 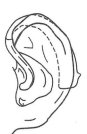

Power Mold:
Some feedback problems have as their origin the movement of the jaw as it affects the ear canal. This movement causes the seal created by the earmold to break and feedback occurs. The movement in the ear canal can be bypassed by this physical shape. The canal portion of a shell mold is reduced to the tubing size for part of the canal length.

 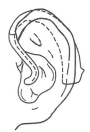

Tragus Configuration:
The anatomy of the ear tells us that there is only one part of the external ear canal area that can be stretched. This is the tragus area. By taking a mold and expanding the girth of the canal in the tragus area and running the mold itself up over the tragus, we can create a tighter seal that does not cause discomfort to the client, while eliminating feedback in many cases.

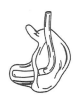 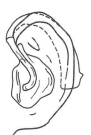

Macrea Antifeedback:
This mold is different from all other molds in that it is "hollowed" out and has two tubes leading into the canal. Tube No. 1 carries the sound from the aid into the ear canal. Tube No. 2 carries the sound in the ear canal through an acoustic damper into the large resonating cavity of the Macrea mold. This mold still often allows full utilization of the volume control range on many instruments. It must be stated that this is an experimental mold.

 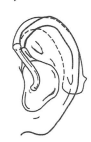

(Courtesy of Microsonic Inc. Reprinted by permission.)

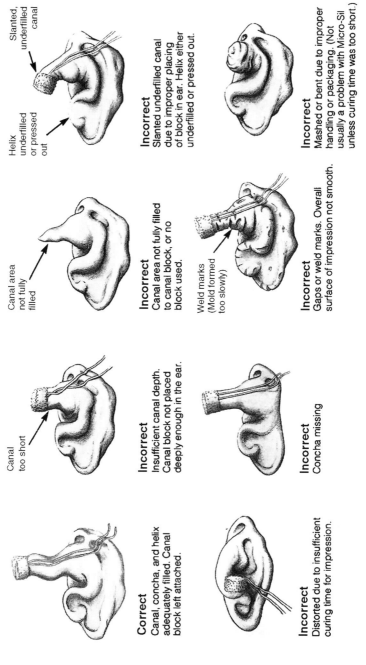

Correct
Canal, concha, and helix adequately filled. Canal block left attached.

Incorrect
Distorted due to insufficient curing time for impression.

Canal too short

Incorrect
Insufficient canal depth. Canal block not placed deeply enough in the ear.

Incorrect
Concha missing

Canal area not fully filled

Incorrect
Canal area not fully filled to canal block, or no block used.

Weld marks (Mold formed too slowly)

Incorrect
Gaps or weld marks. Overall surface of impression not smooth.

Slanted, underfilled canal

Helix underfilled or pressed out

Incorrect
Slanted underfilled canal due to improper placing of block in ear. Helix either underfilled or pressed out.

Incorrect
Mashed or bent due to improper handling or packaging. (Not usually a problem with Micro-Sil unless curing time was too short.)

Fig. 8.7 Several examples of correct and incorrect earmold impressions. (Courtesy of Microsonic Inc. Reprinted by permission.)

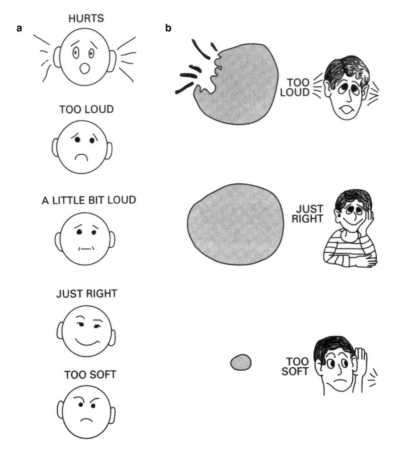

Fig. 8.8 Loudness judgment pictures. (From Valente, M. *Strategies for Selecting and Verifying Hearing Aid Fittings.* New York: Thieme, 1994:43; Kawell, M., Kopun, J., Stelmachowicz, P. (1988), Loudness discomfort levels in children. *Ear and Hearing* 9:33–136; and Skinner, M., Skinner, Margaret W. *Hearing Aid Evaluation,* 1st ed. © 1988. Reprinted by permission of Pearson Education, Inc., Upper Saddle River, NJ.)

Table 8.11 Strategies to assist in hearing instrument retention and acceptance

- Huggie Aids (Huggie Aids Too, Oklahoma City, OK, http://www.huggieaids.com)
- Fishing line/dental floss tied to instrument and safety pin clipped to clothing
- Otoclips/Critter Clips (Adco Hearing Products, Englewood, CO, http://www.adcohearing.com)
- Ear Gear (Ear Gear, Canada, www.gearforears.com)
- Hearing Aid Sweatbands
- Pediatric tone hooks
- Doublestick or toupee tape
- Bonnet with hole cut out for hearing instrument microphone
- Pilot caps by Hanna Andersson (www.hannaandersson.com)
- Ribbon with loops for behind-the-ear (BTE) instruments
- Eyeglass holders
- Sweatbands to hold hearing instruments/earmolds in place
- Orthodontic rubber bands to hold BTE instruments to eyeglasses
- Vests with pockets for body-worn instruments
- Colored hearing instrument cases
- Colored earmolds
- Colored beads on earmold tubing (be aware of choking hazard for young children)
- Decorating hearing instruments with stickers
- Colored Super Seals (JustBekuz Products Co., Colorado, www.justbekuz.com)
- Earwear hearing instrument covers (Ear Gear, Canada, www.gearforears.com)
- SafeNSound security straps and clips (SafeNSound, North Carolina, www.getsafeandsound.com)
- It Stays! body adhesive (Compressionsale, Vernon Hills, Illinois, www.compressionsale.com)

Source: Valente, M., Hosford-Dunn, H., Roeser, R.J. (2008), *Audiology Treatment,* 2nd ed. New York: Thieme. Reprinted by permission.

Table 8.12 Reasons to wear binaural hearing aids

1. Better understanding of speech
2. Better understanding in groups and noise
3. Better directionality
4. Better sound quality
5. Smoother tone quality
6. Binaural loudness summation
7. Better sound identification
8. Prevention of sensory deprivation
9. Improved ease of listening
10. Balanced hearing
11. Greater comfort when loud noises occur
12. Reduced feedback and whistling
13. Tinnitus masking
14. Consumer preference
15. Consumer satisfaction

Source: Kochkin, S. (2000), Binaural hearing aids: the fitting of choice for bilateral loss subjects. http://www.betterhearing.org/research/. Adapted by permission.

Table 8.13   Reasons that people with impaired hearing give for not obtaining or using a hearing aid

- They have poor manual dexterity, and thus find hearing aid controls hard to operate.
- They feel that battery insertion and earmold cleaning are too difficult.
- Earmolds can feel uncomfortable.
- Earmolds may contribute to an accumulation of cerumen in the ear canals.
- External otitis or a skin disorder makes use of earmolds painful.
- Hearing aids, batteries, and repairs are too expensive.
- When amplified, speech and music sound harsh and unpleasant.
- When amplified, many environmental noises are annoying, such as one's own footsteps, traffic, clattering dishes, or a toilet flushing.
- When amplified, sudden loud noises can be frightening, such as a dog barking.
- Continuously amplified background noises are a constant distraction.
- They do not need hearing aids for face-to-face conversation in quiet places, and benefit little from hearing aids in group discussions where considerable background noise and reverberation are present.
- They may notice that distance greatly diminishes the audibility and intelligibility of speech through hearing aids.
- They notice little difference in quality between aided and unaided face-to-face conversation.
- They believe that hearing aids may further damage their hearing.
- They believe that the use of hearing aids may create dependency on hearing for conversation. They feel that this can be a potential problem if their hearing deteriorates further.
- They don't want other people to know that they have a hearing loss.
- They believe that only very deaf people wear hearing aids, and/or they think that others believe this. They don't want anyone to think that they are *deaf*.
- They believe that hearing aids are symbols of a loss of youth and an intact body.
- They believe that only *old* people use hearing aids, and they don't want other people to think that they are old.
- They believe that hearing aids make people appear "different" and thus undesirable.
- They believe that hearing aids make people appear less attractive to the opposite sex.
- They don't want people to treat them as if they were *handicapped*, i.e., patronize them.
- They don't want to admit to themselves (be reminded) that they have a hearing loss.

Source: Erber, N.P. (1996), *Communication Therapy for Adults with Sensory Loss,* 2nd ed. Melbourne, Australia: Clavis Publishing. Reprinted by permission.

Table 8.14   For hearing aid users: Ways to maximize your speech-reading ability in combination with your hearing aid

1. Indicate to the talker in some way that you are hearing impaired.
2. Adjust the communication situation so that noise sources are nearer the talker than to you (all's fair in speech-reading). Reduce noise as much as possible.
3. Look around and become familiar with the situation so that you will know what the talkers are referring to.
4. Watch the talker's lips, not his or her eyes. Look around only during pauses (there are plenty of them) and change of talkers. You can see facial expressions and eye movements without leaving the lips.
5. Adjust the situation so that the light is on the talker's face and not yours. Avoid glare and backlighting that obscure the talker's face or cause you to squint or strain to see.
6. Arrive early for situations that are more formal or structured, such as meetings, religious services, classes, or any place where people will be seated, so that you can stake out the best spot. Do not be afraid to move if you made a mistake or if the structure of the group changes. If there is one primary talker, sit so that you can see him or her without strain. Talk to the organizers beforehand about seating, amplifiers, and so on.
7. Learn to relax, even in tough listening situations. Avoid tension. Keep your shoulders down, do not wrinkle your forehead, and so on (one version of this list said, "Work hard at relaxing": that is not what we mean!).
8. Concentrate on phrases and ideas rather than trying to pick out single words.
9. Make an effort to stay current on recent events, news, sports, and so on. The more you know about likely topics of conservation, the better off you are.
10. Interact with the talker of your group to clarify or verify the message when you miss something.
11. Do not wait until you are lost and three sentences behind.

Source: Alpiner, J.G. (2000), *Rehabilitative Audiology,* 3rd ed. Philadelphia: Lippincott Williams & Wilkins. Used by permission.

Table 8.15   ANSI S3.33 tests used to measure the electroacoustic performance of hearing aids

Test	Explanation of Test Result	Gain Setting	AGC	Input (dB SPL)	Frequency	Measure or Calculate	Tolerance
90 dB curve	Coupler SPL as a function of frequency for a 90 dB input SPL	Full on	Min	90	200–5000 Hz	Coupler SPL	Unspecified
Maximum 90 dB	Maximum value of the 90 dB curve	Full on	Min	90	Frequency of maximum	Maximum of OSPL90 curve	+3 dB
HFA-90 dB	Average of the 90 dB values	Full on	Min	90	HFA	Average coupler SPL at HFA frequencies	±4 dB
HFA full-on gain (HFA-FOG)	Average of the full-on gain at the HFA frequencies	Full on	Min	50	HFA	Average gain at FHA frequencies	±5 dB
Reference test gain (RTG)	Average of the gain at the HFA frequencies for a 60 dB input SPL, with gain control at RTS	RTS	Min	60	HFA	Average gain at HFA frequencies	Unspecified
Frequency range	Range between the lowest and the highest frequency at which the frequency response curve is 20 dB below its HFA value	RTS	Min	60	From the lowest frequency (f1) to the highest frequency (2) at which the frequency response curve is 20 dB below its HFA average	Unspecified	
Frequency response curve	Coupler SPL as a function of frequency for a 60 dB input SPL, with gain control at RTS	RTS	Min	60	From the higher of f1 or 200 Hz to the lower of f2 or 5,000 Hz	Coupler SPL or gain	±4 dB from the lesser of 1.25 f1 or 200 Hz to 2 kHz ±6 dB from 2 kHz to the lesser of 4 kHz or 0.8 f2
Total harmonic distortion (THD)	Ratio sum of the powers of all the harmonics to the power of the fundamental	RTS	Min	70 except 65 @ highest frequency	500, 800, 1,600 Hz (HFA) or ½ the SPA frequencies		+3%

(continued on next page)

Table 8.15 (*Continued*)

Test	Explanation of Test Result	Gain Setting	AGC	Input (dB SPL)	Frequency	Measure or Calculate	Tolerance
Equivalent input noise (EIN)	SPL of an external noise source at the input that would result in the same coupler SPL as that caused by all the internal noise sources in the hearing aid	RTS	Min	Off and 50	(Coupler SPL with no input) (HFA gain with a 50-dB input SPL)	+3 dB
Battery current	Electrical current drawn from the battery when the input SPL is 65 dB at 1000 Hz and the gain control is at RTS	RTS	Min	65	1,000 Hz	Battery current	+20%
SPL for an inductive telephone simulator (SPLITS)	For hearing aids with an inductive input coil (T-coil), the coupler SPL as a function of frequency when the hearing aid, with gain control at RTS, is oriented for maximum output on a telephone magnetic field simulator (TMFS); BTE is as flat as possible on test surface, ITE or ITC with face plate as close as possible and parallel to test surface	RTS	Min	TMFS	200–50,000 Hz	Coupler SPL	Unspecified
HFA-SPLITS	Average of the SPLITS in the HFA frequencies	RTS	Min	TMFS	HFA	Average SPLITS value at the HFA frequencies	±6 dB
RSETS	Relative simulated equivalent telephone sensitivity	RTS	Min	TMFS	HFA	HFA-SPLITS minus (RTG + 60)	Unspecified

	Description				Measurement	Tolerance
Input-output curves	For hearing aids with AGF, the coupler SPL as a function of the input SPL, at one or more of 250, 500, 1,000, 2,000, 4,000 Hz, with gain control at RTS	RTS	Max	50–90 in 5 dB steps	One or more of 250, 500, 1,000, 2,000, 4,000 Hz	Coupler SPL versus Input SPL	±5 dB at 50 and 90 dB input SPL when matched at 70 dB input SPL
Attach time	For hearing aids with AGC, the time between an abrupt change from 55 to 90 dB input SPL and the time when the coupler SPL has stabilized to within 3 dB of the steady value for a 90-dB input SPL, at one or more of 250, 500, 1,000, 2,000, 4,000 Hz, with the gain control at RTS	RTS	Max	Step from 55 to 90	Same frequencies used for input-output curves	Time from input step until coupler SPL settles within 3 dB of its steady value for 90 dB input SPL	±5 milliseconds or 50%, whichever is greater
Release time	For hearing aids with AGC, the time between an abrupt change from 90 to 55 dB input SPL and the time when the coupler SPL has stabilized to within 4 dB of the steady value for a 55 dB input SPL, at one or more of 250, 500, 1,000, 2,000, 4,000 Hz, with the gain control at RTS	RTS	Max	Step from 90 to 55	Same frequencies used for input-output curves	Time from input step until coupler SPL settles within 4 dB of its steady value for 55 dB input SPL	±5 milliseconds or 50%, whichever is greater

Abbreviations: AGC, automatic gain control; BTE, behind the ear; HFA, high-frequency average; ITC, in the canal; ITE, in the ear; RTS, reference test setting; SPA, special purpose average; SPL, sound pressure level; TMFS, telephone magnetic field simulator.

Notes: High-frequency average (HFA) is the average of values at 1,000, 1,600, and 2,500 Hz. In all tests, HFA may be replaced by the special purpose average (SPA), the average of values at three frequencies specified by the hearing aid manufacturer that are at ⅓ octave frequencies separated by ⅔ octave.

Reference test setting (RTS) is the setting of the gain control (i.e., volume control, master or overall gain control) required to produce an HFA0 gain within ± 1.5 dB of the HFA–OSPL90 minus 77 dB for a 60-dB input SPL or, if the full-on HFA gain for a 60-dB input SPL is less than the HFA OSPL90 minus 77 dB, the full-on setting of the gain control.

Automatic gain control (AGC) provides the means for controlling gain as a function of signal level. It includes expansion and various forms of compression.

Source: Bill Cole, Etymonic Design, Inc. Used by permission.

Glossary of Hearing Aid–Related Terms

adaptive frequency response (AFR): the category of hearing aid for which the frequency response is adjusted as the input levels are adjusted.

AGC-I: input-controlled AGC.

AGC-O: output controlled AGC.

ALD: assistive listening device. An assortment of devices are intended to improve hearing in specific listening situations, such as personal amplifiers, telephone amplifiers, headphones for television, and so on.

amplitude modulation (AM): Changing the magnitude of a sound wave in relation to the strength of the carrier wave.

anechoic chamber: a specially designed audiometric space containing large wedges made of sound-absorbing material. These wedges cover the walls, floor, and ceiling in their entirety. The room is devised for both maximum sound absorption as well as minimum sound reverberation.

ANSI: American National Standards Institute.

artificial ear: a device specifically designed for the measurement of earphones. This device mimics the acoustic impedance presented by the average human ear and contains a microphone that enables the measurement of the sound pressure developed by the earphone.

auditory evoked response (AER): recording showing an electrical reaction from different sites in the auditory system using a physiologic amplifier and an averaging/summing computer system.

automatic gain compression (AGC): a nonlinear method by which the gain adjusts as a function of altered signal levels.

automatic gain control: hearing aid compression that changes gain automatic in a nonlinear function, or limit the output when the output reaches a specified level.

class A amplifier: power output (hearing aid) amplifier that consumes the peak requirement battery current at all times; this attempt to minimize battery drain is frequently linked with premature high-frequency overload. This kind of amplifier was often used in hearing aids because they were the only ones small enough for the smallest hearing aid.

class B amplifier: power output (hearing aid) amplifier (occasionally referred to as a push-pull) that uses battery current in proportion to the output needed. It typically has 10 times the battery life of the class A amplifier for the same undistorted output.

class D amplifier: a specific design of a hearing aid amplifier that provides a remarkable enhancement in undistorted high-frequency output as compared with the class D amplifier.

contralateral routing of signals (CROS): a hearing aid arrangement that was first developed for patients who have a unilateral hearing loss. At the poorer ear, a microphone is placed that allows the signal to be routed to the better ear and delivered through an "open" ear mold.

coupler: a device that connects one component of a system to another. In acoustics, there are a variety of couplers. Generally 6 cc represents a normal adult human ear for supra-aural earphones and 2 cc for hearing aids and insert earphones.

coupler response for flat insertion gain (CORFIG): a set of correction factors to predict insertion gain from coupler performance; the arithmetic inverse of GIFROC.

CROS-plus: modification of a CROS hearing aid in which the better ear is fit with a traditional CROS hearing aid and the unaidable ear is fit with a power in-the ear instrument.

damper: a device placed in hearing aid ear hooks, ear molds, and receiver tubing to decrease output and smooth peaks; obtainable in various ohm resistances.

desired sensation level (DSL): a technique for hearing aid fitting that is geared mainly for children.

direct audio input (DAI): a circuit contained in certain hearing aids that provides a direct connection to some assistive listening devices, radios, and televisions.

DSL [I/O]: modification of DSL for nonlinear amplification.

earmold: prescriptive coupler that channels acoustic energy from a hearing aid into the ear canal.

FM system: an assistive listening device that contains a microphone, transmitter, and receiver, and transmits the signal by FM radio waves.

frequency modulation (FM): modification of the frequency signal on a carrier wave.

frequency response: hearing aid gain as a function of frequency, representing the output characteristics.

front routing of signal (FROS): hearing aid built into eyeglasses with the microphone near the front of the eyeglass temple. The signal is sent to the amplifier and then to the ear.

full dynamic range compression: a specific hearing aid/amplification device feature that compresses amplified output levels into a much narrower range than that of the input levels. The compression occurs over an input range from ~40 to 90 dB sound pressure level (SPL).

full on gain (FOG): the gain of a hearing aid with the volume control turned to maximum.

functional gain: the difference in a patient's aided and unaided thresholds for speech or toned signals obtained in a sound field.

gain: an increase in the amplitude or energy of an electrical signal with amplification, or the difference between the input and output signal. In vestibular assessment, the ratio of actual eye movement to desired eye movement; Output – Input = Gain.

HA-1 type coupler: a device correlating with the most current ANSI requirements for coupling earphones to the level meter for audiometer calibration; a standard direct access (2-cc) coupler for testing in-the-ear and in-the-canal hearing aids or, with a custom earmold attachment, behind-the-ear hearing aids.

HA-2 type coupler: a standard 2-cc coupler for testing hearing aids that are not integrated into an earpiece (e.g., behind-the-ear, body, and eyeglass hearing aids) that includes a standard earmold simulator.

HAC: hearing aid consultation.

HAE: hearing aid evaluation.

HAPI: see **Hearing Aid Performance Inventory.**

harmonic distortion: additional spurious frequencies (nonlinearities) in the output signal that are not contained in the input signal but that are related to the fundamental frequency; expressed as a percentage of the total signal at the point of measurement.

HCL: highest comfortable listening level that is useful in the selection and setting of the maximum output of hearing aids.

HE: hearing evaluation.

hearing aid: an electronic instrument that is designed to amplify and deliver sound to an ear.

hearing aid effect: the negative attitude/feelings that hearing aid users think others have of their hearing aid use.

Hearing Aid Performance Inventory: a self-assessment scale of the overall benefit a hearing aid user is receiving.

Hearing Industries Association (HIA): an organization of hearing aid manufacturers.

high-frequency average (HFA): the average of the response values in dB at 1,000, 1,600, and 2,500 Hz, in accordance with the ANSI S3.22.

high-frequency CROS (HICROS): a hearing aid arrangement.

input compression: compression amplification, with the degree of reduction in amplification dependent on the input level as well as the kneepoint in the input-output function; a form of AGC-I.

insertion gain: the difference in the SPL produced by the hearing aid at a specific point in the ear canal and the SPL at the same point in the ear canal without the hearing aid. The difference between the two recordings (an *unaided equalization reference* and an *aided frequency response)* is called the hearing aid insertion gain. This term was originated by Ayers in a 1953 publication.

in situ: Latin origin: in position; measurement of performance made within the actual ear.

intermodulation (IM) distortion: additional frequencies that result when two frequencies occur (are presented to the ear) simultaneously.

in-the-canal hearing aid (ITC): a hearing aid that is inserted deep in the ear canal to improve cosmetic appearance.

in-the-ear hearing aid (ITE): a hearing aid the fits entirely in the structures of the pinna and ear canal.

ipsilateral routing-of-signal (IROS): method of fitting high frequency hearing loss with an open-mold or tube fitting.

K-amp: a hearing circuit with automatic signal processing; named after Mead Killion.

KEMAR: an acronym for Knowles Electronics Manikin for Acoustic Research. The manikin integrates the Zwislocki occluded ear simulator in the ear canal, and is used for in-situ hearing aid performance measurements that more accurately approximate hearing aid performance in real life.

kneepoint (compression threshold): the position on the input/output curve where the slope deviates from unity (a one-to-one relation between input and output); this signifies the point at which nonlinearity starts.

microphone: an electronic apparatus designed to transducer an acoustic signal (a sound) into an electrical signal.

microphonic: the electric potential generated by a transducer that changes a vibration into electrical energy. The alternating potential produced by the cochlea in response to a stimulating sound is an aural, or cochlear, microphonic.

MINICROS: CROS system with tube running directly from the receiver to the ear, in contrast to an earmold.

MULTICROS: CROS system that can be switched to a BICROS system multi-memory, which is a hearing aid that has the capability to store multiple "listening programs" for the user to access.

NBS-9A: device meeting current ANSI specifications for coupling the earphone to a sound level meter for audiometer calibration.

peak clipping: distortion of a waveform that results from amplifier saturation.

PMC: programmable multichannel system for hearing aid fitting.

Prescription of Gain and Output (POGO): hearing aid prescription algorithm based on half-gain rule above 500 Hz and reduction of gain at lower frequencies.

POGO II: a modification of POGO; suitable for more severe hearing loss.

polar directivity pattern: a graph that demonstrates relative amplitude output as a function of the angle of sound incidence from a directionally sensitive apparatus.

probe microphone: a tiny microphone that is often attached to a soft, small tube that is inserted into the external ear canal to determine sound intensity level close to the eardrum. The probe microphone communicates with equipment for recording sound characteristics.

REAR: real ear aided response; the SPL, as a function of frequency, at a specified measurement point in the ear canal for a specified sound field with the hearing aid in place and turned on. This measurement can be provided either in SPL or as gain in decibels relative to the stimulus level. It enables the audiologist to use the patient's ear as a coupler, as well as to make fitting decisions in accordance with these measurements. There are no definite guidelines for setting the hearing aid volume control wheel (VCW) for REAR measures. This is dependent on what hearing aid feature the audiologist wants to measure. The insertion gain approach is popular now, so the most common use of the REAR is currently to provide a reference point for the insertion gain calculation (the REUR is subtracted from the REAR to obtain the insertion gain value).

RECD: real ear coupler difference; the difference, in decibels and as a function of frequency, between the outputs of a hearing aid measured in a real ear versus a 2-cc coupler. The RECD measurement resolves several of the issues regarding correcting from the 2-cc coupler to the real ear.

receiver: a hearing aid component that transduces electrically amplified sound to acoustic energy.

receiver tubing: tubing that extends from the hearing aid receiver to the medial tip of a custom hearing aid. Receiver tubing tends to become occluded with cerumen.

reference test gain: the acoustic gain of a hearing aid as measured in a hearing-aid test box. The gain control of the aid is programmed to amplify an input signal of 60-dB SPL to a level 17 dB below the saturation sound pressure level (SSPL) 90 value. The average values at 1000, 1600, and 2500 Hz determine the reference test gain.

REIG: real-ear insertion gain; the value, in decibels, of the REIR at a certain frequency.

REIR: real-ear insertion response; the difference, in decibels as a function of frequency, between the REUR and the REAR measurements taken at the same measurement point in the same sound field. It is the amount of gain delivered to a patient wearing a hearing aid that he or she did not have before the hearing aid fitting (the REUR was previously present). The REIR is the electroacoustic equivalent (or close equivalent) of functional gain.

release time: in a compression hearing aid, the amount of time required for nonlinear processing to reach the steady state value.

REM: rapid eye movement.

REOR: real-ear occluded response; the SPL, as a function of frequency, at a specified point in the ear canal for a specified sound field, with the hearing aid in place and turned off. This can be expressed either in SPL or as gain in decibels relative to the stimulus level. Although the REOR may be very similar to the REUR at some frequency regions for open-ear fittings, for most hearing aid or earmold styles the REOR will fall substantially below the REUR. For earmold or hearing aid styles that fit tightly enough to cause attenuation, the REOR reflects this aspect, along with the alteration of the REUR. REORs usually become smaller as the size of the earmold or hearing aid placed in the ear becomes larger. The REOR is helpful in selecting an acoustically appropriate sound delivery system.

RESR: real-ear saturation response; a function of frequency specified in SPL, at a specified measurement point in the ear canal with the hearing aid in place and turned on. The measurement is obtained with the stimulus level sufficiently intense as to operate the hearing aid at its maximum output level. The RESR is especially critical for children and nonresponsive patients, when the maximum output of the hearing aid must be not only comfortable but also safe. There are several different input signals that can be used when conducting probe-microphone measurements. Most commonly, the choice is between speech-spectrum–shaped noise or warble tones. RESR values can vary significantly as a function of the input stimulus.

REUR: real-ear unaided response; the output as a function of frequency in SPL at a specified point in the unoccluded ear canal for a specified sound field. REUR can be expressed either in SPL or as a gain in dB relative to the stimulus level. The most common clinical use of the REUR is to serve as a reference value for calculation of insertion gain.

saturation (hearing aids): the condition caused by peak clipping in a hearing aid that prevents an increase in input sound pressure level from producing the same change in output sound pressure level.

saturation sound pressure level (SSPL): the maximum power output of a hearing aid; indicates the greatest SPL output from the receiver of a hearing aid.

screw-set: method used to adjust the gain of hearing aids when the volume control wheel is not present.

signal-to-noise ratio (SNR): the ratio of the signal relative to a corresponding noise, where the signal and noise may be electric energy, electric power, voltage, current, and the acoustical correlates thereof, i.e., sound energy, sound pressure, and sound particle velocity, especially. Also, the ratio of an electrical signal (e.g., AER) to background (nonresponse) electrical activity (noise). An SNR of 2:1 is usually required for confident clinical identification of electrophysiologic recordings (such as an auditory brainstem response).

simplex procedure: an adaptive procedure designed to maximize speech recognition scores by estimating the electroacoustic settings on more than one dimension of a hearing aid.

telecoil: a coil contained within a hearing aid to detect magnetic energy such as that produced by telephone receivers.

transducer: an electroacoustic device that converts energy from one form to another. An example is an earphone that converts electrical energy to acoustic energy (sound).

VCW: volume control wheel on the hearing aid.

vent: an earmold opening (e.g., 1- or 3-mm diameter) traveling from the lateral location to the medial tip of an earmold or hearing aid; the purpose is pressure equalization and sound transmission.

9

Psychosocial Aspects/Rehabilitation

Table 9.1 Eight stages of the helping relationship

Stage	Goals
Entry	1. Open an avenue for assistance from the audiologist. 2. Lay the groundwork for trust. 3. Enable the patient to define his problems related to his hearing impairment.
Clarification	1. Define the client's specific problems as related to his hearing impairment. 2. Get a better feel for how the client sees his hearing impairment and its effect on his general life situation.
Structure	1. Determine if the audiologist has the skills necessary to meet the client's needs. 2. Identify the agency and the type of help offered, and the qualifications and limitations of the audiologist. 3. Arrange the appointment time, decide on any fees to be charged, and specify any restrictions that are to be imposed.
Relationship	A turning point in the process. The client and audiologist either continue to build the relationship through mutual agreement or the relationship is terminated by either party.
Exploration	1. Outline the strategies for intervention. 2. Explore the client's feelings. 3. Outline the alternatives of action.
Consolidation	1. The client decides on a course of action. 2. The client's feelings are clarified. 3. The client will practice new skills.
Planning	1. Formulate plans for termination and having the patient continue alone. 2. Complete the referral plans (agencies are contacted and applications are completed).
Termination	1. Summarize the accomplishments. 2. End the helping relationship: a. Termination b. Referral c. The promise of follow-up d. The offer of "stand-by" help

Source: Brammer, L., as cited in Wylde, M. A. The remediation process: psychologic and counseling aspects. In: Alpines, J.G. (ed.), *Handbook of Adult Rehabilitative Audiology,* 2nd ed. Baltimore: Williams & Wilkins, 1982. Reprinted by permission.

Table 9.2   World Health Organization (WHO) definitions of impairment, disability, and handicap

Impairment: Any loss or abnormality of a psychological or anatomic structure or function.

Disability: Any restriction or inability (resulting from an impairment) to perform an activity in the manner or within the range considered normal for a human being.

Handicap: Any disadvantage for a given individual, resulting from an impairment or a disability, that limits or prevents the fulfillment of a role that is normal (depending on age, sex, and social and cultural factors) for that individual.

Source: World Health Organization. (1980). International classification of impairments, disabilities and handicaps. Geneva: WHO Press. Used by permission.

Table 9.3   International Classification of Functioning, Disability and Health definition of terms

Health condition: An alteration or attribute of the health status; it may be a disease (acute or chronic), disorder, injury, or trauma.

Functioning: An umbrella term encompassing all body functions, activities, and participation.

Disability: An umbrella term for impairment, activity limitations, or participation restrictions.

Body functions: The physiological functions of body systems (including psychological functions).

Body structures: Anatomic parts of the body such as organs, limbs, and their components.

Impairments: Problems in body function or structure as a significant deviation or loss; may be temporary or permanent; progressive, regressive, or static; intermittent or continuous. The deviation from the population norm may be slight or severe and may fluctuate over time.

Activity: The execution of a task or an action by an individual; used in the broadest sense to capture everything that an individual does, at any level of complexity, from simple activities to complex skills and behaviors.

Activity limitation: Difficulties an individual may have in executing activities; refers to a difficulty in the performance, accomplishment, or completion of an activity at the level of the person.

Participation: Involvement in a life situation.

Participation restriction: Problems an individual may experience in involvement in life situations.

Contextual factors: The complete context of an individual's life and living. They include two components: environmental factors and personal factors. Both types of factors may have an impact on the individual with a health condition and that individual's health and health-related states.

Environmental factors: Makeup of the physical, social, and attitudinal environment in which people live and conduct their lives. These factors are external to individuals and can have positive or negative influence on the individual's performance as a member of society, or on an individual's capacity to execute actions or tasks, or on the individual's health and health-related states. Environmental factors are classified according to individual or societal level:

Individual level: The immediate environment of the individual, including settings such as home, workplace, and school. Included at this level are the physical and material features of the environment that an individual comes face to face with, as well as direct contact with others, such as family, acquaintances, peers, and strangers.

Societal level: Formal and informal social structure, services, and overarching approaches or systems in the community or society that have an impact on individuals. This level includes organizations and services related to the work environment, community activities, government agencies, communication and transportation services, and informal social networks, as well as laws, regulations, formal and informal rules, attitudes, and ideologies.

Personal factors: The particular background of an individual's life and living. Personal factors are composed of features of the individual that are not part of a health condition or health states. These factors may include gender, race, other health conditions, fitness, lifestyle, habits, upbringing, coping styles, social background, education, profession, past and current experience, overall behavior pattern and character style, individual psychological assets, and other characteristics, all or any of which may play a role in disability at any level.

Source: http://www3.who.int/icf/icftemplate.cfm?myurl=introduction.html%20&mytitle =Introduction. Reprinted by permission of the World Health Organization.

Table 9.4   Major components of communication therapy

I. Interview client
 A. Characteristics and effects of hearing/vision loss
 B. Related medical/personal factors
 C. Previous use of sensory aids
 D. Previous rehabilitation or communication therapy
 E. Reasons for attending clinic: information, hearing-aid orientation, learn lipreading/
    listening, telephone use, conversational fluency, stress reduction
 F. Discuss nature of typical "problem conversations": partner, conversational format,
    and context:
    1. Who? (e.g., family member, friend, coworker, shop assistant)
    2. What? (e.g., topic, content, vocabulary, language, structure)
    3. Why? (e.g., give/get information, maintain friendship, gossip)
    4. Where? (e.g., home, factory, meeting, acoustic/optical distractions)
    5. How long? (e.g., brief contact, narrative, long discussion)
 G. Administer self-assessment questionnaire (e.g., HHIE-S)
 H. Informally note conversational fluency and level of stress
 I. Describe clinic and typical procedures
II. Screen client's speech-perception abilities and discuss
 A. Visual (e.g., letter chart; face perception)
 B. Auditory (e.g., audiometry, word-identification; high-frequency word list)
 C. Auditory-visual (e.g., SENT-IDENT)
III. Conduct conversation(s) with the client (e.g., TOPICON), playing the role of a typical
    partner. Assess conversational fluency; note instances and causes of communication
    breakdown; discuss effects of topic and client's use of strategies.
Provide instant therapy
    Establish optimal conditions and note effects of the following factors on conversational
        performance:
    Good amplification
    Good environment
    Short distance
    Skilled partner
Situation management
    Choice of partner
    Distance
    Use of sensory aid(s)
    Control of environmental distracters (e.g., noise, reverberation, glare)
    Selection of setting for conversation
Partner training
    Communication partner's role
    Clear speech and language
    Semantic strategies
    Proactive contribution to conversation
    Cooperation
Client training
    Auditory and visual skills
    Use of hearing aids, telephone, and other devices
    Language knowledge and use; meta-communication
    Communication practice
    Problem identification and problem-solving; use of self-help strategies

Table 9.4 (*Continued*)

Observe real conversations (if possible) between client and frequent partners
    Application of newly learned skills
    Discuss conversational occurrences and outcomes

Abbreviations: HHIE-S, Hearing Handicap Inventory for Elderly—Screening; Sent-Ident, sentence identification; Topicon, topical conversation.
Source: Erber, N.P. (1996), *Communication Therapy for Adults with Sensory Loss,* 2nd ed. Clifton Hill, Australia: Helosonics. Reprinted by permission.

Table 9.5 The thirteen commandments for communicating with hearing-impaired older adults

1. Speak at a slightly greater than normal intensity.
2. Speak at your normal rate, but not too rapidly.
3. Do not speak to the elderly person at a greater distance than 6 feet but no less than 3 feet.
4. Encourage the elderly person to concentrate on the speaker's face for greater visibility of lip movements, facial expression, and gestures.
5. Do not speak to the elderly person unless you are visible to him or her (e.g., not from another room while he or she is reading the newspaper or watching TV).
6. Do not force the elderly person to listen to you when there is a great deal of environmental noise. That type of environment can be difficult for a younger, normally hearing person. It can, on the other hand, be defeating for the hearing impaired elderly.
7. Never, under any circumstances, speak directly into the person's ear. Not only can the person not take advantage of visual clues, but the speaker may be causing an already distorting auditory system to distort the speech signal further. In other words, clarity may be depressed as loudness is increased.
8. If the elderly person does not appear to understand what is being said, rephrase the statement rather than simply repeating the misunderstood words. An otherwise frustrating situation can be avoided in that way.
9. Do not over-articulate. Over-articulation not only distorts the sounds of speech, but also the speaker's face, thus making the use of visual clues more difficult.
10. Arrange the room (living room or meeting room) where communication will take place so that no speaker of listener is more than 6 feet apart and all are completely visible. Using this direct approach communication for all parties involved will be enhanced.
11. Include the elderly person in a discussion about him or her. Hearing-impaired persons sometimes feel quite vulnerable. This approach will help alleviate some of those feelings.
12. In meetings or any group activity where there is a speaker presenting information (church meetings, civic organizations, etc.), make it mandatory that the speakers(s) use the public address system. One of the most frequent complaints among elderly persons is that they may enjoy attending meetings of various kinds but all too often the speaker for whatever reason tries to avoid using a microphone. Many elderly persons do not assert themselves by asking a speaker who has just said, "I am sure that you can all hear me if I do not use the microphone," to *please* use it. They then begin to avoid public or organizational meetings if they cannot hear what the speaker is saying. This point cannot be stressed enough.
13. Above all, treat elderly persons as adult. They deserve that respect.

Source: Hull, R.H. (1980). The thirteen commandments for talking to the hearing impaired older person. *Journal of the American Speech and Hearing Association,* 22, 427. Reprinted by permission.

Table 9.6   Steps in conversational problem-solving

1. Recognize that a conversational disfluency has occurred.
2. Identify the source of the difficulty.
3. Select, request, or apply an appropriate corrective strategy to overcome the problem.
4. Judge the effectiveness of the strategy (e.g., partner's slowed speech).
5. Confirm that the correct message was received (e.g., "Did you say . . .?").
6. If the message was received correctly, continue the conversation.
7. If the strategy failed to resolve the difficulty, consider why it failed (e.g., source of difficulty misjudged; or strategy not applied correctly).
8. Request/apply the strategy appropriately, or
9. Request/apply an alternative strategy.
10. Return to step number 4.

Source: Erber, N.P. (1996), *Communication Therapy for Adults with Sensory Loss,* 2nd ed. Australia: Helosonics. Reprinted by permission.

Table 9.7   Some reasons that a client may not request clarification from a communication partner

The client
- is not aware of the effects of the sensory loss on conversational fluency.
- does not recognize when communication difficulties have occurred.
- faces well-developed meta-communication abilities and thus cannot think about or discuss conversational problems in a logical and coherent manner.
- feels that communication partners are responsible for resolving any difficulties that occur.
- can describe the conversational problem, but seems unwilling or unable to do anything about it, feels incapable, helpless, or depressed.
- knows that a general conversational problem exists, but is unable to identify specific sources of difficulty.
- lacks confidence, perhaps as the result of previous errors in identifying sources of conversational difficulty.
- generally lacks assertiveness, and feels uncomfortable about asking another person to help or to change conversational behavior.
- feels that particular situations and contexts are not appropriate for the application of clarification procedures that might disrupt conversations.
- believes that partners will respond negatively to any requests for clarification (e.g., with exaggerated mouth movements, shouting, lack of empathy or cooperation, patronizing attitude, ridicule, disgust).
- feels that most members of society do not accept (a) telling others about one's problems, confusions, or insecurities; (b) describing the faults of others, particularly communication partners; (c) discussing "conversation" in the middle of a conversation (i.e., meta-communication).
- is unable to generalize "known" principles or clarification to specific conversational situations.

Source: Erber, N.P. (1996), *Communication Therapy for Adults with Sensory Loss,* 2nd ed. Australia: Helosonics. Reprinted by permission.

Table 9.8   Example topic areas for ongoing counseling

- Lifestyle changes (e.g., stress management; adequate sleep; limit alcohol, caffeine, and tobacco; avoid silence by maintaining safe levels of background noise; engage in meaningful activities and hobbies; benefits of regular exercise)
- Informational counseling about hearing, hearing loss, hearing loss prevention
- Refocusing attention on the task (diverting attention away from tinnitus onto other tasks)
- Reassurance about the lack of a serious underlying cause (based on medical clearance for treatment program provided by otolaryngologist)
- Realistic expectations and perspectives about treatment outcome
- Promotion of relaxation including the use of relaxation exercise
- Benefits of sound therapy
- Ways to make tinnitus take on less importance
- Lack of quality control of information on the Internet
- Improving sleep patterns (e.g., www.sleepfoundation.org)
- Actively listen to patient
- Provide patients with hope

Source: Montano, J.J and Spitzer, J.B. (eds.), *Adult Audiologic Rehabilitation* (p. 430). Copyright © 2009 Plural Publishing, Inc. All rights reserved. Used with permission.

Table 9.9   Components of auditory training (AT) programs

	Bottom-Up AT	Top-Down AT	Feedback	Communication Strategies	Adaptive	Video	Data Retrieval	Remote Access
LACE™		•	•	•	•		•	•
CasperSent		•	•			•	•	
CATS		•	•	•		•	•	
CAST	•		•		•		•	
SPATS	•		•		•		•	
Seeing/Hearing Speech		•	•		•	•	•	
Conversation Made Easy	•	•	•			•		

Abbreviations: LACE, Listening and Communication Enhancement; CasperSent, Computer-Assisted Speech Perception Testing and Training at Sentence Level; CAST, Contrasts for Auditory and Speech Training; SPAT, Speech Perception Assessment and Training System; Seeing/Hearing Speech, Seeing and Hearing Speech Auditory Training.
Note: Bullets indicate that the training program includes this aspect of aural rehabilitation.
Source: Montano, J.J. and Spitzer, J.B. (eds.), Adult Audiologic Rehabilitation (p. 278). Copyright © 2009 Plural Publishing, Inc. All rights reserved. Used with permission.

Table 9.10   Desirable psychosocial objectives for audiological rehabilitation (AR) groups

- Develop more realistic expectations related to hearing loss and amplification.
- Adopt a more positive and proactive mindset.
- Recognize the commonality of members' needs and problems and develop a sense of connectedness.
- Realize that their feelings related to hearing loss are normal and valid.
- Develop a comfortable relationship with amplification.
- Broaden a repertoire and improve the use of communication strategies.
- Improve attending strategies and speech-reading skills.
- Work toward a more appropriate degree of assertiveness.
- Increase familiarity with resources for independent coping with hearing loss.
- Improve social skills.
- Develop improved problem-solving ability: be aware of one's choices and make choices wisely.
- Make specific plans for behavioral change, and make an ongoing commitment to those changes.
- Increase self-acceptance, self-confidence, self-respect, self-esteem, and achieve a new view of oneself and others.
- Reduce stress.
- Utilize hearing conservation strategies.
- Assume personal responsibility for managing hearing loss.
- Increase self-monitoring and regulating speech.
- Develop an understanding of the behavioral affective, behavioral, cognitive, and social effects of hearing loss on self, family, etc.
- Develop the ability to explain communication needs to others.
- Develop a support system outside the group.
- Internalize the shared responsibilities of communicating with others.
- Identify resources within their extended families and communities.

Source: Montano, J.J. and Spitzer, J.B. (eds.), *Adult Audiologic Rehabilitation* (p. 294). Copyright © 2009 Plural Publishing, Inc. All rights reserved. Used with permission.

Table 9.11   Characteristics of effective counselors

Personality	*Character Strengths*	*Professional*
Patient	Self-awareness	Empathy
Warm personality	Cultural awareness	Warmth and caring
Good listener	Ability to analyze own feelings	Openness
Perceptive and sensitive	Ability to serve as a model	Positive regard and respect
Likes people	Altruism	Concreteness and specificity
Nonthreatening demeanor	Strong sense of ethics	Communication competence
Sense of humor	Responsible	Intentionality
Desire to help		
Positive attitude		
Problem solver		

Source: Montano, J.J. and Spitzer, J.B. (eds.), *Adult Audiologic Rehabilitation* (p. 204). Copyright © 2009 Plural Publishing, Inc. All rights reserved. Used with permission.

Table 9.12 Self-assessment inventories: Summary of handicap aspects assessed

	Inventory/Approach											
Handicap Aspect	HHS	HMS	SHI	Denver	Sanders	Stephens	HPI-A	SAC/SOAC	HHIE	M-A	HPI	CPHI
Speech communication	X	X	X	X	X	X	X	X	X	X	X	X
General speech		X	X	X	X	X	X	X	X	X	X	X
Home/family				X	X							X
Vocational/work				X	X				X	X	X	X
Social				X	X				X	X	X	X
1 on 1, sm. grp, lg. grp.									X		X	
Special communications	X	X	X		X	X	X	X	X		X	X
With and w/out visual cues											X	
Avg. and adverse conditions	X										X	X
Telephone/TV/radio	X										X	X
Emotional/personal/psych. rx.		X		X		X	X	X	X	X		X
Response to auditory failure												X
Acceptance of self/loss		X										X
Use of hearing aid												
Effect on activities/need												
Discouragement/embarrassment												X
Anger/stress/anxiety											X	X
Withdrawal/introversion and Neuroticism											X	X

Inventory/Approach

Handicap Aspect	HHS	HMS	SHI	Denver	Sanders	Stephens	HPI-A	SAC/SOAC	HHIE	M-A	HPI	CPHI
Opinion/behavior of others		X			X	X		X				
Family relations												
Work performance												
Societal response												
Nonspeech Communication	X	X			X	X		X			X	
Intensity/localization	X	X									X	
Doorbell/phone bell												
Warnings/traffic												
Related symptoms					X			X				
Tinnitus/fluctuation/tolerance		X										

Abbreviations: HPI, Hearing Performance Inventory; CPHI, Communication Profile for the Hearing Impaired; HHIE, Hearing Handicap Inventory for Elderly; SAC/SOAC, Self Assessment of Communication; HPI-A, Hearing Problem Inventory-Atlanta; HMS, Hearing Measurement Scale; HHS, Hearing Handicap Scales; SHI, Subjective Hearing Impairment; Sanders, Profile Questionnaire for Rating Communicative Performance in Various Environments; Denver. Denver Scale of Communication Function; M-A, The McCarthy-Alpiner Scale of Hearing Handicap; Stephens, International Outcome Inventory.

Source: Introduction to Aural Rehabilitation, 2nd ed. (pp. 390–391), by R.L. Schow and M.A. Nerbonne, 1980. Austin, TX: PRO-ED. Copyright 1980 by PRO-ED, Inc. Reprinted by permission.

Table 9.13 Examples of psychoanalytic ego defenses manifested in reactions to disability

Defense Mechanism	Definition	Example
Repression	Forcing intrapsychic conflicts, painful experiences, and disturbing memories out of conscious awareness	Person with a visible congenital disability repressing feelings of shame and embarrassment triggered by early life reactions of others
Projection	Externalizing unconscious forbidden ideas, needs, and impulses, and attributing them to other people or environmental conditions	Blaming others for onset of disability, or attributing lack of progress in rehabilitation to staff incompetence rather than one's own lack of effort
Rationalization	Using after-the-fact, false reasons to offset negative emotional consequences	Person who gradually loses hearing and attributes lack of participation to boredom, lack of interest, or fatigue
Sublimation	Adopting useful, socially acceptable behaviors to express forbidden and socially unacceptable wishes and impulses	Anger and desire to retaliate against and uncaring society channeled into artistic endeavors
Reaction formation	Substituting and expressing responses and feelings that are exact opposites of those that are deemed verboten or unacceptable	Replacing initial feelings of aversion and rejection toward a child born with a severe disfigurement with overly demonstrative affection and protectiveness
Regression	Reverting to childlike behaviors first exhibited during an earlier developmental stage	A recently disable person whose temper tantrums are activated when needs are not immediately gratified or who daydreams rather than pursues treatment
Compensation	Seeking to excel in functionally related activities or behaviors to make up for disability-generated loss	Person who lost sight at an early age and has achieved success as a musician
Denial	Resolution of emotional conflict and reduction of anxiety by refusing to perceive, accept, or acknowledge threatening aspects of external reality	Failure to perceive or acknowledge effects of hearing impairment on job performance
Displacement	Shifting energy toward a less intimidating or more accessible object or person to reduce anxiety	Blaming others for not speaking clearly rather than admit to having a hearing problem

Sources: Adapted from Cubbage and Thomas (1989), Livneh and Siller (2004), and Livneh and Cook (2005).
Source: Montano, J.J and Spitzer, J.B. (eds.), *Adult Audiologic Rehabilitation* (p. 191). Copyright © 2009 Plural Publishing, Inc. All rights reserved. Used with permission.

Table 9.14 Comparison of self-report questionnaires to assess domains in the psychological system*

est	Contents	Ratings	Sections	H	P	B	E	S
PHAB	24 statements	7-point scale (always–never)	4 subscales	✓	✓	✓		
OSI	Patient selects up to 5 listening situations	5-point scale (degree of change)	16 categories	✓	✓	✓		
PHI	145 items	5-point scale (agree–disagree)	4 subscales	✓				
CHO	15 items	7-point scale (not at all–tremendously)	4 subscales				✓	
HABP	24 questions (minimum)	5-point scale	6 subscales	✓	✓	✓		✓
ANA	11 questions	3-point scale	4 subscales	✓			✓	
API	64 statements	5-point scale (help–hinders)	4 subscales		✓			
ASS	34 items	5-point scale						✓
AUQ	11 questions with subquestions	4-point scale						✓
HIA	25 items	3-point scale (yes–no)	2 subscales	✓	✓	✓		
HIA-S	10 items	3-point scale (yes–no)	2 subscales	✓	✓	✓		
HIE	25 items	3-point scale (yes–no)	2 subscales	✓	✓	✓		
HIE-S	10 items	3-point scale (yes–no)	2 subscales	✓	✓	✓		
PI	158 situations	5-point scale (always–never)	6 subscales	✓				
PI-R	90 situations	5-point scale (always–never)	6 subscales	✓				
OI-HA	7 items	5-point scale						✓
HAB	66 statements	7-point scale (always–never)	7 subscales	✓	✓	✓		
HAP	66 statements	7-point scale (always–never)	7 subscales		✓			
IPSL	74 questions	7-point scale (always–never)	6 subscales	✓				
ADL	15 items	7-point scale (not at all–tremendously)	4 subscales + 1 global					✓
HAPI	38 items	5-point scale (helps–hinders)	4 subscales		✓			

Abbreviations: APHAB, Abbreviated Profile of Hearing Aid Benefit; COSI, Client Oriented Scale of Improvement; CPHI, Communication Profile for the Hearing Impaired; ECHO, Expected Consequences of Hearing Aid Ownership; GHABP, Glasgow Hearing Aid Benefit Profile; HANA, Hearing Aid Needs Assessment; HAPI, Hearing Aid Performance Inventory; HASS, Hearing Aid Satisfaction Survey; HAUQ, Hearing Aid User's Questionnaire; HHIA, Hearing Handicap Inventory for Adults; HHIA-S, Hearing Handicap Inventory for Adults–Screener; HHIE, Hearing Handicap Inventory for the Elderly; HHIE-S, Hearing Handicap Inventory for the Elderly–Screener; HPI, Hearing Performance Inventory; HPI-R, Hearing Performance Inventory–Revised; IOI-HA, International Outcome Inventory for Hearing Aids; PHAB, Profile of Hearing Aid Benefit; PHAP, Profile of Hearing Aid Performance; PIPSL, Performance Inventory for Profound and Severe Loss; SADL, Satisfaction with Amplification in Daily Life; SHAPI, Shortened Hearing Aid Performance Inventory.

Checkmarks indicate if the questionnaire evaluates handicap (H), aided performance (P), aided benefit (B), expectations (E), and/or satisfaction (S).

Table 9.15 Self-report instruments for assessing hearing handicap

Instrument	Author(s)	Target Population	Assessment Focus	Items	Time (min.)
Hearing Handicap Scale (HHS), 1964	High et al	Adult	Speech communication Environmental sounds Warning signals	20 (2 forms)	5
Hearing Measurement Scale (HMS), 1970	Noble and Atherly	Adult	Speech hearing Nonspeech acuity Localization Reaction to handicap Speech distortion Tinnitus Social effects Personal reaction to loss	53	10–40
Social Hearing Handicap Scale (SHI), 1973	Ewertson and Birk-Nelsen	Adult	Specific listening Situations	21	5
Denver Scale of Communication Function, 1974	Alpiner et al	Adult	Family Social Vocational General communication	25	15
Profile Questionnaire for Rating Communication Performance, 1982	Sanders	Adult	Home Business Social environments	22	15
Denver Scale of Communication Function of Senior Citizens (DSSC), 1976	Zarnoch and Alpiner	Seniors	Attitude toward peers Socialization Communication Specific situations	35	15

Source: Katz, J. (1994). *Handbook of Clinical Audiology*, 4th ed. Philadelphia: Lippincott Williams & Wilkins. Reprinted by permission.

Table 9.16   Information on computer applications for speech perception training

Dynamic Audio Video Interactive Device (DAVID)
   Donald G. Sims
   Department of Communication Research
   National Technical Institute for the Deaf
   Rochester Institute of Technology
   Rochester, NY 14623–0887
Computer-Assisted Speech Perception Evaluation and Training (CASPER)
   Nancy Plant
   c/o Arthur Boothroyd
   City University Graduate Center
   Department of Speech and Hearing Sciences
   33 West 42nd Street
   New York, NY 10036
Auditory-Visual Laser Videodisc Interactive System (ALVIS)
   Lennart L. Kopra
   c/o Department of Communication Sciences and Disorders
   University of Texas at Austin
   CMA 7.202
   Austin, TX 78712
Computerized Laser Videodisc Programs for Training Speechreading and Assertive
   Communication Behaviors
   Richard S. Tyler
   Department of Otolaryngology
   Head and Neck Surgery
   University of Iowa Hospitals
   Iowa City, IA 52242
Computer-Aided Speechreading (CAST)
   M.-K. Pichora-Fuller,
   School of Audiology and Speech Sciences
   University of British Columbia
   5804 Fairview Avenue
   Vancouver, BC V6T 1W5
   Canada
Computer-Assisted Tracking Simulation (CATS)
   James J. Dempsey
   Department of Communication Disorders
   Southern Connecticut State University
   501 Crescent Street
   New Haven, CT 06515–1355
Sound and Beyond
   Cochlear Americas
   400 Inverness Parkway
   Englewood, CO 80112
   www.cochlearamericas.com
Learning to Lipread: An Introductory Course
   M. J. Allen
   P.O. Box 412
   Marden, SA 5070, Australia
   sales@lipread.com.au

(*continued on next page*)

Table 9.16 (*Continued*)

Seeing and Hearing Speech
  Sensimetrics Corporation
  48 Grove Street
  Somerville, MA 02144–2500
  www.sens.com
Conversation Made Easy
  CID Publications
  4560 Clayton Avenue
  St. Louis, MO 63110
Listening and Auditory Communication Enhancement (LACE)
  NeuroTone Inc.
  2317 Broadway, Suite 205
  Redwood city, CA 94063
  www.lacecentral.com

Source: Valente, M., Hosford-Dunn, H., Roeser, R.J. (2007), *Audiology Treatment,* 2nd ed. New York: Thieme. Reprinted by permission.

10
Deafness

Table 10.1 Forms of manual and spoken communication

Nonverbal Communication: Natural Gestures, Facial Expression, Body Movements, Body Language, Pantomime

Artificial Pedagogical Systems, Invented for Educational Purposes

American Sign Language (ASL)	Pidgin Sign English (PSE)	Signed English	Linguistics of Visual English (LOVE)	Signing Exact English (SEE 2)	Seeing Essential English (SEE 1)	Finger Spelling	Cued Speech	English
Independent language visual manual mode; own grammar; own syntax; signs are meaning based; has dialects, regionalisms, slang, and puns; can be written; wide range of vocabulary covering	A combination of elements from ASL and the sign systems, ranging from the more ASL-like (occasionally called Ameslish) to the more English-like (sometimes called CASE—Conceptually Accurate Signed	Signed in accordance with English grammar, but signs are meaning based; specially invented sign markers for important affixes in English; invented by Borastein; used widely in education	Essentially the same as SEE 2, but has a method of writing each sign; used in education; invented by Wampler; usage is diminishing	Signs are word based; special signs for all affixes in English; signed in strict accordance with English; invented by Zawolkow, Pfetzing, and Gustason; widely used in education; very influential	Signs are based on word roots (morphemes) (trans/port/a/tion); an extreme form of word-based signs; invented by Anthony; not popular in U.S., but still common in Iowa and Colorado schools for	Manual representation of the written language; one hand shape for each letter of alphabet; used to borrow English words into ASL; when used with speech and speech-reading, it is called the Rochester Method	Employs 8 hand shapes in 4 positions on the face, and used in conjunction with lip movements to enable a deaf person to lip-read more easily; based on sound with the syllable as the basic unit; devised by Orin Cornett at	Independent language; aural-oral mode: own grammar; own syntax; words are meaning based; contains dialects, regionalisms, slang, and puns; can be written; wide range of vocabulary covering minute differences in meaning; may borrow from

minute
differences
in meaning;
may borrow
from other
languages;
is verbal,
but also
makes use
of nonver-
bal
elements

English);
usually
contains
few if any
sign
markers
(see Signed
English), yet
makes
frequent
use of
finger-spell-
ing English
words; used
in conjunc-
tion with
speech in
interpreting
and college
teaching;
signs are
meaning
based

the deaf;
signs for all
affixes

other
languages; is
verbal, but
also makes use
of nonverbal
elements

Gallaudet
College

Source: Introduction to Aural Rehabilitation, 2nd ed. (p. 156), by Schow R.L. and Nerbonne, M.A., 1980. Austin, TX: PRO-ED. Copyright 1980 by PRO-ED, Inc. Reprinted by permission.

Table 10.2   Speech-reading tests for children: Chronological listing

Date Developed	Title of Test	Author(s)	Content Format
1949	Cavender Test of Lipreading Ability	Cavender	Sentences
1957	Costello Test of Speech-Reading	Costello	Words Sentences
1959	Semi-Diagnostic Test	Hutton, Curry, and Armstrong	Words
1964	Craig Lipreading Inventory	Craig	Words Sentences
1968	Butt Children's Speechreading Test	Butt and Chreist	Questions Commands
1970	Diagnostic Test of Speechreading	Myklebust and Neyhaus	Words Phrases Sentences

Source: Introduction to Aural Rehabilitation, 2nd ed. (p. 141), by Schow R.L. and Nerbonne, M.A., 1980. Austin, TX: PRO-ED. Copyright 1980 by PRO-ED, Inc. Reprinted by permission.

Table 10.3   Speech-reading tests for adults: Chronological listing

Date Developed	Title of Test	Author(s)	Content Format
1946	How Well Can You Read Lips?	Utley	Words Sentences Stories
1957	A Film Test of Lipreading	Taaffe	Sentences
1967	Multiple-Choice Test of Lipreading	Donnelly and Marshall	Sentences
1971	Barley-CID Sentences	Barley	Sentences
1976	Lipreading Screening Test	Binnie, Jackson, and Montgomery	CV-Syllables
1978	Denver Quick Test of Lipreading Ability	Alpiner	Sentences

Source: Introduction to Aural Rehabilitation, 2nd ed. (p. 141), by Schow R.L. and Nerbonne, M.A., 1980. Austin, TX: PRO-ED. Copyright 1980 by PRO-ED, Inc. Reprinted by permission.

Table 10.4 Denver Quick Test of lip-reading ability

The *Denver Quick Test* is designed to measure adult ability to speech-read 20 common everyday sentences. Sentences are presented "live" or taped by the tester and are scored on the basis of meaning recognition. No normative data are available to which individual scores may be compared; however, when the Quick Test was given without acoustic cures to 40 hearing-impaired adults, their scores were highly correlated (0.90) with their results on the *Utley Sentence Test.*

1. Good morning.
2. How old are you?
3. I live in (state of residence).
4. I only have one dollar.
5. There is somebody at the door.
6. Is that all?
7. Where are you going?
8. Let's have a coffee break.
9. Park your car in the lot.
10. What is your address?
11. May I help you?
12. I feel fine.
13. It is time for dinner.
14. Turn right at the corner.
15. Are you ready to order?
16. Is this charge or cash?
17. What time is it?
18. I have a headache.
19. How about going out tonight?
20. Please lend me 50 cents.

Source: Alpiner, J. (ed.), *Handbook of Adult Rehabilitative Audiology.* Baltimore: Lippincott Williams & Wilkins, 1982:18–79. Reprinted by permission.

Table 10.5   Utley Test of lip-reading ability

This test, commonly referred to as the "Utley Test," consists of three subtests: Sentences (Forms A and B), Words (Forms A and B), and stories accompanied by questions that relate to each of the stories. Utley (1946)* demonstrated that the Word and Story subtests are positively correlated with the Sentence portion of the test; therefore, these are the stimuli most often used and associated with the Utley Test. Utley evaluated her viewers' responses by giving one point for each word correctly identified in each sentence. A total of 125 words are contained in the 31 sentences on each form (Forms A and B). Consequently, a respondent's score may range from 0 to 125 points. Utley suggested that homophonous words not be accepted when scoring the sentence subtest.

Utley administered the sentence subtest to 761 hearing-impaired children and adults, and the following descriptive statistics summarize her findings:

	Form A	Form B
Range	0–84	0–89
Mean	33.63	33.80
SD	16.36	17.53

Practice sentences:
1. Good morning.
2. Thank you.
3. Hello.
4. How are you?
5. Goodbye.

Utley Sentence Test, Form A:
1. All right.
2. Where have you been?
3. I have forgotten.
4. I have nothing.
5. That is right.
6. Look out.
7. How have you been?
8. I don't know if I can.
9. How tall are you?
10. It is awfully cold.
11. My folks are home.
12. How much was it?
13. Good night.
14. Where are you going?
15. Excuse me.
16. Did you have a good time?
17. What did you want?
18. How much do you weigh?
19. I cannot stand him.
20. She was home last week.
21. Keep your eye on the ball.
22. I cannot remember.
23. Of course.
24. I flew to Washington.
25. You look well.
26. The train runs every hour.
27. You had better go slow.
28. It says that in the book.
29. We got home at six o'clock.
30. We drove to the country.
31. How much rain fell?

*Utley, J. (1946). A test of lipreading ability. *J. Speech Hear. Disord.* 10(10):109–116.
Source: Introduction to Aural Rehabilitation, 2nd ed. (p. 141), by Schow R.L. and Nerbonne, M.A., 1980. Austin, TX: PRO-ED. Copyright 1980 by PRO-ED, Inc. Reprinted with permission.

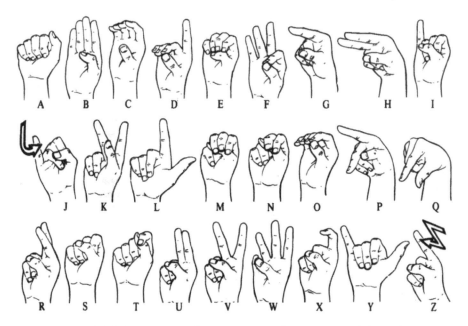

Fig. 10.1 Manual alphabet: American. (From Bess, F.H. and Humes, L.E. *Audiology—The Fundamentals*. Baltimore: Lippincott Williams & Wilkins, 1990:214. Reprinted by permission.)

11
Organizations and Publications

Organizations

Academy of Dispensing Audiologists—http://www.audiologist.org
Academy of Rehabilitative Audiology—http://www.audrehab.org
Acoustic Neuroma Association—http://www.anausa.org
Acoustical Society of America—http://asa.aip.org
Alexander Graham Bell association for the Deaf—http://nc.agbell.org/net community/page.aspx?pid=348
American Academy of Audiology—http://www.audiology.org/Pages/default .aspx
American Academy of Otolaryngology–Head and Neck Surgery—http://www .entnet.org
American Association of the Deaf-Blind—http://www.aadb.org
American Deafness and Rehabilitation Association—http://www.adara.org
American Hearing Research Foundation—http://www.american-hearing.org
American Otological Society—http://www.americanotologicalsociety.org
American Society for Deaf Children—http://www.deafchildren.org
American Speech-Language-Hearing Association—http://www.asha.org
American Speech-Language-Hearing Foundation—http://www.ashfoundation .org/default.htm
American Tinnitus Association—http://www.ata.org
Association for Research in Otolaryngology—http://www.aro.org
Association of Late-Deafened Adults—http://www.alda.org
Audiological Resource Association—http://www.audresources.org
Audiology Foundation of America—http://www.audfound.org
Better Hearing Institute—http://www.betterhearing.org
Center for Hearing and Communication (former name: New York League for the Hard of Hearing)—http://www.chchearing.org
Convention of American Instructors of the Deaf—http://www.caid.org

Council on Education of the Deaf—http://www.deafed.net/pagetext.asp?hdn
pageid=58
The Caption Center—http://www.icdri.org/dhhi/ccowgbh.htm
Deafness Research Foundation—http://www.drf.org
Dogs for the Deaf, Inc.—http://www.dogsforthedeaf.org
Hearing Dog Resource Center—http://www.dcara.org/index.php?option=com
_mtree&task=viewlink&link_id=2274&itemid=27
Hearing Education Awareness for Rockers—http://www.hearnet.com
Hearing Industries Association—http://www.hearing.org
Helen Keller National Center for Deaf-Blind Youths and Adults—http://www
.hknc.org
International Hearing Dog, Inc.—http://www.pawsforsilence.org/home.html
International Hearing Society—http://ihsinfo.org/ihsV2/Home/index.cfm
National Association for the Deaf—http://www.nad.org
National Bands for Certification in Hearing Instrument Sciences—http://www
.nbc-his.com
National Captioning Institute—http://www.ncicap.org
National Hearing Conservation Association—http://hearingconservation.org
National Information Center on Deafness—http://www.wvdhhr.org/wvcdhh/
Community %20 Conn/national_information_center_on_d.htm
National Institute on Deafness and Other Communication Disorders—http://
www.nidcd.mih.gov
New England Assistance Dog Service—http://www.neads.org
Parents' Section of the Alexander Graham Bell Association for the Deaf—http://
agbell.org/NetCommunity/Page.aspx?pid=784
Registry of Interpreters for the Deaf—http://www.rid.org
Self Help for Hard of Hearing People, Inc.—http://hearingloss.org
Sertoma Intl./Foundation—http://www.sertoma.org
Service Dog Center—http://www.servicedogcenter.org
Texas Hearing and Service Dog—http://www.servicedogs.org

Publications

Acta Otolaryngological—http://informahealthcare.com/oto
Advance for Speech-Language Pathologists and Audiologists—http://speech
-language-pathology-audiology.advanceweb.com
American Academy of Otolaryngology–Head and Neck Surgery Bulletin—http://
www.entnet.org/educationandresearch/bulletin.cfm
American Annals of the Deaf—http://gupress.gallaudet.edu/annals
American Journal of Audiology: A Journal of Clinical Practice—http://aja.asha
.org
American Journal of Otolaryngology–Head and Neck Medicine and Surgery—
http://www.amjoto.com
American Journal of Otology—http://www.amjoto.com

American Speech-Language-Hearing Association—http://www.asha.org

Annals in Otolaryngology-Rhinology-Laryngology—http://wwwannals.com

Annals of Otology, Rhinology, and Laryngology—http://www.annals.com

Archives of Otolaryngology–Head and Neck Surgery—http://archotol.ama-assn .org

Audecibel—(now goes by the name of International Hearing Society) http:// ihsinfo.org/ihsV2/home/index.cfm

Audiology Today—http://www.audioloyg.org/resources/audiologytoday/pages/ default.aspx

Australian and New Zealand Journal of Audiology—http://www.audioloyg.asn .au/anzja.htm

Ear and Hearing—http://journals.lww.com/ear-hearing/pages/default.aspx

Ear Nose and Throat Journal (ENT Journal)—http://www.entjournal.com/ME2/ Default.asp

Hearing Health—http://www.drf.org/magazine

Hearing Journal (The)—http://journals.lww.com/thehearingjournal/pages/ default.aspx

Hearing Research—http://www.elseview.com/wps/find/journaldescription.cws _home/506060/description

Hearing Review (The)—http://www.hearingreview.com

International Journal of Audiology—http://www.internationaljournalof audiology.com

International Journal of Pediatric Otorhinolaryngology—http://www.ijporl online.com

Journal of the Academy of Rehabilitative Audiology (JARA)—http://www .audrehab.org/jara.htm

Journal of the Acoustical Society of America—http://scitation.aip.org/jasa

Journal of the American Academy of Audiology—http://www.audiology.org/ resources/journal/pages/default.aspx

Journal of the American Deafness and Rehabilitation Association—http://www .adara.org

Journal of Audiology Medicine—http://iapa-onlin.org/publications/journal-of -audiol-medicine/

Journal of Laryngology and Otology—http://www.jlo.co.uk

Journal of Otolaryngology—http://www.amjoto.com

Journal of Sound and Vibration—http://www.elseview.com/wps/find/journal description.cws_home/622899/description#description

Journal of Speech and Hearing Disorders—archived in JSLHR: http://jshd/asha .org/archive

Journal of Speech and Hearing Research—http://jslhr.asha.org

Language Speech and Hearing Services in the Schools—http://ishss.asha.org

Laryngoscope—http://onlinelibrary.wiley.com/journal/10.1002/(issn)1531 -4995

NSSHLA Journal—http://www.nsslha.org/publications/onlinonly/

Otolaryngologic Clinics of North America—http://www.oto.theclinics.com

Seminars in Hearing—http://www.thieme.com/index.php?page=shop.product
_details&flypage=flypage.tpl&product_id=906&category_id=90&option=com
_virtuemart&itemid=53
SHHH Journal—http://www.hearingloss.org/aboutus/index.asp
Sign Language Studies—http://gupress.gallaudet.edu/SLS.html
Sound and Vibration—(S&V)—http://www.sandv.com/home.htm
Tinnitus Today—http://www.ata.org/about-ata/news-pubs/tinnitus-today
Volta Review—http://agbell.org/NetCommunity/Page.aspx?pid=501

Index

Note: Page references followed by *f* or *t* indicate figures and tables, respectively.